Perspectives
in Behavioral Medicine

EATING REGULATION
AND DISCONTROL

Perspectives in Behavioral Medicine

EATING REGULATION AND DISCONTROL

Edited by

Herbert Weiner
University of California

Andrew Baum
Uniformed Services University of Health Sciences

Ψ **Psychology Press**
Taylor & Francis Group

New York London

First Published by

Lawrence Erlbaum Associates, Inc., Publishers
365 Broadway
Hillsdale, New Jersey 07642

Transferred to Digital Printing 2009 by Psychology Press
270 Madison Ave, New York NY 10016
27 Church Road, Hove, East Sussex, BN3 2FA

Library of Congress Cataloging in Publication Data

Eating regulation and discontrol.

(Perspectives in behavioral medicine ; v. 5)
Based on a conference held in Reston, Va., 1986.
Includes bibliographies and index.
1. Digestive organs—Congresses. 2. Ingestion—
Regulation—Congresses. 3. Gastrointestinal system—
Diseases—Congresses. I. Weiner, Herbert. II. Baum,
Andrew. III. Series: Perspectives on behavioral
medicine ; v. 5. [DNLM: 1. Appetite Disorders—
congresses. 2. Feeding Behavior—physiology—congresses.
3. Neuroregulators—physiology—congresses.
WM 175 E149 1986]
QP145.E27 **1988** 612'.3 87-19635
ISBN 0-89859-928-8

Publisher's Note
The publisher has gone to great lengths to ensure the quality of this
reprint but points out that some imperfections in the original may
be apparent.

CONTENTS

LIST OF CONTRIBUTORS   ix
PREFACE   xi

1

REGULATION OF GASTRIC SECRETION—
NEURAL MECHANISMS   1
  Frank P. Brooks
Intramural Nervous Control,   *1*
Extrinsic Nervous Control,   *7*
Central Nervous Control of Gastric Secretion,   *15*
References,   *24*

2

REGULATION OF GASTRIC SECRETION
Humoral Mechanisms   33
  N. W. Bunnett and J. H. Walsh
Introduction,   *33*
Stimulants of Gastric Acid Secretion Gastrin,   *34*
Gastrin-Releasing Peptide,   *36*
Other Stimulatory Peptides,   *40*
Humoral Inhibitors of Gastric Acid Secretion,   *40*
Other Inhibitory Peptides,   *43*
Conclusions,   *44*
References,   *45*

3

NEURAL MODELS OF THE CONTROL
OF FOOD INTAKE   49
Donald Novin
General Models of Feeding, *49*
Neural Substrates of Feeding, *53*
Acknowledgments, *55*
References, *56*

4

HUMORAL MECHANISMS IN THE CONTROL
OF EATING AND BODY WEIGHT   59
Gerard P. Smith
Therapeutic Implications, *62*
Summary, *63*
Acknowledgments, *63*
References, *64*

5

FUNCTION OF OPIOID PEPTIDES
IN THE BRAIN AND GUT   67
Allen S. Levine and John E. Morley
Distribution of Opioid Peptides, *67*
Thermoregulation, *71*
Respiration, *72*
Opioid Effects of the Cardiovascular System, *73*
Opioid Effects on Immune Function, *76*
Sexual and Reproductive Function, *78*
Opioid Effects on the Gastrointestinal Tract, *81*
Opioids and Feeding, *85*
Memory, *87*
Exorphins, *87*
References, *88*

6

CENTRAL NERVOUS SYSTEM ACTION OF NEUROPEPTIDES
TO INDUCE OR PREVENT EXPERIMENTAL
GASTRODUODENAL ULCERATIONS   101
Yvette Taché
Brain Damage and Gastric Pathogenesis, *101*
Brain Neuropeptides, *102*

CNS Action of Neuropeptides
to Prevent Gastric Duodenal Ulcerations,   105
Central Nervous System Action of Neuropeptides
    to Produce Gastric Ulceration,   107
Peptides Found Inactive
    to Influence Gastric Mucosa,   108
Conclusions,   109
Acknowledgments,   109
References,   109

7

OPIOID, α $_2$-NORADRENERGIC
AND ADRENOCORTICOTROPIN SYSTEMS
OF HYPOTHALAMIC PARAVENTRICULAR NUCLEUS   113
    Sarah Fryer Leibowitz
PVN Opiate System,   114
PVN α_2-Noradrenergic System,   117
PVN Opiate and α_2-Noradrenergic Systems
    in Relation to Glucocorticosteroids,   119
Interaction Between PVN Opiate-α_2-Noradrenergic
    Receptor Systems,   120
PVN Opiate α_2-Noradrenergic-Adrenocorticotropin
    System: Role in Nutritional Homeostasis, Under
    Normal Conditions and After Acute Food
    Deprivation and Stress,   123
References,   129

8

THE FUNCTIONAL BOWEL DISORDERS   137
    Herbert Weiner
Introduction,   137
Irritable Bowel Syndrome,   138
Incidence and Prevalence of IBS,   139
Functional Disturbances of the Esophagus,   140
Functional Disturbances of the Stomach,   144
Functional Disturbances of the Colon,   146
Conclusion,   153
References,   155

9

PEPTIC ULCER DISEASE
Are Some Regulatory Disturbances
Acquired During Postnatal Development?   163
   Sigurd H. Ackerman
The Ontogeny of Responsiveness
   to Parietal Cell Agonists,   *165*
The Ontogeny of Basal and Maximal Acid Output,   *168*
Premature Weaning
   and Experimental Stress Ulcer,   *171*
Conclusion,   *172*
References,   *173*

10

DISCONTROL OF APPETITE AND SATIETY—
SOCIAL AND PSYCHOLOGICAL FACTORS IN OBESITY
What We Don't Know   175
   C. Peter Herman
Social Influence,   *179*
Externality,   *182*
Stress,   *183*
Conclusions,   *184*
References,   *186*

11

THE REGULATION OF BODY WEIGHT
AND THE TREATMENT OF OBESITY   189
   Albert J. Stunkard
The Psychogenic Explanation,   *189*
The Somatogenic Hypothesis:
   The Regulation of Body Weight,   *190*
Implications for Behavior Therapy
   and Pharmacotherapy,   *201*
Summary,   *204*
References,   *205*

AUTHOR INDEX   207

SUBJECT INDEX   226

LIST OF CONTRIBUTORS

SIGURD H. ACKERMAN, Ph.D.   New York Hospital-Cornell Medical Center, 21 Bloomingdale Rd., White Plains, NY 10605

ANDREW BAUM, Ph.D.   Department of Medical Psychology, USU School of Medicine, 4301 Jones Bridge Rd., Bethesda, MD 20814-4799

FRANK BROOKS   Department of Physiology, University of Pennsylvania, Philadelphia, PA 19104

N. W. BUNNETT   Department of Surgery, The University of Washington, Seattle, WA 98195

C. PETER HERMAN   Department of Psychology, University of Toronto, Toronto, Ontario, CANADA M5S 1A1

ALLEN S. LEVINE   VA Medical Center, Neuroendocrine Research Laboratory, 54th & 48th Ave. S., Minneapolis, MN 55417

SARAH F. LIEBOWITZ, Ph.D.   The Rockefeller University, 1230 York Ave., New York, NY 10021-6399

JOHN E. MORLEY, Ph.D.   Director of Geriatric Research Education and Clinical Center, Veterans Administration Medical Center (11E), 16111 Plummer St., Sepulveda, CA 91343

DONALD NOVIN   Psychology Department, University of California, Los Angeles, CA 90024

GERARD P. SMITH, Ph.D.   Department of Psychiatry, Cornell University Medical College, The New York Hospital-Westchester Division, 21 Bloomingdale Rd., White Plains, NY 10605

ALBERT STUNKARD, Ph.D.   Department of Psychology, University of Pennsylvania, Philadelphia, PA 19104

YVETTE TACHÉ   Center for Ulcer Research, Wadsworth Veterans Administration Center, School of Medicine, University of California, Los Angeles, CA 90024

HERBERT WEINER   School of Medicine, University of California, Los Angeles, CA 90024

PREFACE

Why should physicians or behavioral scientists be interested in the gut? This question may seem strange: They always have been! Dyspepsia, overeating, loss of appetite, anorexia nervosa, diarrhea, constipation, incontinence, or abdominal pain are common symptoms in many diseases, or are symptoms per se. Additionally, the gut reflects fear, distress, depression, or elation as one of its many functions.

The gourmet and the gourmand, the vegetarian or dieter are well-known types. Cultures vary enormously in their interest in, and emphasis on food. The French learned from the Chinese how to make appetizing sauces! The thought, sight, smell, and sound of food and cooking elicit a variety of secretory and motility changes in the stomach. These are preparatory, purposive responses mediated and orchestrated by the brain. Babies learn continence; oldsters seem to unlearn it.

In the past the emphasis of physiologists was mainly on studying motility, secretion, digestion, absorption, and excretion. Several major advances have recently occurred to alter this limited point of view; they consist of a huge increase in understanding the organization and function of the enteric nervous system; in the realization that the gut participates in immune responses and may produce antibodies as a first line of defense against ingested viruses, bacteria, parasites, or toxins; and finally in the discovery that a large number of hormones present in, and secreted by the stomach, intestine, and pancreas are also present in the brain. They play a role in every aspect of the gut's functioning—appetite, food intake, satiety, secretion, motility, and the regulation of immune function (where they act as modulators, etc.)

This meeting was arranged to acquaint behavioral scientists with these revelations. Consider such subtle effects as that of vertigo on diminishing gastric motility or those of restraint in increasing motility, leaving acid secretion unchanged but including mucosal erosion.

The conference considered the role of neural discharge in regulating gastric secretion and motility (Brooks). Whence the discharge? One of the truly surprising discoveries is that thyrotropin-releasing-hormone (TRH) is highly concentrated in the dorsal motor nucleus of the vagus nerve. TRH injected thereabouts increases vagally mediated gastric motility, acid secretion, causes bicarbonate secretion to decline, and produces gastric erosions (Taché). These effects are opposed by centrally administered bombesin, corticotrophin releasing hormone (CRH), the calcitonin gene-related peptides (CGRP) and the opioid peptides (Levine and Morley). Inhibiting somatostatin released locally by cysteamine induces duodenal erosions in rats, in part by reducing duodenal bicarbonate secretion.

The regulation of hunger, food intake, and satiety is of a complexity that defies the imagination. Cholecystokinin seems to induce satiety peripherally when the stomach is distended with food by a vagal afferent mechanism (Smith). The vagus also mediates an increase in glucose content in hepatic veins following a meal to induce satiety (Novin). On the other hand, peptides such as NPY in the paraventricular nucleus of the hypothalamus may determine the food the animal selects to eat. While the regulation of carbohydrate intake is not only neurally but also hormonally mediated (e.g., by tryptophane). It is also abundantly clear that a number of peptides and classical neurotransmitters are involved in the regulation and mediation of food intake (Leibowitz).

This book presents information about what happens when such complex regulatory mechanisms come unstuck (Herman), what are the development antecedents of some regulatory disturbances in the stomach (Ackerman), and whether they can be treated (Stunkard) by pharmacological, behavioral, or social means to restore their proper functioning.

Finally, this writer appealed to behavioral scientists to study the functional bowel disorders with the knowledge and concept so far acquired. These disorders are major sources of distress and disability. They are extremely common. They are illnesses not only of the gut but of the persons faced with characteristic personal problems that life engenders.

Herbert Weiner, M.D.
School of Medicine
UCLA

Perspectives
in Behavioral Medicine

EATING REGULATION
AND DISCONTROL

1

REGULATION OF GASTRIC SECRETION— NEURAL MECHANISMS

Frank P. Brooks
University of Pennsylvania

The importance of neural mechanisms in the regulation of gastric secretion has passed through at least three cycles. In Pavlov's time, nerves were considered to be of primary importance as demonstrated in conscious dogs with esophagostomies (sham feeding) and in the comparison of the responses of vagally innervated (Pavlov) gastric fundic pouches to those of vagally denervated (Heidenhain) pouches. Then came the pioneering experiments of Bayliss and Starling and Edkins in the role of hormonal regulation, culminating in the purification and isolation of gastrin by Gregory and his associates. Hormones became the dominant factors, including hormones released by nerve stimulation (e.g., gastrin). We are now in a third phase in which the same substance may play a role in the regulation of gastric secretion as a classical hormone, a neurotransmitter, a neuromodulator, and a paracrine messenger.

I have reviewed the subject on several occasions in the past (Brooks, 1965, 1967, 1968, 1975, 1977, 1981). The number of publications on the subject has increased substantially recently, as indicated by the approximately 20 related abstracts submitted for presentation during Digestive Disease Week in 1985. In this review, I will consider nervous regulation of gastric exocrine and endocrine secretion by nerves within the wall of the stomach, by extrinsic nerves, and by the brain.

INTRAMURAL NERVOUS CONTROL

Structure

The structural basis for the innervation of secretory cells in the stomach is still incompletely understood. Light microscopic studies show bare nerve endings in close contact with parietal cells in rabbits (Hanker, Tapper, & Ambrose, 1977).

In the cat, nerve endings reached only the basal half of the fundic glands (Kyosola, Veyola, & Richardt, 1975). More recently, electron micrographs showed no nerve axons or varicosities closer than 100 nM to parietal cells in the opossum (Seelig, Schlusselberg, & Woodward, 1983); and similar findings have been reported for rat mucosal epithelial cells (Crocket, Doyle, & Joffee, 1981) and rhesus monkey parietal cells (Lechago & Barajas, 1976). The latter were stained for acetylcholinesterase. It is interesting that in salivary glands an electrical intracellular response to single parasympathetic nerve impulses was seen only when the gap between nerve endings and secretory cells was about 20nM (Garrett, 1974). Cholinergic nerve endings have also been demonstrated in contact with gastrin cells (Lechago & Barajas, 1981).

Recent immunohistochemical studies have identified regulatory peptides such as substance P, vasoactive intestinal polypeptide (VIP), enkephalins, and the gastrin-cholecystokinin (CCK) peptides near gland cells. Cell bodies in the myenteric plexus of the stomach contained immunoreactive substance P, VIP, and enkephalins (Schultzberg et al., 1980). The submucosal plexus is poorly developed in the stomach. Gastrin-releasing polypeptide is reported to be present in nerve endings in the pyloric antrum. Nerve endings with vesicles consistent with neuropeptides have been found within 200–300 nm of gastrin cells (Lechago & Barajas, 1981).

Cellular Physiology of H^+ Secretion

The development of relatively pure parietal and chief cell preparations has made it possible to examine the role of neurotransmitters acting on gastric secretory cells. Acetylcholine stimulated the accumulation of acid in the canaliculi of isolated parietal cells. The effect was blocked by atropine (Soll, 1980). Saturable, temperature-dependent binding of [3H]QNB(Quinuclidinyl benzilate—an anticholinergic), to rat parietal cells in vitro has been demonstrated, which is consistent with the presence of cholinergic receptors (Ecknauer, Thompson, Johnson, & Rosenfeld, 1980). The second messenger in stimulus-secretion coupling appears to be calcium, rather than cyclic AMP (Soll, 1981).

The accumulation of H^+ in parietal cells in response to acetylcholine, histamine, or gastrin was blocked by H_2 antagonists such as cimetidine (Soll, 1981). There are two hypotheses to account for this: one, proposed by Soll, is based on potentiation between receptors for the three stimulants (Soll, 1982); the other proposes that acetylcholine and gastrin release histamine (Lorenz, Mohri, Reimann, Troidl, Rohde, & Barth, 1980). In non-rodent mammals, the mucosal source of histamine appears to be a mastlike cell (Lorenz, Thon, Barth, Neugebauer, Reimann, & Kusche, 1983). Histamine release in response to nerve stimulation has yet to be established. Figure 1.1 shows the interactions between receptors on the parietal cell, while Figure 1.2 illustrates the role of histamine as a common mediator.

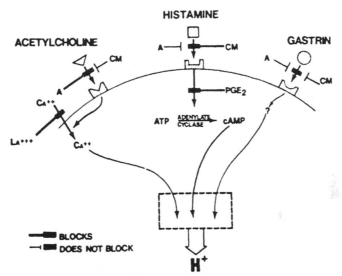

FIGURE 1.1   Receptors on the parietal cell mediating stimulation of acid secretion. Cimetidine (CM), a histamine 2 antagonist, blocks stimulation by histamine,
acetylcholine, and gastrin; atropine (A) blocks only the action of acetylcholine.
The second messenger for acetylcholine and gastrin is probably calcium, while
that for histamine is cyclic AMP. Prostaglandin E_2 blocks the activation of cAMP
by histamine and thereby inhibits acid secretion. Calcium is able to stimulate acid
secretion by penetrating the parietal cell membrane. This is blocked by lanthanum.
(From Soll, A. H. (1981). Physiology of isolated canine parietal cells: Receptors
and effectors regulating function. In L. R. Johnson (Ed.), *Physiology of the gastrointestinal tract*, pp. 673–691. New York: Raven Press.

A calcium-calmodulin complex in the parietal cell may determine levels of
calcium-dependent protein kinases which are thought to influence the availability
of potassium ions for the exchange of H^+ for K^+ at the canalicular membrane,
powered by the $H^+ - K^+$ ATPase or proton pump (Walker, Vinik, Heldsinger,
& Kaveh, 1983).

Similar results have been obtained with isolated fundic glands (Berglindh,
1977). It is interesting that glands from human stomachs after vagotomy
accumulated H^+ at a reduced sensitivity to both histamine and carbachol (Leth,
Elander, Fellenius, Haglund, & Olbe, 1981).

Nervous Stimulation of Acid Secretion in the Isolated Stomach

Electrical field stimulation of the isolated mouse stomach stimulated acid secretion. It was blocked by tetrodotoxin and reduced by atropine and hexamethonium,
a ganglionic cholinergic blocker (Angus & Black, 1978). Mucosal preparations

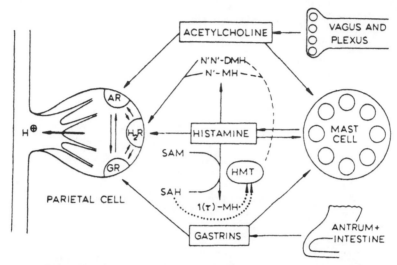

FIGURE 1.2   Stimulants to acid secretion by the parietal cell. Histamine released from mast cells is accorded the central role in this model of the control of acid secretion. Both acetylcholine and gastrin release histamine from mast cells as well as occupying receptors on the parietal cell. The metabolism of histamine is indicated. AR = acetylcholine receptor; $H_2 R = H_2$ receptor; GR = gastrin receptor; $N^1 N^1 - DMH = N^2 N^2 - $ methyl histamine; $N^1 - MH = N^2$ methyl histamine; SAM = S-adenosylhomocysteine; 1 $(r) - MH = r$ methyl histamine; HMT = histamine methyl transferase acting as agonist or releaser,   → acting as an inhibitor   → acting either as an activator or inhibitor depending on the condition. (From Lorenz, W., Troidl, H., & Barth, H. (1975). Stimulus-secretion coupling in the human and canine stomach: Role of histamine. In R. M. Case & H. Goebel (Eds.), *Stimulus secretion coupling in the gastrointestinal tract* (p. 179). Lancaster, PA: MTP Press Ltd.

from rat stomach responded similarly (Baird & Main, 1978). These results are consistent with stimulation of acid secretion by cholinergic neurons in the myenteric plexus.

Pepsinogen and Intrincis Factor Secretion

Rabbit gastric mucosa in organ culture responded to acetylcholine by increasing secretion of pepsinogen and intrinsic factor. The effect was blocked by atropine (Kapadia & Donaldson, 1978). In the isolated fundic gland preparation from rabbits, both acetylcholine and the β-adrenergic agonist isoproterenol stimulated the release of pepsinogen in a dose-related manner. Isoproterenol was without effect on gastric acid secretion (Koelz, Hersey, Sachs, & Chew, 1982). The former's effect was blocked by atropine and the latter by propranolol. Cholinergic binding sites on chief cells in isolated gastric glands have been demonstrated with QNB (Culp, Wolosin, Soll, & Forte, 1983). Similar results were obtained with canine chief cells in primary monolayer culture (Sanders, Amirian, Ayalon, & Soll, 1983).

Alkaline Secretion from Surface Epithelial Cells of the Stomach

Amphibian gastric fundic mucosa secrete bicarbonate actively in vitro in response to carbachol (Flemstrom, 1977). This appears to be the result, in part, of a chloride-bicarbonate exchange at the luminal membrane (Flemstrom & Garner, 1982).

Cholinergic and Adrenergic Control of Secretion in Vivo

Cholinergic and adrenergic transmitters can be given by close intra-arterial or by intravenous injection to determine the pharmacologic actions of these agents. On the other hand, anticholinergics or antiadrenergic drugs can be given by a variety of routes and the extent to which they inhibit nerve-mediated secretion determined. Stable analogues of acetylcholine are potent stimulants of acid secretion in animals but not in man. Beta-adrenergic agonists given intravenously stimulate acid secretion, probably secondary to the release of gastrin (Geumei, Issa, El-Gendi, & Abd-El-Samie, 1969).

The secretion of a bicarbonate-rich fluid with an otherwise similar composition to an ultrafiltrate of plasma can be obtained in dogs after the close intra-arterial injection of acetylcholine (Altimirano, 1963). Mucus secretion was also stimulated (Flemstrom, 1977).

Gastrin and Somatostatin Secretion

Antral mucosa from rats in organ culture released immunoreactive gastrin into the medium in response to carbachol in a dose-related manner (Harty & McGuigan, 1980). It was blocked by atropine. The incorporation of ^{3}H-tryptophane into gastrin also increased in response to carbachol (Harty & McGuigan, 1980). At the same time, the release of somatostatin was reduced by carbachol. The presence of antibodies to somatostatin increased the gastrin released in response to carbachol by 69% (Wolfe, Reel, & McGuigan, 1984). Somatostatin reduced carbachol-induced release of gastrin (Harty, Maico, & McGuigan, 1981). Both norepinephrine and isoproterenol released gastrin and inhibited the release of somatostatin, suggesting parallel cholinergic and β-adrenergic control of gastrin and somatostatin release (Spindel, Harty, & McGuigan, 1984).

Gastrin-releasing peptide (GRP) released gastrin in this preparation. GRP appears to mediate gastrin release in response to β-adrenergic stimulation (Wolfe, Reel, Short, & McGuigan, 1984). Gamma-aminobutyric acid (GABA) released gastrin apparently by releasing acetylcholine from nerve endings (Harty & Franklin,

1983). Adenosine, on the other hand, inhibited the release of gastrin in response to carbachol (Harty & Franklin, 1984). However, carbachol had no effect on gastrin secretion by isolated canine antral mucosal cell cultures (Sugano, Park, Soll, & Yamada, 1984).

Use of the whole stomach in vitro permits a clear distinction between secretion into the vascular compartment and release into the lumen. Gastrin secretion by isolated perfused rat stomachs was increased by methacholine. Seventy-nine percent was secreted into the venous effluent and 21% into the lumen. The effect was blocked by atropine. The secretion of somatostatin was reduced in a reciprocal fashion (Saffouri, Weir, Bitar, & Makhlouf, 1980). Bombesin released gastrin and somatostatin into the venous effluent. Figure 1.3 shows a proposed model for the nervous control of gastrin and somatostatin secretion (Du Val, Saffouri, Weir, Walsh, Arimura, & Mahklouf, 1981). There is controversy over the role of ganglionic receptors in the cholinergic control of gastrin and somatostatin secretion. One group of investigators reported that nicotinic receptor stimulation caused the secretion of both gastrin and somatostatin. Atropine completely blocked only the latter (Schubert & Makhlouf, 1982). An antiserum to

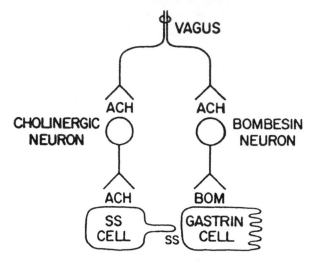

FIGURE 1.3   Model of the neurohumoral control of gastrin secretion. Vagal efferent impulses release acetylcholine which transmits impulses to both a cholinergic inhibitory neuron to somatostatin-secreting cells and a bombesin-like neuron which stimulates gastrin secretion. Somatostatin paracrine secretion inhibits gastrin release. Therefore, vagal stimulation stimulates gastrin secretion by direct cholinergic excitation and by inhibiting the paracrine secretion of somatostatin. (From DuVal, J. W., Saffouri, B., Weir, G. C., Walsh, J. H., Arimura, H., & Mahklouf, G. M. (1981). Stimulation of gastrin and somatostatin secretion from the isolated rat stomach by bombesin. *American Journal of Physiology, 241, (Gastrointestinal and Liver Physiology, 4)* G242–G247).

bombesin reduced gastrin release by two thirds in response to a nicotine ganglionic agonist (Schubert, Walsh, & Makhlouf, 1983). The other group found that hexamethonium, a nicotinic receptor blocker, had no effect on bombesin-induced gastrin release but blocked the release of somatostatin. They concluded that no ganglionic receptors were involved in carbacholine-induced release of gastrin or the inhibition of somatostatin release (Martindale, Kauffman, Levin, Walsh, & Yamada, 1982).

Electrical field stimulation of sheets of rat antral mucosa in Ussing chambers released gastrin and somatostatin on the luminal side. The effect was insensitive to atropine. DMPP (1,1dimethyl-4-phenylpiperazinium) had similar effects which were blocked by hexamethonium (Schubert, Saffouri, & Makhlouf, 1984). The physiological significance of luminal gastrin and somatostatin is unknown. There is evidence, therefore, for vagal noncholinergic release of gastrin (with GRP as a possible neutrotransmitter). There is also evidence for vagal cholinergic inhibition of somatostatin release. Local cholinergic nervous control can be either excitatory or inhibitory to gastrin release. Adrenergic local control is excitatory for gastrin and inhibitory for somatostatin release. The role of nerve cells in the enteric plexus is controversial, and the solution awaits intracellular recordings from these cells.

Extrinsic Nervous Control

The extrinsic innervation of the stomach is supplied by the vagi and splanchnic nerves. The most striking feature of the abdominal vagi is that a majority of nerve fibers are unmyelinated afferents (Morrison, 1977). There may be almost as many afferent fibers in the thoracic-derived splanchnic nerves, but most are myelinated.

The function of vagal afferents with respect to gastric acid is best illustrated by acid secretion mediated by vago-vagal reflexes. In anesthetized cats, electrical stimulation of the central cut end of one vagal trunk resulted in the stimulation of acid secretion (Harper, Kidd, & Scratcherd, 1959). Compared to contractions of the stomach, the acid secretory response was more difficult to demonstrate, possibly because of the presence of more junctions in the pathway (Table 1.1) (Brooks & Carr, 1975).

Mechanoreceptors, osmoreceptors, and chemoreceptors have been demonstrated in single afferents in the vagi (Paintal, 1973). Their physiologic significance in the regulation of gastric acid secretion is less certain. Inhibition of acid secretion by an enterogastric reflex is thought to contain an afferent limb originating in the duodenal bulb (Konturek & Johnson, 1971).

Examination by radio-immunoassays have shown the presence of immunoreactive CCK, gastrin, substance P, somatostatin, VIP, and metenkephalin in the vagus nerves (Lundberg et al., 1978; Rehfeld & Lundberg, 1983). All but

TABLE 1.1
Vagal Stimulation and Basal Gastric Acid Secretion

Afferent Stimulation
26 stimulations in 13 cats
1 increased secretion > 0.0500 mEq/15 min
Efferent Stimulation
56 stimulations in 14 cats
36 increased secretion > 0.0500 mEq/15 min
Mean 0.1931 ± 0.0200 SEM mEq/15 min

Note: From Carr & Brooks, unpublished data.

enkephalin appeared to be in afferent fibers (Lundberg et al., 1979). The nodose ganglion contained a large number of substance P and moderate numbers of VIP reactive cell bodies. Ligation of the vagus nerve indicated the axoplasmic flow of the peptides occurred toward the periphery (Dockray, Gregory, Tracy, & Zhu, 1981). The physiological significance of peptides in axons is unknown.

Electrical stimulation of efferent vagal fibers in anesthetized animals produces different effects depending on the parameters of stimulation. In the ex-vivo perfused dog stomach stimulation at 5 msec pulses, 4 Hz and 1mAmp increased acid outputs, gastric blood flow, and release of gastrin (Lanciault, Shaw, Urquhart, Adair, & Brooks, 1975). If the antrum was excluded, no acid secretory response occurred until a subthreshold dose of gastrin was added to the perfusate (Adair, Shaw, Urquhart, & Brooks, 1974). A similar preparation with pig antrum showed that HCl in the lumen of the antrum increased somatostatin release and decreased the release of gastrin. Vagal stimulation increased gastrin output and decreased somatostatin release (Holst, Jensen, Knuhtsen, Nielsen, & Rehfeld, 1983).

In intact cats and dogs, electrical efferent vagal stimulation stimulates acid secretion, gastric blood flow, and gastrin release into the blood (Bauer, 1977; Bonfils, Mignon, & Rozé, 1979; Lanciault, Bonoma, & Brooks, 1973; Sjodin, 1971). In the cat, acid output approaches maximal pentagastrin-stimulated values (Figure 1.4). Plasma gastrin levels correlated with acid output (Figure 1.5). Stereological analysis indicates that vagal stimulation converts the ultrastructure of parietal cells from a resting to a stimulated pattern (Zalewsky, Bauer, Moody, & Brooks, 1977). The overriding importance of vagal stimulation is shown by the occurrence of maximal acid output despite the simultaneous release of glucagon, somatostatin, and VIP, all of which are inhibitors of acid secretion (Brooks, 1981). Paradoxically, there is a vagal inhibition of gastrin release, independent of antral pH (Olbe, Logan, Goto, Pappas, & Walsh, 1984). An interesting phenomenon of unknown physiological significance was the release of gastrin and somatostatin into the lumen of the stomach during vagal stimulation (Degertikin et al., 1984; Uvnäs-Wallensten, 1977; Uvnäs-Wallensten, Efendic, & Luft, 1977).

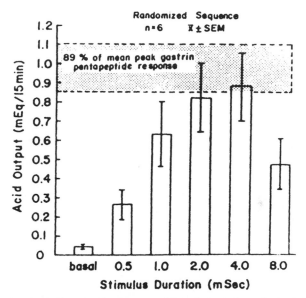

FIGURE 1.4   Acid outputs in response to bilateral cervical vagal stimulation in six cats anesthetized with chloralose-urethane. Stimulation with bipolar platinum electrodes was at 5 Hz and 1 mAmp, while the pulse duration was varied from 0.5 to 8 msec. Note maximum acid output at 4 msec approached maximum acid output obtainable with pentagastrin intravenously in similar cats. (From Brooks, F. P. (1981). Neural factors regulating gastric function. In Weiner, M. A. Hofer, & A. S. Stunkard (1981) *Brain, behavior, and bodily disease* (p. 90). New York: Raven Press.

Electrical stimulation in the above experiments is almost certainly not physiologic. In the sheep's parotid gland, electrical activity recorded from single units in post-ganglionic parasympathetic nerves during reflex-induced secretion showed a pattern of action potentials in doublets or triplets rather than a continuous regular discharge (Carr, 1977). A comparison of bursts with continuous stimulation of vagal efferents was carried out in anesthetized ferrets. Bursts at 10 times the continuous frequency of stimulation but for a tenth of the length of time were also compared with bursts at a frequency obtained from recordings of vagal efferents during reflex-induced secretion. Acid secretion was less during natural bursts and even lower during high-frequency stimulation than during continuous low-frequency stimulation (Grundy and Scratcherd, 1982). Stimulation of the left cervical vagal trunk elicited larger acid outputs than that of the right. Fatigue of the response began to appear after three hours of stimulation in the dog and cat (Bauer, 1977; Cumming, Greetham, & Percival, 1969).

There is also evidence for vago-sympathetic reflex stimulation of acid secretion when an α-adrenergic receptor blockade was established (Tansy, Probst, & Martin, 1975).

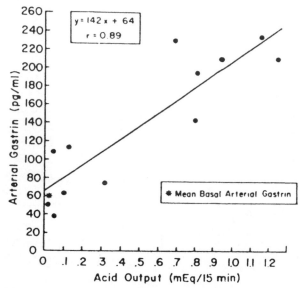

FIGURE 1.5   Correlation between acid output and immunoreactive gastrin levels in femoral arterial blood in five anesthetized cats during electrical stimulation of efferent vagal fibers just below the diaphragm. Note that the actual level of gastrin prior to electrical stimulation when acid output was <0.1 mM/15 min was very close to the extrapolated level at zero acid output. (From Brooks, F. P. (1981). Neural factors regulating gastric function. In H. Weiner, M. A. Hofer, and A. S. Stunkard *Brain, behavior, and bodily disease* (p. 90). New York: Raven Press.

Vagal Stimulation in Conscious Subjects

Vagal stimulation can be exerted under these conditions by sham feeding, insulin hypoglycemia, or glucocytopenia produced by 2-deoxy-D-glucose. Sham feeding for a sufficiently long period can produce maximal acid outputs (Preshaw & Webster, 1967). Resection of the antrum and duodenal bulb reduced the acid secretory response to sham feeding. It could be restored by a subthreshold dose of gastrin (Olbe, 1964).

Sham Feeding

For human studies, sham feeding can be modified by a "chew-and-spit" technique. By this method, sham feeding accounted for a third of the acid output in response to a meal; distention and chemostimulation by means of small peptides and amino acids accounted for the rest (Richardson, Walsh, Cooper, Feldman, & Fordtran, 1977). Intragastric titration to a pH of 2.5 abolished gastrin release and reduced acid output in response to sham feeding by 50%. This finding suggests that the acid secretion during vagal stimulation is mediated equally by a direct effect on parietal cells and by the release of gastrin (Feldman & Walsh,

1980). However, in patients with duodenal ulcer after surgical resection of the antrum and duodenal bulb (the major sources of gastrin), sham feeding-induced acid secretion was reduced by 61% (Knutson & Olbe, 1974). It was not restored to its preoperative level by subthreshold doses of gastrin or pentagastrin. Rather the effect was additive (Knutson & Olbe, 1974). These results suggest that the permissive role of gastrin in mediating vagal stimulation of acid secretion in man is less important than in dogs.

Proximal gastric vagotomy in duodenal ulcer patients almost abolished the acid secretory response to modified sham feeding and prevented the rise in serum gastrin. Atropine reduced acid output but failed to prevent the rise in gastrin (Stenquist, Rehfeld, & Olbe, 1979). Vagotomy abolishes acid secretion during sham feeding in animals. These results suggest that there is a non-cholinergically mediated release of gastrin which is active during vagal stimulation. There is also a vagal cholinergic inhibition of gastrin release.

In conscious human subjects, inhibition of gastrin release in response to sham feeding can be divided into two mechanisms: one related to intragastric pH and the other to a cholinergic vagal inhibitory mechanism (Micali et al., 1984). Paradoxically, sham feeding increased the release of somatostatin into gastric content (Degertekin et al., 1984). Inhibition of the acid secretory response to sham feeding by antral acidification could be reduced by pretreatment with indomethacin, suggesting a role for prostaglandins in mediating inhibition of gastrin release (Befrits, Samuelsson, & Johansson, 1984). Finally, anticipated feeding, such as watching or smelling food preparation, can stimulate acid secretion without a detectable rise in plasma gastrin (Moore & Motoki, 1979). This indicates a direct nervous pathway to the parietal cell.

Hypoglycemia and Glucocytopenia

Insulin hypoglycemia is a more potent stimulus to acid secretion in man than is sham feeding. When the hypoglycemia is produced by the intravenous infusion of insulin, a steady state can be achieved and acid output approaches maximal secretory levels (Farooq & Isenberg, 1975). The stimulating effect of insulin is due to the hypoglycemia-activating glucose receptors in the hypothalamus, globus pallidus, and medulla, which in turn relay nerve impulses to the dorsal motor nucleus of the vagus. There is both a threshold of hypoglycemia and a dose response to insulin (Baron, 1979; Spencer & Grossman, 1971). There is characteristically a delay in the acid-secretory response after the intravenous injection of insulin with the onset of acid secretion following the nadir of the blood glucose. Recordings from vagal efferents in the rat show an approximate doubling of the frequency of spontaneous action potentials in the gastric vagus nerve after insulin (Hirano & Niijima, 1980).

In man, insulin hypoglycemia also stimulates gastric acid secretion by way of vagal efferents to the stomach. However, insulin hypoglycemia can still release gastrin after an anatomically complete vagotomy, probably by adrenergic pathways. This may account for the difficulty in interpretation of the completeness of vagotomy with slight increases in acid output after insulin.

Stimulation of acid gastric secretion by 2-deoxy-D-glucose is based on the production of glucocytopenia in the same cells stimulated by insulin hypoglycemia. In comparison with insulin hypoglycemia, the acid secretory response in dogs has a shorter lag phase (Figure 1.6) (Brooks & Grossman, 1969).

The significance of hypoglycemia in the physiological control of acid secretion is uncertain, but a comparison of acid outputs with blood glucose during blood sugar levels of 35–40 mg showed maximal acid outputs. From 59–110 mg per dl there was an inverse relationship, and from 110 mg per dl and greater there was no effect (Moore, 1980).

Another nervous mediated mechanism for the stimulation of gastric acid secretion is the reflex release of gastrin by distention of the antrum or of the corpus by local or vago-vagal reflexes (Debas, Walsh, & Grossman, 1975; Grossman, 1962).

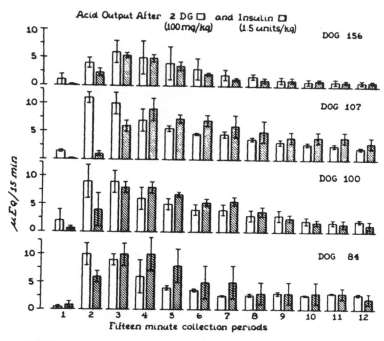

FIGURE 1.6   Acid output after 2-deoxy-D-glucose (2 DG) and insulin. (In this figure, the units on the ordinate should be mEq/15 min.) (From Brooks, F. P., & Grossman, M. I. (1969). Vagal stimulation of bile flow in conscious dogs. In S. Y. Botelho, F. P. Brooks, & W. B. Shelley. (Eds.), *Exocrine glands* (p. 261). Philadelphia: University of Pennsylvania Press.

The Effects of Vagotomy

In dogs, the effect of vagotomy was to shift the dose response of acid secretion to histamine and gastrin to the right while acetylcholine-like agents shift it to the left (Figure 1.7) (Emas & Grossman, 1967; Hirschowitz, 1977). Converting a vagally innervated fundic pouch to a vagally denervated pouch reduced the percent of maximal acid secretory response during a meal from 67 to 33% (Helander, Svensson, & Emas, 1979). In cats, vagally denervated pouches contained smaller parietal cells and a lower volume density of parietal cells than vagally innervated mucosa (Helander et al., 1979).

The effect of truncal vagotomy in man was also to reduce the sensitivity of parietal cells to histamine (Elder et al., 1972; Rosato & Rosato, 1971). The inhibiting effect of fat in the duodenum and of glucagon was also dependent on intact vagi (Kihl & Olbe, 1980; Olsen, Kirkegaard, Holst, & Christiansen, 1982). The effect of fat may be mediated by the release of neurotensin. Neurotensin inhibited acid secretion in vagally innervated but not denervated fundic pouches in dogs (Anderson, Chang, Folkers, & Rosell, 1976; Anderson, Rosell, Sjodin, & Folkers, 1980).

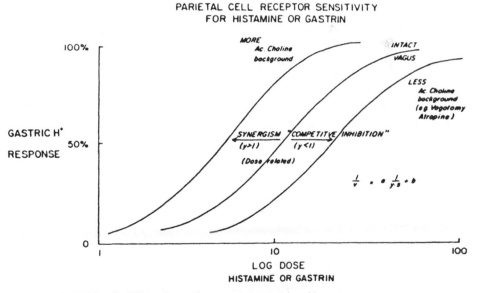

FIGURE 1.7   Effect of truncal vagotomy on gastric acid secretory response to varying doses of histamine or gastrin in conscious dogs. The sensitivity of the parietal cells to histamine and gastrin is reduced by vagotomy or atropine and increased by bethanechol. (From Hirschowitz, B. I. (1977). The vagus and gastric secretion. In F. P. Brooks & P. W. Evers (Eds.), *Nerves and the gut* (pp. 96–118). Thorofare, NJ: Charles B. Slack Inc.

The Role of the Splanchnic Nerves
in the Regulation of Gastric Acid Secretion

In cats, splanchnic nerve electrical stimulation inhibited vagally stimulated acid secretion by 40% and blood flow by 70% (Reed & Sanders, 1971; Reed, Sanders, & Thorpe, 1977). It also reduced the response to histamine and pentagastrin.

Epinephrine in low doses caused an increase in acid output in man and an increase in serum gastrin. Higher doses increased gastrin levels but had no effect on gastric acid output (Christensen & Stadil, 1976). Norepinephrine in higher doses inhibited acid output. Propranolol, an β-adrenergic antagonist, blocked the effects of epinephrine on gastrin release and acid output (Stadil & Rehfeld, 1973). Distention-induced release of gastrin in man appears to be mediated by β-adrenergic pathways (Peters, Walsh, Ferrari, & Feldman, 1982).

Regulation of Pepsinogen
and Intrinsic Factor Secretion

Insulin hypoglycemia in dogs is a more potent stimulus to pepsinogen secretion than either histamine or a meat meal (Long & Brooks, 1965). It is also a potent stimulant in man (Hengels, Fritsch, & Samloff, 1983). Electrical efferent vagal stimulation increases pepsinogen secretion in the cat and ferret (Andrews, Scratcherd, & Wynne, 1976; Reed & Sanders, 1971). The secretion of intrinsic factor responded in parallel with that of acid initially, but then faded while acid secretion maintained a plateau (Vatu, 1975).

Neuropeptides and Neurotransmitters in Vivo

Acetylcholine is a well-recognized muscarinic neurotransmitter in the vagal control of gastric acid secretion. Atropine is a typical example of an anticholinergic muscarinic antagonist acting at the level of cholinergic receptors on secretory cells. Hexomethionium is the prototype of an anticholinergic agent acting on nicotinic cholinergic receptors on parasympathetic ganglia. Recent studies have shown that there are subclasses of muscarinic receptor antagonists: One (M_1) on secretory cells and the other (M_2) on ganglion cells (Feldman, 1984). Pirenzepine is probably an example of an M_2 antagonist.

Enkephalins

Enkephalins are present in the myenteric plexus (Polak, Bloom, Sullivan, Facer, & Pearse, 1977). Since the opiate antagonist naloxone reduces basal acid output and the response to sham feeding in man, opioid neuropeptides may play a role in mediating normal responses (Feldman & Cowley, 1982).

Nervous Control of Gastric Mucosal Blood Flow

Direct microscopic visualization of mucosal blood flow makes its possible to record the diameter of blood vessels in vivo. In cats it has been shown that electrical vagal stimulation increased blood flow while splanchnic stimulation reduced it. The neurotransmitter released during splanchnic stimulation is norepinephrine; that released by the vagus is unknown (Guth & Smith, 1977). Blood flow and gastric acid secretion after splanchnic stimulation were reduced in parallel (Blair et al., 1975).

Vagal stimulation also increased the permeability of capillaries (Jansson, Lundgren, & Martinson, 1970). Electrical field stimulation of strips from dog gastric arteries in vitro reduced the contractile response to norepinephrine. The response was blocked by atropine, suggesting a cholinergic innervation (Van Hee & Vanhoutte, 1978). Electrical vagal stimulation of perfused stomachs decreased the perfusion pressure. Vagotomy in general reduces gastric mucosal blood flow. There is some controversy over how long the effect lasts (Bell & Battersby, 1968; Delaney, 1967; Hunter, Goldstone, Vella, & Way, 1979; Knight, McIsaac, & Fielding, 1978; Nakamura, Ishi, Kusano, & Hayshi, 1974).

Central Nervous Control of Gastric Secretion

There is a rapidly developing fund of information regarding control at the levels of the medulla, the hypothalamus, and the limbic system. One of the older experimental tools is to determine the effect of transecting the brain at different levels. We found that decortication in cats decreased acid output in response to electrical efferent vagal stimulation (Figure 1.8). Basal plasma gastrin and gastrin release in response to vagal stimulation was increased modestly. It is interesting that sensory deprivation by blinding (Schapiro, Britt, & Dohrn, 1973; Schapiro, Wruble, Britt, & Bell, 1970; Schapiro, Wruble, Britt, & Bell, 1970a) destruction of the inner ear (Schapiro, Gross, Nakamura, Wruble, & Britt, 1970), or sectioning of the olfactory stalks (Schapiro, Britt, Gross, & Gaines, 1971) in conscious dogs also depressed the acid secretory response to vagal stimulation. In contrast to decortication midcollicular decerebration had no effect on acid output during electrical efferent vagal stimulation but markedly increased the concentration of gastrin in the blood (Figure 1.9) (Feng, Aronchick, & Brooks, 1983).

One of the important new techniques is the use of horseradish peroxidase to trace nervous pathways between the stomach and the brain. Yamamoto and his colleagues injected HRP into the wall of the stomach of cats and found labeling of cells in the dorsal motor nucleus of the vagus (DMV) and the nucleus of the tractus solitarius (Yamamoto, Satomi, Ise, & Takahushi, 1977). Kalia and Mesulam traced vagal afferents from the nodose ganglion to the nucleus ambiguus and the nucleus retroambigualis in the cat (Kalia & Mesulam, 1980). They also compared the projection of vagal efferents from the larynx, tracheobronchial

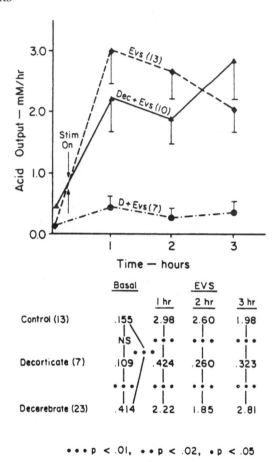

FIGURE 1.8   Diamond-shaped points indicate acid output in response to bilateral electrical efferent cervical vagal stimulation (EVS) in anesthetized cats with gastric fistulae. Parameters of stimulation were 5 Hz, 1 mAmp, and a pulse duration of 4 msec. Basal gastric content was collected for one hour before beginning stimulation. Solid triangles indicate acid output when a midcollicular decerebration was performed prior to collecting gastric content. Solid circles indicate acid output when a cerebral decortication had been performed. Numbers in parentheses indicate number of cats. (From Feng, H. S., Aronchick, C. A., & Brooks, F. P. (1983). Decortication and decerebration effects compared on efferent electrical vagal stimulation of the stomach in cats. *Clinical Research*, *31*, 530A.

tree, pulmonary parenchyma, heart, and gastrointestinal tract to the dorsal motor nucleus and were unable to detect the localization of cell bodies in relation to the site of termination of axons (Kalia & Mesulam, 1980).

Gillis and his associates used the dye-fast blue to trace efferent vagal pathways to the medulla of the cat. Injections into the corpus or fundus of the stomach labeled only cell bodies in the DMV and the nucleus retroambigualis, while

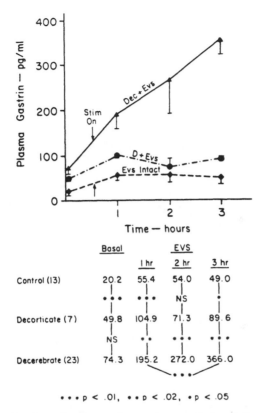

$$\bullet \bullet \bullet\ p < .01,\quad \bullet \bullet\ p < .02,\quad \bullet\ p < .05$$

FIGURE 1.9   Plasma immunoreactive gastrin concentrations before and during bilateral electrical efferent cervical vagal stimulation (EVS) in anesthetized cats with gastric fistulae. Parameters of stimulation as in Figure 8. Symbols indicate control cats (diamond-shaped points), decerebrate cats (solid triangles), and decorticate cats (solid circles). (From Feng, H. S., Aronchick, C. A., & Brooks, F. P. (1983). Decortication and decerebration effects compared on efferent electrical vagal stimulation of the stomach in cats. *Clinical Research, 31*, 530A.

injections into the antrum or pylorus were followed by labeling of cell bodies only in the DMV. There were fewer cells labeled in the right nucleus than in the left. Similarly, with corpus and fundic injections fewer cells were labeled on the right in the DMV and only those in the left nucleus retroambigualis were labeled (Pagani, Norman, & Gillis, 1984. Figure 1.10) shows a cross section of the brain stem at the level of the vagal nuclei (Pagani, Norman, Kasbekar, & Gillis, 1984).

After demonstrating central projections from the antrum and pylorus with fast blue, the same sections were examined by immunocytologic methods and substance P, 5-hydroxytryptamine and avian pancreatic polypeptide immunoreactivity was found in nerve fibers adjacent to the cell bodies and dendrites of cells

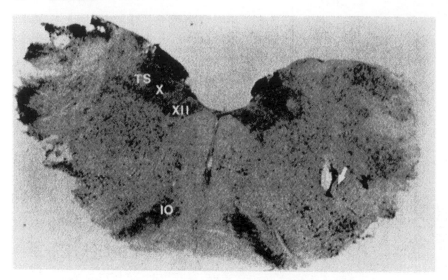

FIGURE 1.10   Coronal section of brain stem passing through nucleus ambiguus (indicated by *arrow*), tractus solitarius (TS), dorsal motor nucleus of vagus (X), hypoglossal nucleus (XII), and inferior olivary nucleus (IO). Lesion site (L) marks site of electrical stimulation located 4.0 mm beneath dorsal surface of brain stem. (From Pagani, F. D., Norman, W. P., Kasbekar, D. K., & Gillis, R. A. (1984). Effects of stimulation of nucleus ambiguus complex on gastroduodenal function. *American Journal of Physiology, 9, (Gastrointestinal and Liver Physiology* 3): G253–G262.

labeled with fast blue. Positive immunoreactivity was found in the area for CCK and dynorphin but not for neurotensin, enkephalin, GABA, or corticotropin-releasing factor (CRF). These results suggest that the substances detected could function as neurotransmitters (Gillis, Skirboll, Norman, & Pagani, 1984). Substance P-like immunoreactivity was localized to punctate varicosities in the periphery of the DMV in cats. Some made synaptic contact with the cell bodies of neurons in the DMV (Maley & Elde, 1981).

Coil and Norgren incubated the cut central stump of the dorsal and ventral vagal trunks below the diaphragm in HRP and found bilateral labeling in the rat of about a third of the cells in the rostral portion of the nucleus ambiguus. Incubation of the ventral trunk labeled the DMV on the left side, while that of the dorsal trunk resulted in bilateral labeling (Coil & Norgren, 1979).

These results take on more physiologic significance when we consider the effect of electrical stimulation of the vagal nuclei. Stimulation of the DMV produced increases in the number and amplitude of phasic antral contractions in 17 of 30 cats, but increases in acid output were seen in only 7 of 37 15-minute collections in 25 cats. Increases in both acid secretion and antral contractions were seen in 5 cats (Lombardi, Feng, & Brooks, 1982). Similar studies reported no increases in titratable acidity but an increase in pepsinogen secretion during stimulation of the DMV (Ormsbee et al., 1982). In both studies, stimulation of the cervical efferent vagi produced increases in both acid output and antral contractions.

Stimulation of the nucleus ambiguus increased antral phasic contractions and possibly bicarbonate secretion, but not the secretion of pepsinogen (Pagani, Norman, Kasbekar, & Gillis, 1984). On the basis of the failure of retrograde labeling of cell bodies in the nucleus ambiguus from antral and pyloric injections of fast blue, it seems likely that the neurons in the nucleus act indirectly to stimulate contractions, possibly by way of the DMV. Failure of high frequency (>50 H$_2$) stimulation to produce contractions is consistent with multiple synapses in the pathway (Pagani et al., 1984).

The above experiments were conducted in anesthetized cats. Wyrwicka and Garcia stimulated the DMV in conscious cats with chronically implanted electrodes and noted an increase in acid output in 8 of 14 cats where the tips of the electrodes were found to be in the DMV (Wyrwicka & Garcia, 1979).

There is evidence for a GABA neuromodulating or transmitting system in the nucleus ambiguus of the cat with inhibition of antral contractions by GABA agonists (muscimol) and stimulation by GABA antagonists (bicuculline) when injected into the nucleus (Williford et al., 1981). No information is available in cats on effects on acid secretion, but intracerebroventricular (ICV) injection of muscimol in rats stimulated acid secretion by a cholinergically mediated pathway. The effect was reversed by bicuculline (Levine, Morley, Kneip, Grace, & Silvis, 1981). A stable analogue of GABA, beta-cp-chlorphenyl-gamma aminobutyric acid (a lipophilic, GABA mimetic), is a potent stimulus to acid secretion in the rat after subcutaneous infection. Its effect is blocked by atropine or vagotomy (Goto & Debas, 1983, Figure 1.11) shows a dose response of acid output.

The hypothalamus has been implicated in the nervous control of gastric acid secretion for many years. In rats, acid secretion could be increased or decreased by electrical stimulation in the lateral or ventromedial areas of the hypothalamus (Brooks, 1967). Later studies showed that the response was not homogeneous throughout the ventromedial hypothalamus (Ishikawa, Zagata, & Osumi, 1983). Feeding or satiety behavior respectively could be elicited by stimulation in these areas (Brooks, 1967). Attempts to confirm these observations in cats resulted in dissociation between feeding behavior and acid secretion (Wyrwicka, 1978). Comparable ventromedial hypothalamic lesions in rats increased basal acid secretion and food intake but not in cats (Wyrwicka, 1978). Subsequent studies have confirmed the effect of ventromedial lesions on acid secretion and extended them to an increased response to sucrose (Weingarten & Powley, 1980).

The hypothalamus is also involved in a control system relating glucose homeostasis to acid secretion. In cats, 2-deoxy-D-glucose injected into the lateral hypothalamus stimulated gastric acid output much as did electrical stimulation. The effect was blocked by electrolytic lesions in the lateral hypothalamus. Reflex loops mediating acid secretion in response to diminished availability of glucose

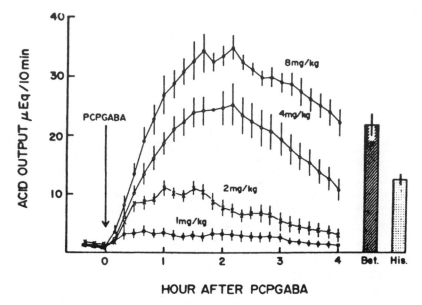

HOUR AFTER PCPGABA

FIGURE 1.11   Acid response of the rat stomach to graded doses of beta-(p-chlorophenyl)-gamma-aminobutyric acid given subcutaneously. Each point represents mean (± SE) 10-min acid output in eight rats. The maximal 10-min acid responses to bethanechol (Bet) 1 mg/kg and to histamine (His) 10 mg/kg are shown as bars for comparison. (From Goto, Y., & Debas, H. T. (1983). GABA-mimetic effect on gastric acid secretion: Possible significance in central mechanisms. *Digestive Disease and Science 28*, 56–60.

originate in the liver, medulla, median forebrain bundle, and hypothalamus with efferent pathways via the DMV and the globus pallidus (Figure 1.12) (Kadekaro, Timo-Iaria, de Lourdes, & Vicentini, (1980).

Hypothalamic stimulation in rats with simultaneous recordings from the DMV have defined an excitatory pathway for gastric acid secretion from the lateral hypothalamus to the DMV (Shiraishi, 1980). Neurons responding to deoxyglucose coincident with a fall in gastric pH accounted for over half of all neurons responding to deoxyglucose (Shiraishi & Simpson, 1982). Direct projections from the amygdaloid to the dorsal motor nucleus of rats have also been demonstrated (Takeuchi, Matsushima, Matsushima, & Hopkins, 1983). Other evidence for an organized central nervous system responding to insulin hypoglycemia comes from the demonstration of increased utilization of glucose in the nucleus of the solitary tract, the DMV, the medial forebrain bundle, the superior olivary nucleus, and the interstitial nucleus of the stria terminalis in the rat (Kadekaro, Savaki, & Sokaloff, 1980). Intraventricular injections of labeled insulin showed selective binding over the median eminence and in the ventral arcuate nucleus (van Houten & Posner, 1980).

FIGURE 1.12   A system for the role of glucose homeostasis in the control of gastric acid secretion. Glucoreceptors are located in the medulla, midbrain, hypothalamus, globus pallidus, and in the liver. Four reflex loops are illustrated: (1) from the median forebrain bundle via the dorsal nucleus, (2) from the hypothalamus and globus pallidus via the lateral hypothalamus or the mesencephalon to the dorsal motor nuclei of the vagus, (3) from the liver via the lower brain stem, and (4) from the lower brain stem via the dorsal motor nuclei of the vagi. H (hypothalamus), MD (mesodiencephalic transition), R (rhomboencephalon), GH (hypothalamic receptor), GL (liver glucoreceptors) GR (rhomboencephalic glucoreceptors), GP (globus pallidus). (1) Hypothalamo-hypothalamic relay, (2) Hypothalamo-pallidal loops with hypothalamic relay (2a) and direct hypothalamo-pallidal loops (2b). (3) Hepato-rhombo-encephalic loop (with a probably ascending pathway to the hypothalamic center). (4) Rhomboencephalic loop. S (stomach). Interrupted lines represent pathways whose location and whose synaptic relays are unknown. (From Kadekaro, M., Timo-Iaria, C., & de L. M. Vicentini, M. (1977). Control of gastric secretion by the central nervous system. In F. P. Brooks & P. W. Evers (Eds.), *Nerves and the gut* (pp. 377–429). Thorofare, NJ: Charles B. Slack Inc.

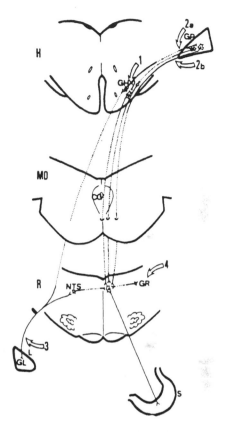

Attempts are now in progress to define putative neurotransmitters in the hypothalamus by injecting minute amounts of the material into the brain substance or into the cerebral ventricles. Excitation of gastric acid secretion has been reported after the injection of pentagastrin into the lateral hypothalamus and the medulla in rats (Evered, Minty, & Tepperman, 1982; Tepperman & Evered, 1980). The injection of tetragastrin into the lateral hypothalamus was associated with an increased frequency of electrical discharges in the hypothalamus (Simpson & Shiraishi, 1980). Injection of CRF into the paraventricular hypothalamus in pylorus-ligated rats reduced acid output (Gunion & Taché, 1984).

A number of peptides alter gastric secretion when injected into the cerebral ventricles or the cisterna magna. In rats, intracisternal bombesin inhibited acid secretion after pyloric ligation (Lesiege & Taché, 1983). The effect appears to be neurally mediated, in part, by α-2 receptors through the spinal sympathetic innervation of the stomach. Gastrin-releasing peptide (mammalian bombesin) has a similar effect (Taché, Marki, Rivier, Vale, & Brown, 1981). (see also Dr. Taché's chapter). In anesthetized cats, ICV bombesin inhibited acid secretion in response to efferent electrical stimulation of the cervical vagi (Aronchick,

Feng, Brooks, & Chey, 1983). In conscious dogs, ICV bombesin inhibited pentagastrin and meal-stimulated acid secretion (Pappas, Hamel, Debas, & Taché, 1984). When given intravenously, bombesin stimulated acid secretion in these species.

CRF inhibited acid secretion given intravenously to cats and dogs (Taché, Goto, Gunion, Rivier, & Debas, 1984). Given into the cerebral ventricles of conscious dogs, it also inhibited acid secretion mediated in part by parasympathetic ganglia, opioids, and vasopressin (Lenz, Hester, Webb, & Brown, 1984). Thyrocalcitonin (Morley, Levine, & Silvis, 1981) and calcitonin-gene related peptide injected into the cisterna magna or cerebral ventricular system inhibit acid secretion in pylorus-ligated rats or conscious dogs (Lenz, Vale, Rivier, & Brown, 1984; Lenz, Webb, Hester, Rivier, & Brown, 1984; Taché et al., 1984).

Prostaglandin E_2 given ICV inhibited acid secretion in anesthetized rats (Puururen, 1983). By comparison, norepinephrine inhibited acid output in rats. It also blocked the stimulating effect of electrical stimulation of the lateral hypothalamus (Osumi, Aibara, Sakae, & Fujiwara, 1977).

In contrast, a thyrotropic-releasing hormone analogue injected intracisternally in rats produced a dose-dependent increase in acid secretion (Schubert & Makhlouf, 1982). The effect was partially blocked by vagotomy.

Without knowing the site of action or the fate of peptides injected into the cerebrospinal fluid, it is difficult to interpret the functional significance of these results. They do provide preliminary evidence for identifying potentially important neuromodulators and neurotransmitters in the central nervous system.

Behavioral Factors in the Central Nervous Control
of Gastric Acid Secretion

We have reviewed these in the past (Brooks, 1967; Smith & Brooks, 1970). Certainly the relation of the control of acid secretion and such carefully controlled functions as food intake and glucose homeostasis have added much to our knowledge of both the control of gastric secretion and feeding behavior. I will mention only two recent preliminary reports in healthy human subjects. Cold stress had an initial depressing effect on acid secretion followed by a rebound after removing the cold stress (Thompson, Richardson, & Malagelada, 1983) (Figure 1.13). This is reminiscent of the observations in monkeys subjected to avoidance conditioning (Polish, Brady, Mason, Thach, & Niemeck, 1962).

Hypnotically induced sensations of eating an ideal meal produced a threefold increase in acid output, while inducing an avoidance of thinking about food when hungry reduced both basal acid output and pentagastrin-stimulated acid output (Klein & Spiegel, 1984). When confirmed, this report will be a welcome advance over the negative results of the past (Hall, Herb, Brady, & Brooks, 1967).

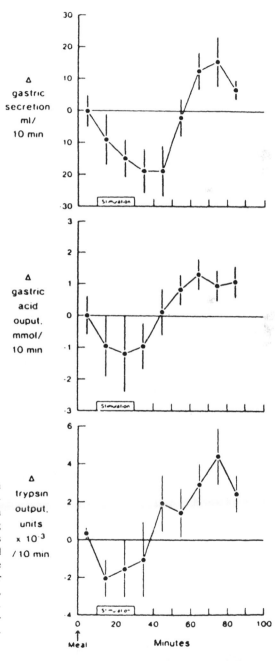

FIGURE 1.13   Noxious stimulation and gastric acid and pancreatic protease secretion in nine normal human subjects. Painful stimuli (immersing the hands in ice water) first inhibits acid secretion during a meal followed 50 minutes later by an overshoot above baseline. Trypsin follows a similar pattern. (From Thompson, D. G., Richelson, E., & Malagelada, J-R. (1983). Perturbation of upper gastrointestinal function by cold stress. *Gut, 24,* 277–283.

In summary, nervous control of acid secretion has been evaluated at the intramural, extrinsic, and brain levels. The recognition of new neurotransmitters and nervous pathways has already led to recognition of discrete sensory and motor systems. The attraction of new investigators to the field bodes well for future research.

REFERENCES

Adair, L. S., Shaw, S. E., Urquhart, S., & Brooks, F. P. (1974). Permissive role of gastrin in vagally mediated acid secretion. *The Physiologist, 17,* 169.

Altamirano, M. (1963). Alkaline secretion produced by intra-arterial acetylcholine. *Journal of Physiology (London), 168,* 787–803.

Andersson, S., Chang, D., Folkers, K., & Rosell, S. (1976). Inhibition of gastric acid secretion in dogs by neurotensin. *Life Sciences, 19,* 367–370.

Andersson, S., Rosell, S., Sjodin, L., & Folkers, K. (1980). Inhibition of acid secretion from vagally innervated and denervated gastric pouches by (Glu^4)-neurotensin. *Scandinavian Journal of Gastroenterology, 15,* 253–256.

Andrews, P. L. R., Scratcherd, T., & Wynne, R. D. A. (1976). The vagal stimulation of gastric acid, pepsin, and motility in the anesthetized ferret. *Journal of Physiology (London), 259,* 9–10P.

Angus, J. A., & Black, J. W. (1978). Production of acid secretion in the mouse isolated stomach by electrical field stimulation. *British Journal of Pharmacology, 62,* 460P.

Aronchick, C., Feng, H. S., Brooks, F. P., & Chey, W-Y. (1983). Bombesin in the 4th ventricle of cats inhibits vagally stimulated antral contractions and acid secretion. *Gastroenterology, 84,* 1093.

Baird, A. W., & Main, I. H. M. (1978). Characterization of acid secretory responses of the rat isolated gastric mucosa to electrical field stimulation. *British Journal of Pharmacology, 64,* 445–446P.

Baron, J. H. (1979). *Clinical tests of gastric secretion.* New York: Oxford University Press.

Bauer, R. F. (1977). Electrically induced vagal stimulation of gastric acid secretion. In F. P. Brooks & P. W. Evers (Eds.), *Nerves and the gut* (pp. 86–95). Thorofare, NJ: Charles B. Slack, Inc.

Befrits, R., Samuelsson, K., & Johansson, C. (1984). Gastric acid inhibition by antal acidification mediated by endogenous prostaglandins. *Gastroenterology, 86,* 1023.

Bell, P. R. F., & Battersby, C. (1968). Effect of vagotomy on gastric mucosal blood flow. *Gastroenterology, 54,* 1032–1037.

Berglindh, T. (1977). Potentiation by carbachol and aminophylline of histamine and dc-cAMP induced parietal cell activity in isolated gastric glands. *Acta Physiologica Scandinavica, 99,* 75–84.

Blair, E. L., Grand, E. R., Reed, J. D., Sanders, D. J., Sanger, G., & Shaw, B. (1975). The effect of sympathetic nerve stimulation on serum gastrin, gastric acid secretion and mucosal blood flow responses to meat extract stimulation in anesthetized cats. *Journal of Physiology (London), 253,* 493–504.

Bonfils, S., Mignon, M., & Rozé, C. (1979). Vagal control of gastric secretion. *International Review of Physiology, 19,* 59–106.

Brooks, F. P. (1967). Central neural control of acid secretion. In C. F. Code (Ed.), *Handbook of physiology. Section 6: Alimentary canal. Volume II: Secretion* (pp. 805–826). Washington, DC: American Physiological Society.

Brooks, F. P. (1968). Central inhibition of gastric secretion. In L. S. Semb & S. Myren (Eds.), *The physiology of gastric secretion* (pp. 338–344). Baltimore: Williams and Wilkins Co.

Brooks, F. P. (1975). The role of the brain in the control of gastric secretion. In M. H. F. Friedman (Ed.), *Functions of the stomach and intestine* (pp. 207–220). Baltimore: University Park Press.

Brooks, F. P. (1977). Nervous control of gastrointestinal function: Neurophysiological considerations. In G. B. Jerzy-Glass (Ed.), *Progress in gastroenterology* (Vol. III, pp. 373–394). New York: Grune and Stratton, Inc.

Brooks, F. P. (1981). Neural factors regulating gastric function. In H. Weiner, M. A. Hofer, & A. S. Stunkard (Eds.), *Brain, behavior and bodily disease* (pp. 87–97). New York: Raven Press.

Brooks, F. P., & Carr, D. H. (1975). Gastric acid and motor responses to electrical stimulation of afferent and efferent fibres in the cat's vagus. *Journal of Physiology (London), 250*, 17–18P.

Brooks, F. P., & Davis, R. A. (1965). The nervous control of gastric secretion. In W. S. Yamamoto & J. R. Brobeck (Eds.), *Physiological controls and regulations* (pp. 295–307). Philadelphia: W. B. Saunders Co.

Brooks, F. P., & Grossman, M. I. (1969). Vagal stimulation of bile flow in conscious dogs. In S. Y. Botelho, F. P. Brooks, & W. B. Shelley (Eds.), *The exocrine glands* (pp. 253–275). Philadelphia: The University of Pennsylvania Press.

Carr, D. H. (1977). Reflex-induced electrical activity in single units of secretory nerves to the parotid gland. In F. P. Brooks & P. W. Evers (Eds.), *Nerves and the gut* (pp. 79–85). Thorofare, NJ: Charles B. Slack, Inc.

Christensen, K. C., & Stadil, F. (1976). Effect of epinephrine and norepinephrine on gastrin release and gastric secretion of acid in man. *Scandinavian Journal of Gastroenterology, 37*, 87–92.

Coil, J. D., & Norgren, R. (1979). Cells of origin of motor axons in the subdiaphragmatic vagus of the rat. *Journal of the Autonomic Nervous System, 1*, 203–210.

Crocket, A., Doyle, D., & Joffe, S. N. (1981). Electron microscopy of gastric mucosal innervation in rats. *Experientia (Basel), 37*, 270–271.

Culp, D. J., Wolosin, J. M., Soll, A. H., & Forte, J. G. (1983). Muscarinic receptors and guanylate cyclase in mammalian gastric glandular cells. *American Journal of Physiology, 245 (Gastrointestinal and Liver Physiology, 8*, G760–G768.

Cumming, J. D., Greetham, R. B., & Percival, H. G. (1969). The exhaustion of gastric acid secretion during prolonged experiments on anaesthetized dogs. *Journal of Physiology (London), 169*, 61–62P.

Debas, H. T., Walsh, J. H., & Grossman, M. I. (1975). Evidence for oxyntopyloric reflex for release of antral gastrin. *Gastroenterology, 68*, 687–690.

Degertekin, H., Ertan, A., Akdamar, K., Groot, K., Kodaira, H., Godiwala T., Mather, F., & Arimura, A. (1984). Luminal release of gastric somatostatin-like immunoreactivity in response to various stimuli in man. *Gastroenterology, 86*, 1059.

Delaney, J. P. (1967). Chronic alterations in gastrointestinal blood flow induced by vagotomy. *Surgery, 62*, 155–158.

Dockray, G. J., Gregory, R. A., Tracy, H. S., & Zhu, W-Y. (1981). Transport of cholecystokinin-octapeptide-like immunoreactivity toward the gut in afferent vagal fibers in cat and dog. *Journal of Physiology (London), 314*, 501–511.

Du Val, J. W., Saffouri, B., Weir, G. C., Walsh, J. I., Arimura, A., & Mahklouf, G. M. (1981). Stimulation of gastrin and somatostatin secretion from the isolated rat stomach by bombesin. *American Journal of Physiology, 241 (Gastrointestinal and Liver Physiology, 4)*, G242–G247.

Ecknauer, R., Thompson, W. J., Johnson, L. R., & Rosenfeld, G. C. (1980). Isolated parietal cells: [3H]QNB binding to putative cholinergic receptors. *American Journal of Physiology, 239 (Gastrointestinal and Liver Physiology, 2)*, G204–G209.

Elder, J. B., Gillespie, G., Campbell, E. H. G., Gillespie, J. E., Crean, G. P., & Kay, A. W. (1972). The effect of vagotomy on the lower part of the acid dose-response curve to pentagastrin in man. *Clinical Science, 43*, 193–200.

Emas, S., & Grossman, M. I. (1967). Effect of truncal vagotomy on acid and pepsin responses to histamine and gastrin in dogs. *American Journal of Physiology, 212*, 1007–1017.

Evered, M. D., Minty, F. M., & Tepperman, B. L. (1982). Brain sites where pentagastrin affects gastric secretion and motility. *Federal Proceedings, 41*, 1508.

Farooq, O., & Isenberg, J. I. (1975). Effect of continuous intravenous infusion of insulin versus rapid intravenous injection of insulin on gastric acid secretion in man. *Gastroenterology, 68*, 683–686.

Feldman, M. (1984). Inhibition of gastric acid secretion by selective and nonselective anticholinergics. *Gastroenterology, 86*, 361–366.

Feldman, M., & Cowley, Y. M. (1982). Effect of an opiate antagonist (naloxone) on the gastric acid secretory response to sham feeding, pentagastrin, and histamine in man. *Digestive Disease and Science, 27*, 308–310.

Feldman, M., & Walsh, J. H. (1980). Acid inhibition of sham feeding-stimulated gastrin release and gastric acid secretion: Effect of atropine. *Gastroenterology, 78*, 772–776.

Feng, H. S., Aronchick, C. A., & Brooks, F. P. (1983). Decortication and decerebration effects compared on efferent electrical vagal stimulation of the stomach in cats. *Clinical Research, 31*, 530A.

Flemstrom, G. (1977). Active alkalinization by amphibian gastric fundic mucosa in vitro. *American Journal of Physiology, 233 (Endocrinal Metabolism and Gastrointestinal Physiology, 2)*, E1–E12.

Flemstrom, G., & Garner, A. (1982). Gastroduodenal HCO_3 transport characteristics and proposed role in acidity regulation and mucosal protection. *American Journal of Physiology, 242 (Gastrointestinal and Liver Physiology, 5)*, G183–G193.

Garrett, J. R. (1974). Innervation of the salivary glands, morphological considerations. In N. A. Thorn & O. H. Petersen (Eds.), *Secretory mechanisms of exocrine glands* (Alfred Benzon Symposium VII, pp. 17–27). Copenhagen: Munksgard.

Gemuei, A., Issa, I., El-Gindi, M., & Abd-El-Samie, Y. (1969). Beta-adrenergic receptors and gastric acid secretion. *Surgery, 66*, 663–668.

Gillis, R. A., Skirboll, L., Norman, W. P., & Pagani, F. P. (1984). Evidence for substance P (SP), 5-hydroxyptamine (5-HT), and avian pancreatic polypeptide (APP) in fibers innervating cell bodies of vagal preganglionic parasympathetic fibers which project to the stomach. *Gastroenterology, 86*, 1088.

Goto, Y., & Debas, H. T. (1983). GABA-mimetic effect on gastric acid secretion. *Digestive Disease and Science, 28*, 56–59.

Grossman, M. I. (1962). Secretion of acid and pepsin in response to distention of vagally innervated fundic gland area in dogs. *Gastroenterology, 42*, 718–721.

Grundy, D., & Scratcherd, T. (1982). Effect of stimulation of the vagus nerve in bursts on gastric acid secretion and motility in anesthetized ferret. *Journal of Physiology (London), 333*, 451–462.

Gunion, M. W., & Taché, Y. (1984). Intrahypothalamic corticotropin-releasing factor decreases gastric acid output but increases secretion volume. *Gastroenterology, 86*, 1102.

Guth, P. H., & Smith, E. (1977). Nervous regulation of the gastric microcirculation. In F. P. Brooks & P. W. Evers (Eds.), *Nerves and the gut*, (pp. 365–376). Thorofare, NJ: Charles B. Slack, Inc.

Hall, W. H., Herb, R. W., Brady, J. P., & Brooks, F. P. (1967). Gastric function during hypnosis and hypnotically induced gastrointestinal symptoms. *Journal of Psychosomatic Research, 11*, 263–267.

Hanker, J. S., Tapper, E. J., & Ambrose, W. W. (1977). Enzyme cytochemical correlates of the nervous control of the gastric parietal cell. In F. P. Brooks & P. W. Evers (Eds.), *Nerves and the gut* (pp. 65–68). Thorofare, NJ: Charles B. Slack, Inc.

Harper, A. A., Kidd, C., & Scratcherd, T. (1959). Vago-vagal reflex effects on gastric and pancreatic secretion and gastrointestinal motility. *Journal of Physiology (London), 148*, 417–436.

Harty, R. F., & Franklin, P. A. (1983). Cholinergic mediation of GABA-stimulated gastrin release from rat antral mucosa. *Gastroenterology, 84,* 1182.

Harty, R. F., & Franklin, P. A. (1984). Effects of exogenous and endogenous adenosine on gastrin release from rat antral mucosa. *Gastroenterology, 86,* 1107.

Harty, R. F., Maico, D. G., & McGuigan, J. E. (1981). Somatostatin inhibition of basal and carbachol-stimulated gastrin release in rat antral organ culture. *Gastroenterology, 81,* 707–712.

Harty, R. F., & McGuigan, J. E. (1980). Effects of carbachol and atropine on gastrin secretion and synthesis in rat antral organ culture. *Gastroenterology, 78,* 925–930.

Helander, H. T., Svensson, S. O., & Emas, S. (1979). Parietal cell structure and acid secretion in the vagally innervated stomach and the vagally denervated fundic pouch in cats. *Scandinavian Journal of Gastroenterology, 14,* 425–432.

Hengels, K. S., Fritsch, W. P., & Samloff, I. M. (1983). Radioimmunoassay of pepsin I. *Gastroenterology, 84,* 1186.

Hirano, T., & Niijima, A. (1980). Effects of 2-deoxy-D-glucose and insulin on efferent activity in gastric vagus nerve. *Experientia, 36,* 1197–1198.

Hirschowitz, B. I. (1977). The vagus and gastric secretion. In F. P. Brooks & P. W. Evers (Eds.), *Nerves and the gut* (pp. 96–118). Thorofare, NJ: Charles B. Slack, Inc.

Holst, J. J., Jensen, S. L., Knuhtsen, S., Nielsen, O. V., & Rehfeld, J. F. (1983). Effect of vagus, gastric inhibitor polypeptide and HCl on gastrin and somatostatin release from perfused pig antrum. *American Journal of Physiology, 244 (Gastrointestinal and Liver Physiology, 7),* G515–G522.

Hunter, G. C., Goldstone, J., Vella, R., & Way, L. W. (1979). Effect of vagotomy upon intragastric redistribution of microvascular flow. *Journal of Surgical Research, 26,* 314–319.

Ishikawa, T., Zagata, M., & Osumi, Y. (1983). Dual effects of electrical stimulation of ventromedial hypothalamic neurons on gastric acid secretion in rats. *American Journal of Physiology, 245 (Gastrointestinal and Liver Physiology, 8),* G265–G269.

Jansson, G., Lundgren, O., & Martinson, J. (1970). Neurohormonal control of gastric blood flow. *Gastroenterology, 58,* 425–429.

Kadekaro, M., Savaki, H., & Sokoloff, L. (1980). Metabolic mapping of neural pathways involved in gastrosecretory response to insulin hypoglycemia in the rat. *Journal of Physiology (London), 300,* 393–407.

Kadekaro, M., Timo-Iaria, C., de Lourdes, M., & Vicentini, M. (1977). Control of gastric secretion by the central nervous system. In F. P. Brooks & P. W. Evers (Eds.), *Nerves and the gut* (pp. 377–429). Thorofare, NJ: Charles B. Slack, Inc.

Kalia, M., & Mesulam, M. M. (1980a). Brain stem projections of sensory and motor components of the vagus complex in the cat. I. The cervical vagus and nodose ganglion. *Journal of Comparative Neurology, 193,* 435–465.

Kalia, M., & Mesulam, M. M. (1980b). Brain stem projections of sensory and motor components of the vagus complex in the cat. II. Laryngeal, tracheobronchial, pulmonary, cardiac, and gastrointestinal branches. *Journal of Comparative Neurology, 193,* 467–508.

Kapadia, C. R., & Donaldson, R. M., Jr. (1978). Macromolecular secretion by isolated gastric mucosa. *Gastroenterology, 74,* 535–539.

Kihl, B., & Olbe, L. (1980). Fat inhibition of gastric acid secretion in duodenal ulcer patients before and after proximal gastric vagotomy. *Gut, 21,* 1056–1061.

Klein, K. B., & Spiegel, D. (1984). Hypnosis can both stimulate and inhibit gastric acid secretion. *Gastroenterology, 86,* 1137.

Knight, S. E., McIsaac, R. L., & Fielding, L. P. (1978). The effect of highly selective vagotomy on the relationship between gastric mucosal blood flow and acid secretion in man. *British Journal of Surgery, 65,* 721–723.

Knutson, U., & Olbe, L. (1974a). The effect of exogenous gastrin on the acid sham feeding response in antrum-bulb-resected duodenal ulcer patients. *Scandinavian Journal of Gastroenterology, 9,* 231–238.

Knutson, U., & Olbe, L. (1974b). Gastric acid response to sham feeding before and after resection of antrum and duodenal bulb in duodenal ulcer patients. *Scandinavian Journal of Gastroenterology, 9*, 191–201.

Koelz, H. R., Hersey, S. J., Sachs, G., & Chew, C. S. (1982). Pepsinogen release from isolated gastric glands. *American Journal of Physiology, 243 (Gastrointestinal and Liver Physiology, 6)*, G218–G225.

Konturek, S. J., & Johnson, L. R. (1971). Evidence for an enterogastric reflex for the inhibition of acid secretion. *Gastroenterology, 61*, 667–674.

Kyosola, K., Veyola, L., & Richardt, L. (1975). Cholinergic innervation of the gastric wall of the cat. *Histochemistry, 44*, 23–30.

Lanciault, G., Bonoma, C., & Brooks, F. P. (1973). Vagal stimulation, gastrin release, and acid secretion in anesthetized dogs. *American Journal of Physiology, 225*, 546–552.

Lanciault, G., Shaw, J. E., Urquhart, J., Adair, L., & Brooks, F. P. (1975). Response of the isolated perfused stomach of the dog to electrical vagal stimulation. *Gastroenterology, 68*, 294–300.

Lechago, J., & Barajas, L. (1976). The innervation of the oxyntic gastric mucosa. *Gastroenterology, 70*, 965.

Lechago, J., & Barajas, L. (1981). Innervation of rat antral gastrin-producing cells. *Anat. Rec., 200*, 309–314.

Lenz, H. J., Hester, S. E., Webb, V. J., & Brown, M. A. (1984). Corticotropin-releasing factor (CRF): Mechanisms to inhibit gastric acid secretion (GAS) in the dog. *Gastroenterology, 86*, 1158.

Lenz, H. J., Vale, W. W., Rivier, J. E., & Brown, M. R. (1984). Calcitonin gene-related peptide (CGRP), a novel neuropeptide, acts within the brain to inhibit gastric acid secretion (GAS). *Gastroenterology, 86*, 1158.

Lenz, H. S., Webb, V. J., Hester, S. E., Rivier, J. E., & Brown, M. R. (1984). Calcitonin gene-related peptide: Inhibition of gastric acid secretion in the dog. *Gastroenterology, 86*, 1158.

Lesiege, D., & Taché, Y. (1983). Mechanism for intracisternal bombesin-induced inhibition of gastric acid secretion. *Federal Proceedings, 42*, 592.

Leth, R., Elander, B., Fellenius, E., Haglund, U., & Olbe, L. (1981). Effect of antrectomy or proximal gastric vagotomy on ^{14}C-aminopyrine accumulation in isolated human gastric glands. *Scandinavian Journal of Gastroenterology, 16*, 1106.

Levine, A. S., Morley, J. E., Kneip, J., Grace, M., & Silvis, S. E. (1981). Muscimol induces gastric acid secretion after central administration. *Brain Research, 229*, 270–274.

Lombardi, D. M., Feng, H. S., & Brooks, F. P. (1982). Disassociation of secretory and motor responses to stimulation of the dorsal motor nucleus of the vagus in anesthetized cats. *Gastroenterology, 82*, 1120.

Long, J. F., & Brooks, F. P. (1965). The comparative gastric and pepsin response to histamine insulin hypoglycemia and feeding in dogs with vagally innervated gastric pouches. *Quarterly Journal of Experimental Physiology, 50*, 256–262.

Lorenz, W., Mohri, K., Reimann, H. -J., Troidl, H., Rohde, H., & Barth, H. (1980). Intramural mechanisms: Relevance of mast cell concept. In K. H. Holtermuller & J. R. Malagelada (Eds.), *Advances in ulcer disease* (pp. 176–194). Amsterdam: Excerpta Medica.

Lorenz, W. Thon, K., Barth, E., Neugebauer, E., Reimann, H. J., & Kusche, J. (1983). Metabolism and function of gastric histamine in health and disease. *Journal of Clinical Gastroenterology, 5* (Supp. 1), 37–56.

Lundberg, J. M., Hokfelt, T., Kewenter, J., Petterson, G., Ahlman, H., Edin, R., Dahlstrom, A., Nilsson, G., Terenius, L., Uvnäs-Wallensten, K., & Said, S. (1979). Substance P, VIP, and enkephalin-like immunoreactivity in the human vagus nerve. *Gastroenterology, 77*, 468–471.

Lundberg, J. M., Hokfelt, T., Nilsson, G., Terenius, L., Rehfeld, J., Elde, R., & Said, S. (1978). Peptide neurons in the vagus, splanchnic and sciatic nerves. *Acta Physiologica Scandinavica, 104*, 499–501.

Maley, B., & Elde, R. (1981). Localization of substance P-like immunoreactivity in cell bodies of the feline dorsal vagal nucleus. *Neuroscience Letters, 27*, 187–191.

Martindale, R., Kauffman, G. L., Levin, S., Walsh, J. H., & Yamada, T. (1982). Differential regulation of gastrin and somatostatin secretion from isolated perfused rat stomachs. *Gastroenterology, 83*, 240–244.

Micali, B., Albanese, V., Caputo, G., Gioffré, M., Saitta, F. P., & Venuti, A. (1984). Evidence for a pH-dependent mechanism of gastrin release during vagal stimulation by sham feeding. *Gastroenterology, 86*, 1183.

Moore, J. G. (1980). The relationship of gastric acid secretion to plasma glucose in five men. *Scandinavian Journal of Gastroenterology, 15*, 625–632.

Moore, J. G., & Motoki, D. (1979). Gastric secretory and humoral responses to anticipated feeding in five men. *Gastroenterology, 76*, 71–75.

Morley, J. E., Levine, A. S., & Silvis, S. E. (1981). Intraventricular calcitonin inhibits gastric acid secretion. *Science, 214*, 671–672.

Morrison, J. F. B. (1977). The afferent innervation of the gastrointestinal tract. In F. P. Brooks & P. W. Evers (Eds.), *Nerves and the gut* (pp. 297–326). Thorofare, NJ: Charles B. Slack, Inc.

Nakamura, K., Ishi, K., Kusano, M., & Hayshi, S. (1974). Acute and long-term effects of vagotomy on gastric mucosal blood flow. In F. Halle & S. Andersson (Eds.), *Vagotomy: Latest advances with special reference to gastric and duodenal ulcer* (pp. 109–111). New York: Springer-Verlag.

Olbe, L. (1964). Effect of resection of gastrin releasing regions on acid response to sham feeding and insulin hypoglycemia in Pavlov pouch dogs. *Acta Physiologica Scandinavica, 62*, 169–175.

Olbe, L., Logan, D., Goto, Y., Pappas, T. N., & Walsh, J. H. (1984). Evidence for pH-independent vagal inhibition of gastric release. *Gastroenterology, 86*, 1200.

Olsen, P. S., Kirkegaard, P., Holst, S. S., & Christiansen, J. (1982). Vagal control of glucagon-induced inhibition of gastric acid secretion in duodenal ulcer patients. *Scandinavian Journal of Gastroenterology, 17*, 629–632.

Ormsbee, H. S., III, Norman, W. P., Woodward, A. F., Kasbekar, D. K., Hardy, F. E., Jr., Pagani, F. D., & Gillis, R. A. (1982). Selective motor and secretory pathways from the hindbrain to the stomach. *Digestive Disease and Science, 27*, 650.

Osumi, Y., Aibara, S., Sakae, K., & Fugiwara, M. (1977). Central noradrenergic inhibition of gastric mucosal blood flow and acid secretion in rats. *Life Science, 20*, 1407–1416.

Pagani, F. D., Norman, W. P., & Gillis, R. A. (1984). Vagal fibers originating from the dorsal motor nucleus of the vagus and nucleus retroambigualis innervate specific stomach sites. *Gastroenterology, 86*, 1205.

Pagani, F. D., Norman, W. P., Kasbekar, D. K., & Gillis, R. A. (1984). Effects of stimulation of nucleus ambiguus complex on gastrointestinal function. *American Journal of Physiology, 246 (Gastrointestinal and Liver Physiology, 9)*, G253–G262.

Paintal, A. S. (1973). Vagal sensory receptors and their reflex effects. *Physiological Reviews, 53*, 159–227.

Pappas, T. N., Hamel, D., Debas, H. T., & Taché, Y. (1984). Bombesin (BBS) acts in the dog brain to inhibit gastric acid secretion. *Gastroenterology, 86*, 1206.

Peters, M. N., Walsh, J. H., Ferrari, J., & Feldman, M. (1982). Adrenergic regulation of distention-induced gastrin release in humans. *Gastroenterology, 82*, 659–663.

Polak, J. M., Bloom, S. R., Sullivan, S. N., Facer, P., & Pearse, A. G. E. (1977). Enkephalin-like immunoreactivity in the human gastrointestinal tract. *Lancet, 1*, 972–973.

Polish, E., Brady, J. V., Mason, J. W., Thach, J. S., & Niemeck, W. (1962). Gastric contents and occurrence of duodenal lesions in the rhesus monkey during avoidance behavior. *Gastroenterology, 43*, 193–201.

Preshaw, R. M., & Webster, D. R. (1967). A comparison of sham feeding and teasing as stimuli for gastric acid secretion in the dog. *Quarterly Journal of Experimental Physiology, 52*, 37–43.

Puurunen, S. (1983). Inhibition of gastric acid secretion by intracerebroventricularly administered prostaglandin E_2 in anaesthetized rats. *British Journal of Pharmacology, 78*, 131–135.

Reed, J. D., & Sanders, D. J. (1971a). Pepsin secretion, gastric motility, and mucosal blood flow in anaesthetized cat. *Journal of Physiology (London), 216,* 159–170.

Reed, J. D., & Sanders, D. J. (1971b). Splanchnic nerve inhibition of gastric acid secretion and mucosal blood flow in anaesthetized cats. *Journal of Physiology (London), 219,* 555–570.

Reed, J. D., Sanders, D. J., & Thorpe, V. (1971). The effect of splanchnic nerve stimulation in gastric acid secretion and mucosal blood flow in the anaesthetized cat. *Journal of Physiology (London), 214,* 1–13.

Rehfeld, J. F., & Lundberg, J. M. (1983). Cholecystokinin in feline vagal and sciatic nerves: Concentration, molecular form and transport velocity. *Brain Research, 275,* 341–347.

Richardson, C. T., Walsh, J. H., Cooper, K. A., Feldman, M., & Fordtran, J. S. (1977). Studies on the role of cephalic vagal stimulation in the acid secretory response to eating in normal human subjects. *Journal of Clinical Investigation, 60,* 435–441.

Rosato, E. F., & Rosato, F. E. (1971). Effect of truncal vagotomy on acid and pepsin responses to histamine in duodenal ulcer patients. *Annals of Surgery, 173,* 63–66.

Saffouri, B., Weir, G. C., Bitar, K. N., & Makhlouf, G. M. (1980). Gastrin and somatostatin secretion by perfused rat stomach: Functional linkage of antral peptides. *American Journal of Physiology, 231 (Gastrointestinal and Liver Physiology, 1),* G495–G501.

Sanders, M. J., Amirian, D. A., Ayalon, A., & Soll, A. H. (1983). Regulation of pepsinogen release from canine chief cells in primary monolayer culture. *American Journal of Physiology, 245 (Gastrointestinal and Liver Physiology, 8),* G641–G646.

Schapiro, H., Britt, L. G., & Dohrn, R. H. (1973). Sensory deprivation on visceral activity. IV. The effect of temporary visual deprivation on canine gastric secretion. *American Journal of Digestive Diseases, 18,* 573–575.

Schapiro, H., Britt, L. G., Gross, C. W., & Gaines, K. J. (1971). Sensory deprivation on visceral activity. III. The effect of olfactory deprivation of canine gastric secretion. *Psychosomatic Medicine, 33,* 429–435.

Schapiro, H., Gross, C. W., Nakamura, T., Wruble, L. D., & Britt, L. G. (1970). Sensory deprivation on visceral activity. II. The effect of auditory and vestibular deprivation on canine gastric secretion. *Psychosomatic Medicine, 32,* 515–521.

Schapiro, H., Wruble, L. D., Britt, L. G., & Bell, T. A. (1970a). The effect of visual deprivation on canine gastric secretion. *American Journal of Digestive Diseases, 15,* 529–538.

Schapiro, H., Wruble, L. D., Britt, L. G., & Bell, T. A. (1970b). Sensory deprivation on visceral activity. I. The effect of visual deprivation on canine gastric secretion. *Psychosomatic Medicine, 32,* 379–396.

Schubert, M. L., & Makhlouf, G. M. (1982). Regulation of gastric and somatostatin secretion by intramural neurons: Effect of nicotinic receptor stimulation with dimethyl-phenylpiperazinium. *Gastroenterology, 83,* 626–632.

Schubert, M. L., Saffouri, B., & Makhlouf, G. M. (1984). Neural regulation of gastrin and somatostatin secretion in isolated antral sheets. *Gastroenterology, 86,* 1238.

Schubert, M. L., Walsh, J. H., & Makhlouf, J. E. (1983). Bombesin antiserum inhibits neurally stimulated gastrin secretion in the isolated perfused stomach. *Gastroenterology, 84,* 1302.

Schultzberg, M., Hokfelt, T., Nilsson, G., Terenius, L., Rehfeld, J. F., Brown, M., Elde, R., Goldstein, M., & Said, S. (1980). Distribution of peptide and catecholamine containing neurons in the gastrointestinal tract of rat and guinea pig. Immunohistochemical studies with antisera to substance P, vasoactive intestinal polypeptide, enkephalins, somatostatin, gastrin/cholecystokinin, neurotensin and dopamine hydroxylase. *Neuroscience, 5,* 689–744.

Seelig, L. L., Jr., Schlusselberg, D., & Woodward, E. J. (1983). Nerve and smooth muscle relationships with gastric glandular epithelial cells of the opossum. *Gastroenterology, 84,* 1303.

Shiraishi, T. (1980). Effects of lateral hypothalamic stimulation on medulla oblongata and gastric vagal neural responses. *Brain Research Bulletin, 5,* 245–250.

Shiraishi, T., & Simpson, A. (1982). Lateral hypothalamus neuron responses to electro-osmotic 2-deoxy-D-glucose. *Brain Research Bulletin, 8,* 645–651.

Simpson, A., & Shiraishi, T. (1980). Gastrin-related peptide effects in lateral hypothalamus depend on food deprivation. *Brain Research Bulletin, 5,* 153–158.

Sjodin, L. (1971). Electrical stimulation of nerves and secretion from digestive glands. In F. P. Brooks & P. W. Evers (Eds.), *Nerves and the gut* (pp. 1–13). Thorofare, NJ: Charles B. Slack, Inc.

Smith, G. P., & Brooks, F. P. (1970). Brain, behavior and gastric secretion. In G. B. J. Glass (Ed.), *Progress in gastroenterology* (Vol. II, pp. 57–72). New York: Grune and Stratton, Inc.

Soll, A. H. (1980). Secretagogue stimulation of [^{14}C] aminopyrine accumulation by isolated canine parietal cells. *American Journal of Physiology, 238 (Gastrointestinal and Liver Physiology, 1),* G366–G375.

Soll, A. H. (1981a). Extracellular calcium and cholinergic stimulation of isolated canine parietal cells. *Journal of Clinical Investigation, 68,* 270–278.

Soll, A. H. (1981b). Physiology of isolated canine parietal cells: Receptors and effectors regulating function. In L. R. Johnson (Ed.), *Physiology of the gastrointestinal tract* (pp. 673–691). New York: Raven Press.

Soll, A. H. (1982). Potentiating interactions of gastric stimulants on [^{14}C] aminopyrine accumulation by isolated canine parietal cells. *Gastroenterology, 83,* 216–223.

Spencer, J., & Grossman, M. I. (1971). The gastric secretory response to insulin: An "all-or-none" phenomenon? *Gut, 12,* 891–896.

Spindel, E., Harty, R. F., & McGuigan, J. E. (1984). The effects of adrenergic stimulation on human antral gastrin and somatostatin release in vitro. *Gastroenterology, 86,* 1264.

Stadil, F., & Rehfeld, J. F. (1973). Release of gastrin by epinephrine in man. *Gastroenterology, 65,* 210–215.

Stenquist, B., Rehfeld, J. F., & Olbe, L. (1979). Effect of proximal gastric vagotomy and anticholinergics on acid and gastrin responses to sham feeding in duodenal ulcer patients. *Gut, 20,* 1020–1027.

Sugano, K., Park, J. H., Soll, A. H., & Yamada, T. (1984). Gastrin biosynthesis and release: Studies with isolated canine antral mucosal cell cultures. *Gastroenterology, 86,* 1269.

Taché, Y., Goto, Y., Gunion, M., Rivier, J., & Debas, H. (1984). Inhibition of gastric acid secretion in rats and in dogs by corticotropin-releasing factor. *Gastroenterology, 86,* 281–286.

Taché, Y., Goto, Y., & Lauffenburger, M. (1983). Potent central nervous system action of a stabilized TRH analogue, RX 77368, to stimulate gastric secretion in rats. *The Physiologist, 26,* A–50.

Taché, Y., Gunion, M., Lauffenburger, M., Goto, Y., Walsh, J., Debas, H. T., & Rivier, J. (1984). Inhibition of gastric acid secretion by intracerebral injection of calcitonin gene-related peptide (CGRP) in rats. *Gastroenterology, 86,* 1272.

Taché, Y., Marki, W., Rivier, J., Vale, W., & Brown, M. (1981). Central nervous system inhibition of gastric secretion in the rat by gastrin-releasing peptide, a mammalian bombesin. *Gastroenterology, 81,* 298–302.

Takeuchi, Y., Matsushima, S., Matsushima, R., & Hopkins, D. A. (1983). Direct amygdaloid projections to the dorsal motor nucleus of the vagus nerve: A light and electron microscopic study in the rat. *Brain Research, 280,* 143–147.

Tansy, M. F., Probst, S. J., & Martin, J. S. (1975). Evidence of nonvagal neural stimulation of canine gastric acid secretion. *Surgical Gynecology and Obstetrics, 140,* 861–867.

Tepperman, B. L., & Evered, M. D. (1980). Gastrin injected into the lateral hypothalamus stimulates secretion of gastric acid in rats. *Science, 209,* 1142–1143.

Thompson, D. G., Richelson, E., & Malagelada, J. R. (1983). Perturbation of upper gastrointestinal function by cold stress. *Gut, 24,* 277–283.

Uvnäs-Wallensten, K. (1977). Occurrence of gastrin in gastric juice, in central secretion and in antral perfusates of cats. *Gastroenterology, 73*, 487–494.

Uvnäs-Wallensten, K., Efendic, S., & Luft, R. (1977). Vagal release of somatostatin into the antral lumen of cats. *Acta Physiologica Scandinavica, 99*, 126–128.

Van Hee, R. H., & Vanhoutte, P. M. (1978). Cholinergic inhibition of adrenergic neurotransmission in the canine gastric artery. *Gastroenterology, 74*, 1266–1270.

van Houten, M., & Posner, B. I. (1980). Insulin binding sites localized to nerve terminals in rat median eminence and arcuate nucleus. *Science, 207*, 1081–1083.

Vatu, M. H. (1975). Gastric intrinsic factor secretion. *Scandinavian Journal of Gastroenterology, 10*, 337–338.

Walker, W., Vinik, A., Heldsinger, A., & Kaveh, R. (1983). Role of calcium and calmodulin in activation of the oxyntic cell by histamine and carbamylcholine in the guinea pig. *Journal of Clinical Investigation, 72*, 955–964.

Weingarten, H. P., & Powley, T. L. (1980). Ventromedial hypothalamic lesions elevate basal and cephalic phase gastric acid output. *American Journal of Physiology, 239 (Gastrointestinal and Liver Physiology, 2)*, G221–G229.

Williford, D. J., Ormsbee, H. S., Norman, W., Harmon, J. W., Garvey, T. Q., III, Dimirco, J. A., & Gillis, R. A. (1981). Hindbrain GABA receptors influence parasympathetic outflow to the stomach. *Science, 214*, 193–194.

Wolfe, M. M., Reel, G. M., & McGuigan, J. E. (1983). Effects of carbachol on gastrin and somatostatin release in rat antral tissue culture. *Clinical Research, 31*, 477A.

Wolfe, M. M., Reel, G. M., Short, G. M., & McGuigan, J. E. (1984). β-adrenergic stimulation of gastrin release mediated by gastrin-releasing peptide in cultured rat antral mucosa. *Gastroenterology, 86*, 1301.

Wyrwicka, W. (1978). Effects of electrical stimulation within the hypothalamus on gastric acid secretion and food intake in cats. *Experimental Neurology, 60*, 286–303.

Wyrwicka, W. (1979). Changes in gastric acid secretion in ophagic or hyperphagic cats after hypothalamic lesions. *Experimental Neurology, 63*, 293–303.

Wyrwicka, W., & Garcia R. (1979). Effect of electrical stimulation of the dorsal nucleus of the vagus nerve on gastric acid secretion in cats. *Experimental Neurology, 65*, 315–325.

Yamamoto, T., Satomi, H., Ise, H., & Takahushi, K. (1977). Evidence of the dual innervation of the cat stomach by the vagal dorsal motor and medial solitary nuclei as demonstrated by the horseradish peroxidase method. *Brain Research, 122*, 125–131.

Zalewsky, C. A., Bauer, R. F., Moody, F. G., & Brooks, F. P. (1977). Effect of vagal stimulation upon parietal cell ultrastructure. In F. P. Brooks & P. W. Evers (Eds.), *Nerves and the gut* (pp. 41–50). Thorofare, NJ: Charles B. Slack, Inc.

Zalewsky, C. A., Moody, F. G., Allen, M., & Davis, E. K. (1983). Stimulation of canine gastric mucus secretion with intra-arterial acetylcholine chloride. *Gastroenterology, 85*, 1067–1075.

2

REGULATION
OF GASTRIC SECRETION:
Humoral Mechanisms

N. W. Bunnett
University of Washington

J. H. Walsh
*Veterans Administration Medical Center
and UCLA School of Medicine*

INTRODUCTION

The secretion of hydrogen ions from the parietal cell is an integrated response to a vast array of stimulatory and inhibitory agents, which include nutrients, biogenic amines, prostaglandins, and the regulatory peptides. Some of the peptides which affect acid secretion are secreted from endocrine cells into the general circulation, which transports them to the parietal cells. These act as circulating hormones. Other peptides act in a paracrine manner and are secreted into the interstitial fluid to influence adjacent cells. However, most of the peptides in the gut are localized to nerve fibers. These peptides may be released from nerve endings to act on nearby cells, as neurotransmitters, or may be secreted into the circulation and influence more distant targets as neuroendocrine agents. The classification of the peptides on the basis of the mode of delivery to the target cell is not strict, and in many instances convincing evidence for a hormonal, paracrine, neurotransmitter, or neuroendocrine role is lacking. This chapter mainly concerns those peptides of the alimentary tract which act humorally to regulate gastric acid secretion, but reference will be made to the paracrine and neural peptides where appropriate.

A bewildering number of peptides have been isolated from the alimentary tract in recent years, but few are likely to have a physiological role in the regulation of gastric acid secretion. Of these, gastrin and gastrin-releasing peptide (GRP) are stimulants of gastric secretion, and somatostatin is an inhibitor of the parietal cell.

STIMULANTS OF GASTRIC ACID SECRETION GASTRIN

Gastrin is a hormonal peptide and a physiological stimulant of gastric acid secretion (for review see Dockray, 1978; Walsh, 1981).

Localization

Gastrin was originally isolated as a heptadecapeptide from the antral mucosa of the pig (Gregory & Tracy, 1964) and has since been isolated in a number of molecular forms (Gregory, 1982). Hormonal peptides are secreted from endocrine cells. Gastrin has been localized to endocrine cells (G cells) of the antral mucosa and proximal duodenum by immunocytochemistry in man and animals (McGuigan, 1968; Greider, Steinberg, & McGuigan, 1972; Bunnett, 1984). In most species, the G cells are characterized at the ultrastructural level by the presence of vesicular granules (about 200 nm in diameter) that are aggregated in the basal region. A tuft of microvilli projects into the glandular lumen, presumably to sense the gastric contents. Granule release by exocytosis at the base of the cell, in contact with the basal membrane of the antral glands and in close proximity to blood capillaries of the lamina propria, has been observed by electron microscopy (Fujita & Kobayashi, 1981). Mechanisms modulating G-cell function may act at the base of the cell through blood-borne mediators, at the lateral surface through neural and paracrine agents, or at the apex through nutrients from the gastric lumen.

Secretion

Gastrin release into the general circulation has been demonstrated by use of radioimmunoassay. Luminal peptides, amino acids and calcium, circulating bombesin and catecholamines, and activation of nervous reflexes stimulate gastrin secretion into the general circulation (Walsh & Grossman, 1975). Acidification of the antral mucosa below pH3 and certain gastrointestinal peptides, such as somatostatin, inhibit gastrin secretion (Walsh, Richardson, & Fordtran, 1975; Bolman, Copper, & Wells, 1978). Of the food components, peptides and amino acids resulting from protein digestion are the strongest stimulants of gastrin secretion (Elwin, 1974). Of individual amino acids, L phenylalanine and L tryptophan are significantly more potent stimulants of gastrin release and acid secretion than other amino acids in man (Taylor, Byrne, Chrisite, Ament, & Walsh, 1982). Dietary amines may account for about 50% of the postprandial gastrin response in rats. Removal of ammonia and amines from pelleted rat food by lyophilization under alkaline conditions reduced the gastrin response to the food by half; addition of the amine containing condensate back to the freeze-dried food restored the feeding response to normal (Lichtenberger, Graziani, &

Dubinsky, 1982). Analysis of the condensate revealed that it contained ammonia, methylamine, ethylamine, dimethylamine, and a fourth unidentified aliphatic amine, all of which stimulated gastrin release from isolated gastrin cells (Lichtenberger, et al., 1982). In humans, coffee and wine are potent stimulants of gastrin release and acid secretion, but the responses are not entirely caused by caffeine or ethanol (Feldman, Isenberg, & Grossman, 1981; Lenz, Ferrari-Taylor, & Isenberg, 1983). Distention of the stomach with liquid or a balloon results in a minimal secretion of gastrin but does stimulate acid secretion (Soares, Zaterka, & Walsh, 1977). The effects of vagal and cholinergic stimulation on gastrin release are complex. In dogs, activation of vagal cholinergic reflexes by sham feeding or insulin induced hypoglycemia causes a release of gastrin that can be inhibited by a large dose of atropine or by vagal denervation (Csendes, Walsh, & Grossman, 1972; Nilsson, Simon, Yalow, & Berson, 1972; Tepperman, Walsh, & Preshaw, 1972). These data are compatible with cholinergic stimulation of gastrin release, but there is some evidence for a vagal inhibitory mechanism. Low doses of atropine, for example, enhance the gastrin response to feeding in dogs (Impicciatore, Walsh, & Grossman, 1977).

Actions

The most apparent action of gastrin is the stimulation of gastric acid secretion (McGuigan, Isaza, & Landor, 1971; Walsh & Grossman, 1975), and there is evidence that a substantial fraction of the gastric acid response to a protein meal is mediated by circulating gastrin (see section on criteria for a peptide hormone). Gastrin stimulates oxygen consumption, aminopyrine accumulation, and morphological changes in isolated parietal cells in vitro (all of which are consistent with the secretion of acid in vivo), and radiolabeled gastrin binds to isolated canine parietal cells (for review see Soll, 1981).

Catabolism

The action of a circulating hormone can be terminated by its catabolism at the target cell and its clearance from the general circulation. Circulating gastrin 17 has a half life in dogs of about 3 min, but the longer gastrin precursor, gastrin 34, has a longer half life of about 15 min (Straus & Yalow, 1974; Walsh, Debas, & Grossman, 1974). Specific organs do not seem to degrade gastrin, but rather there is a general breakdown across most capillary beds since venous concentrations at most sites are between 20 and 25% lower than arterial concentrations (Strunz, Walsh, & Grossman, 1978). Gastric mucosal cells are able to degrade gastrin 17 into forms that are unable to bind to antigastrin antibodies or cell surface receptors for gastrin 17 (Del Mazo & McGuigan, 1976).

Physiological Importance

It is generally agreed that gastrin is a hormone and a physiologically important stimulant of gastric acid secretion. The peptide is localized in endocrine cells and is secreted into the general circulation after feeding. There have been several attempts to correlate gastric acid secretion with serum gastrin concentrations. The results have been equivocal, showing general correlation between acid stimulation and gastrin release but a poor relation between individual gastrin concentrations and secretory rates (Fordtran & Walsh, 1973; Richardson, Walsh Hicks & Fordtran, 1976). Distention of the stomach causes moderate stimulation of acid secretion that is not correlated with gastrin release. However, when the effects of distention were taken into account and individual responses to graded exogenous doses of gastrin 17 were measured, it was found that the increase in circulating gastrin 17 was sufficient to account for the gastric secretory responses to individual amino acids (Feldman, Walsh, & Wong, 1978). More direct evidence for a physiological role of circulating gastrin was obtained by the demonstration that there was a high degree of correlation between serum gastrin and gastrin 17 responses to graded intragastric concentrations of peptone (Lam, Isenberg, Grossman, Lane, & Walsh, 1980).

GASTRIN-RELEASING PEPTIDE

GRP is a neuropeptide of the brain and alimentary tract and is the mammalian equivalent of the amphibian skin peptide, bombesin (McDonald, et al., 1978). As its name suggests, GRP is a potent stimulant of gastrin release and consequently gastric acid secretion. Although the peptide is confined to nerve fibers where it probably functions primarily as a neurotransmitter, there is some evidence that the peptide can enter the general circulation to influence distant organs. GRP is the neural peptide most likely to have a physiological role in regulation of gastric acid secretion and this peptide is discussed in detail (for review see Walsh, 1981).

Localization

GRP was originally isolated from non-antral mucosa from the pig stomach as a molecule of 27 amino acids (McDonald, et al., 1978) and has been isolated more recently from the canine intestine in 27, 23, and 10 amino acid forms (Reeve, et al., 1983). The highest concentrations of immunoreactive GRP are found in the fundic mucosa (Walsh, Reeve, & Vigna, 1981), and GRP nerves have been stained by immunocytochemistry in the mucosa and muscle layers of the alimentary tract (Dockray, Vaillant, & Walsh, 1979).

Secretion

Once released from a nerve ending, a neurotransmitter diffuses across the synaptic cleft to its target cell. At present it is not possible to study this process in vivo, and for this reason it is very difficult to quantitate the secretion of neuropeptides. There has been some success with measuring the secretion of GRP in gastric venous blood (Knuhtsen, Holst, Knigge, Olesen, & Nielsen, 1984) and in arterial blood (Bloom & Edwards, 1984). In the anesthetized pig, electrical stimulation of the vagal, but not splanchnic, nerves increased the rate of GRP secretion into fundic and antral venous blood, although in only 2 out of the 8 animals studied was there a rise in peripheral venous GRP. Chromatographic analysis of the plasma indicated that most of the secreted peptide was GRP27 and GRP10. The short half life of GRP (1.4 min) suggests that it is unlikely that GRP exerts any significant physiological influences on cells outside the immediate vicinity of the GRP nerves (Knuhtsen, et al., 1984). In the conscious calf, electrical stimulation of the cut ends of the splanchnic nerves causes an increase in the concentration of immunoreactive GRP in arterial plasma (Bloom & Edwards, 1984). In this species, GRP may act as a neurocrine agent secreted from nerves into the blood to act hormonally. The reproduction of the concentrations of immunoreactive GRP in arterial blood by the infusion of the exogenous peptide had no effect on the release of gastrin in the calf but elicited a prompt and large secretion of insulin into the circulation (Bloom & Edwards, 1984). In the calf, GRP may act as a neuroendocrine agent to stimulate insulin secretion. Whether GRP can release gastrin in this way in other species is unknown.

Actions

GRP is a potent stimulant of gastrin secretion and gastric acid release (McDonald, et al., 1978). Intravenous infusions of graded doses of bombesin and canine GRP10, 23, and 27 potently stimulated the secretion of gastrin and acid in conscious dogs (Orloff, et al., 1984; Bunnett, et al., 1985a; see Figure 2.1). In this study, GRP27 was the most potent form of GRP, but this may be related to differences in the rate of inactivation of GRP. There is no good evidence to suggest a direct action of GRP on the mammalian parietal cell, and control of acid secretion by GRP is probably exercised through the regulation of gastrin release.

Catabolism

The action of a neuropeptide may be terminated by its passive diffusion away from the target cell, by its active re-uptake into the nerve ending, or by its enzymatic catabolism. Active uptake mechanisms have not been demonstrated for neuropeptides (Jessell, Iversen, & Kanazawa, 1976; Segawa, Nakata, Yajima,

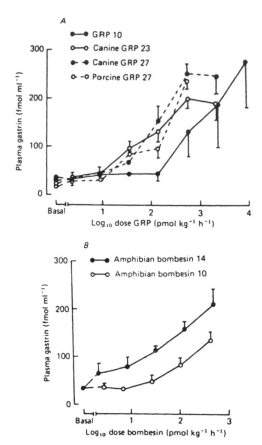

FIGURE 2.1   The effects of intravenous infusions of A, gastrin releasing peptide (GRP) and B, amphibian bombesin on the concentration of immunoreactive gastrin in peripherally sampled venous blood in the conscious dog. Mean ± SEM, n = 6. Reproduced from Bunnett et al., 1985a.

& Kitagawa, 1977), but efficient catabolic pathways inactivate a number of neuropeptides. The enzymatic inactivation of bombesin, neurotensin, and substance P has been examined in the stomach wall of the conscious rat by using a chronically implanted infusion catheter to deliver radiolabeled peptides to the tissue and implanted dialysis fibers to collect catabolites which were fractionated by high pressure liquid chromatography (Bunnett, Reeve, & Walsh, 1983; Bunnett, et al., 1984; Bunnett, Orloff, & Turner, 1985c). These studies have been extended by in vitro experiments, and the catabolic enzymes have been tentatively identified by using selective enzyme inhibitors (Orloff, Turner, & Bunnett, 1986). The carboxyl-terminal decapeptide of GRP, (1–10) GRP27, is catabolized and inactivated in the porcine stomach in vitro by a membrane-associated endopeptidase, endopeptidase EC 3.4.24.11 (enkephalinase"; Bunnett, et al., 1985b; see Figure 2.2). Most neuropeptides that have been studied in this way are catabolized and inactivated very quickly by gastric tissues. One of the reasons why it is so difficult to measure the release of many neuropeptides may be because

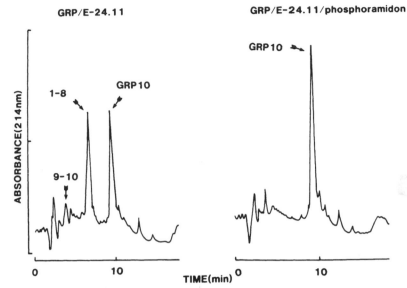

FIGURE 2.2   High pressure liquid chromatography elution profile of gastrin releasing peptide (GRP10) incubated with homogenous porcine endopeptidase-24.11 in the absence and presence of the selective inhibitor phosphoramidon $(10^{-6}M)$. Incubation conditions: $5 \times 10^{-4}M$ enzyme GRP 10; 2ug enzyme; in Tris/HCl (20mM pH 7.4, 200ul total volume); 37°C, 30 min. Peaks were identified by amino acid analysis. Gradient 4.8-50% acetonitrile, 20 min. Reproduced from Bunnett et al., 1985b.

they are degraded within a short time of secretion by peptidase enzymes bound to membranes of the effector cells.

Physiological Importance

GRP is a potent stimulant of gastrin release and acid secretion. It is confined to nerve fibers and released into the circulation by electrical stimulation of the splanchnic and vagal nerves. The rigid criteria which were used to establish acetylcholine as a neurotransmitter have not been met for GRP or any other neuropeptide. Whether GRP can enter the general circulation to act as a phys-iological stimulant of gastrin release or functions locally as a neurotransmitter will require the development of highly sensitive assays and of techniques to examine the secretion of peptides into the interstitial fluid. The problems asso-ciated with the measurement of neuropeptide secretion make it difficult to ascribe a physiological role to GRP, but several lines of indirect evidence suggest that GRP may be an important neurotransmitter regulating gastric acid secretion through the control of gastrin release: (a) GRP has been localized to nerve fibers of the gastric mucosa; (b) electrical stimulation of the vagal nerve stimulates the release of GRP into blood and a concomitant release of gastrin and stimulation of acid secretion; (c) GRP and bombesin are rapidly inactivated by gastric tissues in vivo and in vitro; and (d) GRP potently stimulates the secretion of gastrin and hydrochloric acid.

OTHER STIMULATORY PEPTIDES

Cholecystokinin (CCK)

CCK is structurally related to gastrin, sharing the biologically active carboxyl-terminal sequence of five amino acids with gastrin 17. In man and the conscious dog, a preparation of 95% pure CCK 33 was found to be a weak stimulant of basal gastric acid secretion and a weak inhibitor of gastrin-stimulated acid secretion (Corazziari, Solomon, & Grossman, 1979). However, the dose was too high to suggest a likely physiological effect.

HUMORAL INHIBITORS OF GASTRIC ACID SECRETION

Somatostatin

Somatostatin was discovered in extracts of ovine hypothalami as an inhibitor of growth hormone secretion (Brazeau, et al., 1973). The peptide has since been isolated from the brain and the alimentary tract as peptides of 14 and 28 amino acids (Pradayrol, Jornvall, Mutt, & Ribet, 1980) which are potent inhibitors of several endocrine and exocrine secretions, including gastrin release and gastric acid secretion. Somatostatin is distributed widely throughout the body and may act in a number of ways (for reviews see Walsh, 1981, and Schusdziarra, 1984). The presence of somatostatin in nerve fibers suggests it may act as a neurotransmitter. Somatostatin localization to endocrine-like cells and its release into the circulation suggest a hormonal role. In addition, the localization of somatostatin to the morphologically unusual "paracrine-like" cells of the stomach and pancreas may imply that the peptide has a local action on adjacent cells.

Localization

There is good anatomical evidence that gastric and pancreatic somatostatin may act as a paracrine agent. The somatostatin (D) cells of the stomach and pancreas differ from typical endocrine cells of these organs in that they give off long cytoplasmic processes which are packed with secretory granules and which end with small bulbous expansions on the putative target cells (Larsson, 1981). In the mucosa of the stomach, somatostatin cells give off processes that terminate on parietal cells and gastrin-containing cells. In the pancreatic islets, similar processes terminate on glucagon and insulin cells and also on capillaries. The direct delivery of somatostatin from these processes to the target cell would imply a paracrine function. Release of somatostatin into pancreatic capillaries would suggest a hormonal function.

Whereas the gastric and pancreatic somatostatin cells give off long tail-like processes, the duodenal somatostatin cells resemble the typical endocrine cells of the alimentary tract. The cells are characterized by a triangular flask shape with a luminal connection (Larsson, 1981). Thus, it is possible that duodenal somatostatin is secreted into the general circulation as a circulating hormone. In the intestine, somatostatin is also localized to nerve fibers of the lamina propria, suggesting a neurotransmitter role in this tissue (Larsson, 1981).

Secretion

The secretion of gastric somatostatin has been examined by a variety of in vivo and in vitro techniques. Immunoreactive somatostatin has been measured in vivo in gastric venous blood (Schusdziarra, Harris, Conlon, Arimura, & Unger, 1978). Acidification of the stomach stimulates the secretion of somatostatin into antral venous but not oxyntic venous blood, whereas duodenal acidification releases both antral and oxyntic somatostatin. These data may correlate with morphological observations. In the antrum, somatostatin cells are of the open type because they have contact with the glandular lumen and release may be stimulated by luminal acid. In the oxyntic region, the somatostatin cells do not contact the lumen and cannot respond to acid. Duodenal acidification presumably stimulates oxyntic and antral somatostatin secretion by a nervous reflex.

A new and potentially very useful approach in the study of paracrine and neural secretion in vivo involves the chronic implantation of hollow dialysis tubes into the stomach wall (Bunnett, Walsh, Debas, & Kauffman, 1982; Bunnett, Debas, Walsh, Kauffman, & Golanska, 1983). Molecules can be measured in the dialysate by specific radioimmunoassay. This technique has been used with some success to measure the secretion of prostaglandins and somatostatin in the stomach wall of the conscious dog and rat. It appears that the somatostatin concentrations are severalfold higher in the interstitial fluid than in blood and that somatostatin secretion in the oxyntic region and the antrum is stimulated by feeding and insulin-induced hypoglycemia in dogs (Bunnett, unpublished observation). Although potentially valuable, this technique requires further evaluation.

The isolated and vascularly perfused rat stomach has been used in vitro to examine somatostatin secretion. Gastric somatostatin release is stimulated by infusions of glucagon, theophylline, and dibutyryl cAMP (Chiba, et al., 1978) and also by secretin, bombesin, and pentagastrin, whereas met-enkephalin and substance P inhibit somatostatin secretion (Chiba, et al., 1980a,b). A functional relationship between somatostatin and gastrin release was suggested by the high degree of negative correlation between stimulation of somatostatin output and inhibition of gastrin release during glucagon, secretin, and vasoactive intestinal peptide infusion (Chiba, et al., 1980a,b). A similar inverse relation was found during methacholine infusion where stimulation of gastrin and inhibition of somatostatin were closely linked (Saffouri, Weir, Bitar, & Makhlouf, 1980). Furthermore, in the isolated and vascularly perfused porcine stomach, electrical stimulation of the vagal nerves resulted in a prompt rise in the secretion of gastrin and a concomitant fall in the output of somatostatin, whereas acidification of the lumen had the reverse effect (Holst, et al., 1984).

Although gastric somatostatin may act as a paracrine agent, substantial quantities of the peptide are released into the general circulation. The ingestion of a mixed meal elicits a significant rise in the peripheral venous concentrations of somatostatin in dogs and man (Schusdziarra, 1984). The source of the peripheral increment in somatostatin is probably the stomach and intestine. All three nutrients (carbohydrates, fat, and proteins) release gastric and intestinal somatostatin (Schusdziarra, 1984). In addition, acid is a potent stimulant of duodenal as well as gastric somatostatin release. Acidification of the duodenal bulb stimulates the secretion of somatostatin (Schusdziarra, Rouiller, Harris, & Unger, 1979), and this observation may be of great importance since the proximal duodenum is in contact with gastric contents of low pH. Indeed, duodenal somatostatin may be an important component of the "bulbogastrone mechanism" which describes the inhibition of gastric acid secretion by acidification of the duodenal bulb.

Actions

Practically all gastrointestinal endocrine and exocrine secretions are inhibited by the administration of pharmacologically high doses of somatostatin (for review see Schusdziarra, 1984; Walsh, 1981). Intravenously administered somatostatin is a potent inhibitor of basal, food-stimulated, and neurally stimulated gastrin release and gastrin-stimulated gastric acid secretion. In anesthetized pigs, the infusion of somatostatin into the arterial blood supply to the antrum prevented the increase in gastrin caused by infusions of calcium, parathyroid hormone, and acetylcholine (Bolman, et al., 1978). Somatostatin 14 and its precursor somatostatin 28 potently inhibited gastrin- and bombesin-stimulated acid secretion in conscious dogs (Vaysse, Pradayrol, Susini, Chayvialle, & Ribet, 1981). In man, intravenously administered somatostatin powerfully inhibits gastric acid secretion and gastrin release in both normal subjects and duodenal ulcer patients (M. Mogard, personal communication). Somatostatin does not affect the isolated canine parietal cell or rabbit oxyntic gland, but the reason for this is unknown.

Catabolism

Somatostatin has a short half-life in the general circulation. In the conscious dog, the half life of somatostain 14 and somatostatin 28 is 1.3 and 3.6 min, respectively (Vaysse, et al., 1981). The catabolic fate of somatostatin is unknown.

Physiological Importance

Somatostatin is a physiologically important inhibitor of gastric acid secretion and gastrin release. Anatomical and some physiological evidence suggests that gastric somatostatin may exert a local inhibition of the parietal and gastrin cells. However, gastric and intestinal somatostatin is released into the general circulation after the ingestion of a mixed meal, and the intravenous infusion of somatostatin 14 at rates chosen to duplicate the postprandial elevations in circulating somatostatin-like immunoreactivity inhibits the secretion of gastric acid and gastrin release (Vaysse et al., 1981; M. Mogard, personal communication). These observations support the contention that somatostatin is a circulating hormone but do not exclude its putative role as a paracrine agent and neurotransmitter in some tissues.

OTHER INHIBITORY PEPTIDES

In addition to somatostatin, there are a number of peptides in the small intestine which may be involved in the hormonal inhibition of gastric acid secretion by intestinal acid and fat.

Secretin

Secretin is a hormonal peptide of the small intestine with the primary effect of stimulating pancreatic bicarbonate secretion in response to intestinal acidification (for review see Walsh, 1981). Secretin is a good inhibitor of gastrin-stimulated gastric acid secretion, but there is no convincing evidence that it does so under physiological conditions. In combination with CCK, secretin appears to be a better inhibitor of pentagastrin-stimulated secretion (Henriksen, Jorgensen, & Moller, 1974).

Gastric Inhibitory Peptide

GIP was isolated from impure preparations of CCK and identified by its inhibitory effects on acid secretion from denervated gastric pouches in dogs during the infusion of pentagastrin (Brown, Mutt, & Pederson, 1970). When sensitive immunoassays were developed for the peptide, it was found to be released into the general circulation by intestinal fat (Brown, Dryburgh, Ross, & Dupre, 1975) and was considered a strong candidate for the "enterogastrone," the humoral mechanism by which intestinal fat inhibits gastric acid secretion. However, its physiological importance as a hormonal inhibitor of gastric secretion is now open to doubt in view of its weak effects on acid secretion from the intact, as opposed to the denervated, stomach. In human subjects with intact stomachs, intravenous infusion of GIP produced a very slight inhibition of gastric acid secretion even when the circulating concentrations of the peptide were far higher than those measured after feeding or intraduodenal instillation of fat (Maxwell, et al., 1980). In dogs with gastric fistulas, the intraduodenal instillation of fat produced a complete inhibition of the acid response to liver extract and only a slight elevation in the circulating concentrations of GIP, whereas much higher concentrations of circulating GIP produced by infusion of exogenous peptide resulted in a minor inhibition of acid secretion to the liver extract (Yamagishi & Debas, 1980). Recently, it has been shown that GIP potentiates the release of somatostatin to gastric acidification in the isolated and vascularly perfused pig stomach and that the release of somatostatin in the presence of GIP is easily reversed by vagal stimulation (Holst et al., 1984). This latter observation may explain the potent effects of GIP on the denervated stomach but the weak effects on the intact stomach.

Neurotensin

Neurotensin, a tridecapeptide of the terminal ileum, is released from endocrine cells into the general circulation after the ingestion of fatty meals (Rokeaus, 1982; Hammer, Carraway, & Leeman, 1982). The intravenous infusion of neurotensin inhibits gastric acid secretion (Blackburn, et al., 1980). The correlation between the rise in the circulating concentrations of neurotensin and the inhibition of gastric acid secretion by intraduodenal fat (Rokeaus, 1982) suggests an enterogastrone-like role for the peptide, but the physiological importance of neurotensin in the inhibition of acid secretion is unknown.

CONCLUSIONS

Most of the gastrointestinal peptides affect the secretion of hydrochloric acid by the stomach, but usually only at pharmacologically high doses. Of all of these peptides there is convincing evidence that only gastrin, somatostatin, and GRP are involved in the physiological control of gastric acid secretion. The evidence for gastrin is based on its potent stimulatory effects in vivo and in vitro and on the measurement of immunoreactive gastrin in blood plasma. The evidence for somatostatin and GRP depends on their biological effects and on anatomical studies of somatostatin cells and GRP nerves in the gastric mucosa.

Over the past decade, progress in biochemistry and molecular biology has contributed enormously to our understanding of the regulatory peptides. Several new peptides have been discovered and isolated, and it is likely that many peptides await discovery and that some of these may be involved in the regulation of gastric acid secretion. Similar advances in physiology are required to understand the biological importance of these peptides. Techniques are required to investigate the local release and actions of the peptide and to study the ways in which peptides interact with one another and with other agents at the level of the target cell. Further refinement of the techniques for sampling interstitial fluid in which peptides may be measured and improved methods of cell and nerve culture to examine regulation of peptide secretion in vitro are likely to make important contributions to understanding the physiological importance of the regulatory peptides.

REFERENCES

Blackburn, A. M., Bloom, S. R., Long, R. G., Fletcher, D. R., Christofides, N. D., Fitzpatrick, M. L., & Baron, J. H. (1980, May 10). Effects of neurotensin on gastric function in man. *The Lancet, 1,* 987–989.

Bloom, S. R., & Edwards, A. V. (1984). Characteristics of the neuroendocrine responses to stimulation of the splanchnic nerves in bursts in conscious calves. *Journal of Physiology, 346,* 533–548.

Bolman, R. M., III, Cooper, C. W., & Wells, S. A. (1978). Somatostatin inhibition and reversal of parathyroid hormone-, calcium-, and acetylcholine-induced gastrin release in the pig. *Endocrinology, 103,* 259–266.

Brazeau, P., Vale, W., Burgus, R., Ling, N., Butcher, M., Rivier, J., & Guillemin, R. (1973). Hypothalamic polypeptide that inhibits the secretion of immunoreactive pituitary growth hormone. *Science, 179,* 77–79.

Brown, J. D., Dryburgh, J. R., Ross, S. A., & Dupre, J. (1975). Identification and actions of gastric inhibitory polypeptide. *Recent Progress in Hormone Research, 31,* 487–532.

Brown, J. C., Mutt, V., & Pederson, R. A. (1970). Further purification of a polypeptide demonstrating enterogastrone activity. *Journal of Physiology, 209,* 57–64.

Bunnett, N. W. (1984). The localisation of gastrin-like immunoreactivity (GIR) in the alimentary tract of the sheep. *Quarterly Journal of Experimental Physiology, 69,* 521–529.

Bunnett, N. W., Clark, B., Debas, H. T., del Milton, R. C., Kovacs, T. O. G., Orloff, M. S., Pappas, T. N., Reeve, J. R., Rivier, J. E., & Walsh, J. H. (1985a). Canine bombesin-like gastrin releasing peptides stimulate gastrin release and acid secretion in the dog. *Journal of Physiology, 365,* 121–130.

Bunnett, N. W., Kobayashi, R., Orloff, M. S., Reeve, J. R., Turner, A. J., & Walsh, J. H. (1985b). Catabolism of gastrin releasing peptide and substance P by gastric membrane-bound peptidases. *Peptides, 6,* 277–283.

Bunnett, N. W., Mogard, M., Orloff, M. O., Corbet, H. J., Reeve, J. R., & Walsh, J. H. (1984). Catabolism of neurotensin in interstitial fluid of the rat stomach. *American Journal of Physiology, 9,* G666–G674.

Bunnett, N. W., Orloff, M. S., & Turner, A. J. (1985c). Catabolism of substance P in the stomach wall of the rat. *Life Science,* 599–606.

Bunnett, N. W., Reeve, J. R., & Walsh, J. H. (1983). Catabolism of bombesin in interstitial fluid of the rat stomach. *Neuropeptides, 4,* 55–64.

Bunnett, N. W., Walsh, J. H., Debas, H. T., & Kauffman, G. L. (1982). The measurement of prostaglandins, histamine and peptides in interstitial fluid from the dog stomach. *Regulatory Peptides, 4,* 358.

Bunnett, N. W., Walsh, J. H., Debas, H. T., Kauffman, G. L., & Golanska, E. M. (1983). Measurement of prostaglandin E2 in interstitial fluid from the dog stomach after feeding and indomethacin. *Gastroenterology, 85,* 1391–1398.

Chiba, T., Seino, Y., Goto, Y., Kadowaki, S., Taminato, T., Abe, H., Kato, Y., Matsukura, S., Nozawa, M., & Imura, H. (1978). Somatostatin release from isolated perfused rat stomach. *Biochemical and Biophysical Research Communications, 82*, 731–737.

Chiba, T., Taminato, T., Kadowaki, S., Abe, H., Chihara, K., Goto, Y., Seino, Y., & Fujita, T. (1980a). Effects of glucagon, secretin, and vasoactive intestinal polypeptide on gastric somatostatin and gastrin release from isolated perfused rat stomach. *Gastroenterology, 79*, 67–71.

Chiba, T., Taminato, T., Kadowaki, S., Inoue, Y., Mori, K., Seino, Y., Abe, H., Chihara, K., Matsukura, S., Fujita, T., & Goto, Y. (1980b). Effects of various gastrointestinal peptides on gastric somatostatin release. *Endocrinology, 106*, 145–149.

Corazziari, E., Solomon, T. E., & Grossman, M. I. (1979). Effects of ninety five percent pure cholecystokinin on gastrin-stimulated acid secretion in man and dog. *Gastroenterology, 77*, 91–95.

Csendes, A., Walsh, J. H., & Grossman, M. I. (1972). Effects of atropine and of antral acidification on gastrin release and acid secretion in response to insulin and feeding in dogs. *Gastroenterology, 63*, 257–263.

Del Mazo, J., & McGuigan, J. E. (1976). Degradation of gastrin by gastric mucosal cells. *Journal of Laboratory and Clinical Medicine, 88*, 292–300.

Dockray, G. J. (1978). Gastrin overview. In S. R. Bloom (Ed.), *Gut hormones* (pp. 129–139). Edinburgh: Churchill Livingstone.

Dockray, G. J., Vaillant, C., & Walsh, J. H. (1979). The neuronal origin of bombesin-like immunoreactivity in the rat gastrointestinal tract. *Neuroscience, 4*, 1561–1568.

Elwin, C. E. (1974). Gastric acid responses to antral application of some amino acids, peptides and isolated fractions of a protein hydrolysate. *Scandinavian Journal of Gastroenterology, 68*, 662–666.

Feldman, E. J., Isenberg, J. I., & Grossman, M. I. (1981). Gastric acid and gastrin response to decaffeinated coffee and a peptone meal. *Journal of the American Medical Association, 26*, 248–250.

Feldman, M., Walsh, J. H., & Wong, H. C. (1978). Role of gastrin heptadecapeptide in the acid secretory response to amino acids in man. *Journal of Clinical Investigation, 61*, 308–313.

Fordtran, J. S., & Walsh, J. H. (1973). Gastric acid secretion rate and buffer content of the stomach after eating. Results in normal subjects and in patients with duodenal ulcer. *Journal of Clinical Investigation, 52*, 645–657.

Fujita, T., & Kobayashi, S. (1981). The endocrine cell. In S. R. Bloom & J. M. Polak (Eds.), *Gut hormones* (pp. 90–95), Edinburgh: Churchill Livingstone.

Gregory, R. A. (1982). Heterogeneity of gut and brain regulatory peptides. *British Medical Bulletin, 38*, 271–276.

Gregory, R. A., & Tracy, J. J. (1964). The constitution and properties of two gastrins extracted from hog antral mucosa. Part I. The isolation of two gastrins from hog antral mucosa. Part II. The properties of two gastrins from hog antral mucosa. *Gut, 5*, 103–117.

Greider, M. H., Steinberg, V., & McGuigan, J. E. (1972). Electron microscopic identification of gastrin cell of the human antral mucosa by means of immunocytochemistry. *Gastroenterology, 63*, 572–582.

Hammer, R. A., Carraway, R. E., & Leeman, S. E. (1982). Elevation of neurotensin-like immunoreactivity after a meal. *Journal of Clinical Investigation, 70*, 74–81.

Henriksen, F. W., Jorgensen, S. P., & Moller, S. (1974). Interaction between secretin and cholecystokinin on inhibition of gastric acid secretion in man. *Scandinavian Journal of Gastroenterology, 9*, 735–740.

Holst, J. J., Knuhtsen, S., Jensen, S. L., Fahrenkrug, J., Larsson, L. I., & Nielsen, O. V. (1984). Interrelations of nerves and hormones in the stomach and pancreas. In J. M. Polak, S. R. Bloom, N. A. Wright, & A. G. Butler (Eds.) *Physiology of the gut. Basic science in gastroenterology* (pp. 85–99). Glaxo Research Group Ltd.: Ware, Herts, England.

Impicciatore, M., Walsh, J. H., & Grossman, M. I. (1977). Low doses of atropine enhance serum gastrin response to food in dogs. *Gastroenterology, 72*, 995–996.

Jessell, T. M., Iversen, L. L., & Kanazawa, I. (1976). Release and metabolism of substance P in rat hypothalamus. *Nature, 264*, 81–83.

Knuhtsen, S., Holst, J. J., Knigge, U., Olesen, M., & Nielsen, O. V. (1984). Radioimmunoassay, pharmacokinetics, and neuronal release of gastrin-releasing peptide in anesthetized pigs. *Gastroenterology, 87*, 372–378.

Lam, S. K., Isenberg, J. I., Grossman, M. I., Lane, W. H., & Walsh, J. H. (1980). Gastric acid secretion is abnormally sensitive to endogenous gastrin released after peptone test meals in duodenal ulcer patients. *Journal of Clinical Investigation, 65*, 555–562.

Larsson, L. I. (1981). Somatostatin cells. In S. R. Bloom & J. M. Polak (Eds.), *Gut hormones* (pp. 350–353), Edinbergh: Churchill Livingstone.

Lenz, H. J., Ferrari-Taylor, J., & Isenberg, J. I. (1983). Wine and five percent ethanol are potent stimulants of gastric acid secretion in humans. *Gastroenterology, 85*, 1082–1087.

Lichtenberger, L. M., Graziani, L. A., & Dubinsky, W. P. (1982). Importance of dietary amines in meal-induced gastrin release. *American Journal of Physiology, 243*, G341–G347.

Maxwell, V., Shulkes, A., Brown, J. C., Solomon, T. E., Walsh, J. H., & Grossman, M. I. (1980). Effect of gastric inhibitory polypeptide on pentagastrin-stimulated acid secretion in man. *Digestive Diseases, 25*, 113–116.

McDonald, T. J., Nilsson, G., Vagne, M., Ghatei, M., Bloom, S. R., & Mutt, V. (1978). A gastrin releasing peptide from porcine non-antral gastric tissue. *Gut, 19*, 767–774.

McGuigan, J. E. (1968). Gastric mucosal intracellular localization of gastrin by immunofluorescence. *Gastroenterology, 55*, 315–327.

McGuigan, J. E., Isaza, J., & Landor, J. H. (1971). Relationships of gastrin dose, serum gastrin and acid secretion. *Gastroenterology, 61*, 659–666.

Nilsson, G., Simon, J., Yalow, R. S., & Berson, S. A. (1972). Plasma gastrin and gastric acid responses to sham feeding and feeding in dogs. *Gastroenterology, 63*, 51–59.

Orloff, M. S., Melendez, R. L., Rivier, J., Reeve, J. R., Chew, P., & Debas, H. T. (1984). Serum gastrin and gastric acid output in response to infusion of bombesin and three gastrin releasing peptides in conscious dogs. *Gastroenterology, 86*, 1202.

Orloff, M. S., Turner, A. J., & Bunnett, N. W. (1986). Substance P and neurotensin catabolism in the stomach wall of the rat is sensitive to inhibitors of antiotensin converting enzyme (EC 3.4.15.1). *Regulatory Peptides, 14*, 21–31.

Pradayrol, L., Jornvall, H., Mutt, V., & Ribet, A. (1980). N-terminally extended somatostatin: The primary structure of somatostatin 28. *FEBS Letters, 109*, 55–58.

Reeve, J. R., Walsh, J. H., Chew, P., Clark, B., Hawke, D., & Shively, J. E. (1983). Amino acid sequences of three bombesin-like peptides from canine intestine extracts. *The Journal of Biological Chemistry, 258*, 5582–5588.

Richardson, C. T., Walsh, J. H., Hicks, M. I., & Fordtran, J. S. (1976). Studies on the mechanisms of food stimulated gastric acid secretion in normal human subjects. *Journal of Clinical Investigation, 58*, 623–631.

Rokeaus, A. (1982). Studies on neurotensin as a hormone. *Acta Physiologiea Scandinavia*, Supplement 501.

Saffouri, B., Weir, G. C., Bitar, K. N., & Makhlouf, G. M. (1980). Gastrin and somatostatin secretion by perfused rat stomach: Functional linkage of antral peptides. *American Journal of Physiology, 238*, 495–501.

Schusdziarra, V. (1984). Somatostatin-Physiological and pathophysiological aspects. In J. M. Polak, S. R. Bloom, N. A. Wright, & A. G. Butler (Eds.) *Physiology of the gut. Basic science in gastroenterology* (pp. 69–84). Glaxo Research Group Ltd. Ware, Herts, England.

Schusdziarra, V., Harris, V., Conlon, J. M., Arimura, A., & Unger, R. H. (1978). Pancreatic and gastric somatostatin release in response to intragastric and intraduodenal nutrients and HCl in the dog. *Journal of Clinical Investigation, 62*, 509–518.

Schusdziarra, V., Rouiller, D., Harris, V., & Unger, R. H. (1979). Release of gastric somatostatin-like immunoreactivity during acidification of the duodenal bulb. *Gastroenterology, 79*, 950–953.

Segawa, T., Nakata, Y., Yajima, H., & Kitagawa, K. (1977). Further observation of the lack of active uptake system for substance P in the central nervous system. *Japanese Journal of Pharmacology, 27*, 573–580.

Soares, E. C., Zaterka, S., & Walsh, J. H. (1977). Acid secretion and serum gastrin at graded intragastric pressures in man. *Gastroenterology, 72*, 676–679.

Soll. A. H. (1981). Physiology of isolated canine parietal cells: Receptors and effectors regulating function. In L. R. Johnson (Ed.) (pp. 673–692), New York: Raven Press.

Straus, E., & Yalow, R. S. (1974). Studies on the distribution and degradation of heptadecapeptide, big and big big gastrin. *Gastroenterology, 66*, 936–943.

Strunz, U. T., Walsh, J. H., & Grossman, M. I. (1978). Removal of gastrin by various organs in dogs. *Gastroenterology, 74*, 32–33.

Taylor, I. I., Byrne, W. J., Christie, D. L., Ament, M. E., & Walsh, J. H. (1982). Effect of individual L-amino acids on gastric acid secretion and serum gastrin and pancreatic polypeptide release in humans. *Gastroenterology, 83*, 273–278.

Tepperman, B. L., Walsh, J. H., & Preshaw, R. M. (1972). Effect of antral denervation on gastrin release by sham feeding and insulin hypoglycemia in dogs. *Gastroenterology, 63*, 973–980.

Vaysse, N., Pradayrol, L., Susini, C., Chayvialle, J. A., & Ribet, A. (1981). Somatostatin 28: Biological actions. In S. R. Bloom & J. M. Polak (Eds.) *Gut hormones* (pp. 358–361). Edinburgh: Churchill Livingstone.

Walsh, J. H. (1981). Gastrointestinal hormones and peptides. In L. R. Johnson (Ed.), *Physiology of the gastrointestinal tract* (pp. 54–144). New York: Raven Press.

Walsh, J. H., Debas, H. T., & Grossman, M. I. (1974). Pure human big gastrin. Immunochemical properties, disappearance half time, and acid-stimulating action in dogs. *Journal of Clinical Investigation, 54*, 477–485.

Walsh, J. H., & Grossman, M. I. (1975). Medical progress: Gastrin. *New England Journal of Medicine, 292*, 1323–1424.

Walsh, J. H., Richardson, C. T., & Fordtran, J. S. (1975). pH dependence of acid secretion and gastrin release in normal and ulcer patients. *Journal of Clinical Investigation, 55*, 462–469.

Walsh, J. H., Reeve, J. R., & Vigna, S. R. (1981). Distribution and molecular forms of mammalian bombesin. In S. R. Bloom & J. M. Polak (Eds.), *Gut hormones* (pp. 413–418). Edinburgh: Churchill Livingstone.

Yamagishi, T., & Debas, H. T. (1980). Gastric inhibitory polypeptide (GIP) is not the primary mediator of the enterogastrone action of fat in the dog. *Gastroenterology, 78*, 931–936.

3

NEURAL MODELS
OF THE CONTROL
OF FOOD INTAKE

Donald Novin
Psychology Department
Brain Research Institute
University of California

It has become increasingly clear, at least to me, that we are likely to fail if we continue to look for *the* center for feeding or *the* satiety or hunger signal. Scientists must certainly seek the most parsimonious theories, but evolutionary considerations may mandate redundancy in vital biological functions.

GENERAL MODELS OF FEEDING

It is not possible yet to specify which signals are the critical ones controlling feeding. Indeed, for the reason stated above, there might not be *one* critical signal (Novin, 1983). Nevertheless, there is good evidence that information detected by gustatory, visceral, and brain receptors constitute the major factors in the control of feeding. The idea that there is an integration of a variety of signals and that all of them play some role in feeding control has not, until recently, been a popular notion. In the past, what has been dominant has been homeostatic or set-point theories, both of which give a more prominent place in control to internal events while relegating external factors to a modulatory role (Mayer, 1955). In contrast, incentive models (Toates, 1981) assume that external stimuli (the incentives) have a primary role in eliciting and directing feeding behavior, and internal events "gate" these primary controls.

What is dissatisfying about homeostatic and set-point models as well as incentive models is that they create artificial and perhaps misleading distinctions between the various controlling conditions. In the case of homeostatic models, the basic controls are internal events (e.g., glucose availability, fat storage, hormone levels), whereas food palatability, for example, would be considered a modulating condition.

The most reasonable supposition is that palatability cues are as critical a factor in controlling food intake as any so-called internal or homeostatic variable, but not more so, as incentive models would argue. If there is a real physiological set point against which current conditions are continuously compared, gustatory cues have been shown experimentally (Peck, 1976) to exert powerful effects on where this reference point is established. Thus, until evidence to the contrary is presented, it is best to consider food intake as jointly and interactively controlled by both internal and external factors. For a more extensive review of these arguments, refer to Toates' excellent theoretical paper on hunger models (1981).

Historically, if not logically, the stomach is a good place to start when considering the origin of signals and neural substrates that might control or modulate food intake. Cannon, early in this century (1963), developed the first systematic and empirically based theory of hunger. In his formulation, the empty stomach displayed strong contractions, and these were the basic hunger stimuli. The ingestion of a meal reduced these contractions, and the resultant stomach quiesence was the signal of satiety. Later theorists made assumptions that these signals were neural in origin and likely traveled to the brain over the vagus nerves. The reasons for the ultimate replacement of this theory are more fully outlined in another paper (Novin & VanderWeele, 1976), but primarily it was that newer theories seemed to account for a greater variety of the facts with fewer assumptions and contradictions.

The next major step in the neural modeling of feeding control was the "dual center" hypothesis. In this formulation, the hypothalamus exercised the primary control over feeding. More specifically, there was the ventro-medial hypothalamic nuclei (VMH) that acted as a satiety center inhibiting a lateral hypothalamic area (LHA) feeding center. This theory grew primarily from lesion work on rats and other animals and in part by observation of human cases of naturally occurring brain damage (Stevenson, 1969). Initial observations of experimental lesions in rats and other animals appeared to demonstrate that after VMH lesions, animals would overeat and, as a consequence, become obese. Thus came the notion of the VMH as a satiety center. In contrast, destruction of the LHA resulted in aphagia, in some cases so severe that the animal might starve to death. On the basis of the observation that the effect of destruction of both areas was most like the destruction of the LHA, it was hypothesized that the VMH satiety center operated by inhibiting the LHA. Studies of the effects of electrical stimulation of the brain in behaving animals provided additional and powerful support for the dual center hypothesis. Stimulation of the LHA resulted in increased feeding and hunger motivation, whereas VMH stimulation suppressed food intake. In so far as one would assume that stimulation should have the opposite effects of destruction of the brain area, these results provide powerful support for the theory. For more than a decade this was the leading theory of the neural control of food intake, probably because it was powerful and parsimonious, that is, it made many testable predictions with relatively few assumptions (Stevenson, 1969).

However good the dual center theory was, it seemed there were always facts that could not easily fit into this theoretical framework. It was always assumed that the metabolic effects of the lesions, especially those following VMH destruction, were secondary to the feeding effects of the lesion. However, there were data (Frohman, Goldman, & Bernardis, 1972) showing that there were metabolic effects of the lesion that were primary and independent of the altered feeding. In addition, it was demonstrated that if the animal was made to either gain or lose substantial amounts of weight prior to the production of the lesions, the feeding effects of the lesions were substantially reduced or eliminated (Powley & Keesey, 1970). These observations led to the more currently popular set-point theory (Mrosovsky & Powley, 1977). In this theory there is a predetermined level of body weight, or more specifically adiposity, and a way of measuring deviations from that. Those deviations from a set point activate mechanisms designed to restore conditions as close as possible to the pre-set value. In this scheme, the VMH and LHA do not control food intake directly, rather they set the upper and lower limits, respectively, for body weight (adiposity). Thus, when they are destroyed, new, more extreme levels of body weight are maintained.

The neural and hormonal mechanisms that are presumed to operate in this scheme have not been fully worked out, but one prominent mechanism certainly involves the pancreatic hormones, especially insulin. In this formulation, VMH lesions disinhibit the parasympathetic excitation of the beta cell, and insulin secretion is increased, leading to enhanced lipogenesis. The increased demand for lipid storage can ultimately be met only by increased nutrient intake until a new level of adiposity is achieved. The set-point theory accounts for many new and old observations not compatible with the notion that these hypothalamic structures had as their primary role the direct control of feeding behavior.

Recently, incentive models have become popular (Toates, 1981). In this model of feeding, behavior is not driven by an internal state or need, but rather is stimulated by certain external signals whose strength is modulated by internal states and prior experience with the external signals. In this scheme, such stimuli as the sight, smell, and taste of food become the cause for ingestion. The effectiveness of these stimuli is facilitated or inhibited by past experience with those particular stimuli and gated by concurrent internal states such as stomach distention and glucose availability. Thus, Booth (1977) showed that flavors associated with a calorically concentrated nutrient are preferred early in a meal, well before repletion occurs. In contrast, nearing repletion preferences switch to a flavor previously associated with a calorically diluted nutrient.

Incentive theorists have quite rightly criticized homeostatic models for not taking into account the important effects external factors have in the control of food intake (see Toates, 1981, for a discussion of this point). However, incentive theorists overlook the powerful and direct effects that internal states have in the control of ingestion. With all other conditions held constant, the longer the food deprivation, the stronger is the hunger drive. It would seem hard to argue that this was not the effect of an internal state. Furthermore, Louis-Sylvestre and Le Magnen (1980) have demonstrated that in the relatively undisturbed, ad-libitum feeding rat, every meal was preceded by a small but consistent decrease in blood glucose level, and no such change in internal state occurred without being followed by a spontaneous meal. These data suggest that the internal state, whatever the external stimulation, can be the direct cause of feeding. That is, the external food incentive was present at all times, and this did not predict whether or not the animal would initiate a meal. However, the internal state, namely a fall in the glycemic level, did predict this.

Another issue is that it seems odd to build a theory in which gustatory chemoreceptors are considered to be detecting external stimuli, whereas gastric and gut receptors are monitoring internal events. Both homeostatic and incentive models commit this error. From a topological sense, and more directly in consideration of the embryological origins of these tissues, this distinction is difficult to justify. The alimentary canal is a continuous tube in direct contact with the outside world.

At the moment there is no evidence to make one elevate external factors above internal ones or vice versa in their importance for feeding control. Indeed, in some cases as mentioned above, the distinction might not even be particularly useful or even valid.

Other theories have focussed more narrowly on one or a few aspects of the control of food intake. There have been theories emphasizing one organ, such as stomach, gut, or liver (Carlson, 1980). Other hypotheses have concentrated on the signals that might drive food intake. This has resulted in glucostatic, lipostatic, aminostatic, and caloriestatic theories (Carlson, 1980). Still other formulations emphasize the neurotransmitters involved, such as catecholamines (Liebowitz, 1980) or peptides (Morley & Levine, 1982) or humoral agents that themselves act as signals, such as insulin (Woods, et al., 1984) or cholecystokinin (Smith, Gibbs, & Kulkosky, 1982).

There can be no question that there must be initiating signals capable of activating organs that are differentially sensitive to them. Also, there must be a message system transmitting this information using either humoral agents, the nervous system with its attendant neurotransmitters, or both. It is difficult to formulate a grand theory to encompass these observations because there seem to be no necessary links in the causal chain connecting the initiating signals to the act of ingestion. Thus, the elimination of some presumed important factor has often given small or confusing results. One way to understand this is to recognize that the control of feeding is probably multifactorial and redundant. The multitude of controls may be, in part, due to the nature of the goal object. Unlike thirst, in which the goal object is the intake of water, however it might be mixed with other substances, there is no one substance the ingestion of which is uniquely connected to a hunger drive. Any one of a number of macro- and micronutrients may or may not satiate, depending on a variety of as yet largely unknown variables. Redundancy may partly arise from the complex nature of the ingested material but is probably also derived from the safety factor it provides by having parallel channels of control or modulation of this vital function.

NEURAL SUBSTRATES OF FEEDING

Because of the above considerations, a picture of the neural substrates of feeding can only be painted with broad brushstrokes. One obviously needs to consider a wide variety of receptors, their pathways into and through the brain, and the convergence and integration of this information at several levels of the neuraxis. Much has been discovered recently, but clearly much further study is required.

Certainly, in all higher organisms, all of the five classical senses are involved in the control of feeding. One of these, the gustatory sense, appears from both practical judgment and empirical study to be the most important. In addition, there is evidence that other sensory systems that may influence feeding depend on past association with gustation for their effects on feeding (Rusiniak, Hankins, Garcia, & Brett, 1979).

Many of the details of the gustatory sense, including its innervation and pathways through the brain, have been uncovered. There are several excellent reviews that may be consulted for the details (e.g., Norgren, Grill, & Pfaffman, 1977). Briefly, in the rat, taste sensation is carried to the brain via the Vth, VIIth and Xth cranial nerves. Their first relay is in the anterior portion of the nucleus of the solitary tract (NTS) in the medulla. From here there is a major projection to the parabrachial nucleus (PBN) in the pons. At the pontine level, the pathway bifurcates and reaches both the thalamus and the hypothalamic-limbic system. One stucture that receives much of this input is the hypothalamic paraventricular nucleus, a structure known to be involved in feeding control (Liebowitz, 1980). Finally, gustatory information is represented in the cortex. It should be pointed out that there is evidence in the rat and in higher animals for more direct pathways as from the PBN directly to the cortex bypassing the intervening relays (Lasiter, Glanzman, & Mensah, 1982). Much of the information about these pathways is derived from labeling studies, which clearly outline the connectivity. We have only begun to determine which, if any, of these pathways have functional significance, or what that function might be.

The neural substrates of other inputs into the feeding control system are less well documented. However, we do know that all of the visceral organs hypothesized to be involved in the control of food intake are innervated by both the vagal parasympathetic and the splanchnic sympathetic branches of the autonomic nervous system. In the past these systems had been thought to be largely effector systems, but now it is known that much of their nerve fibers are devoted to sensory functions. The pathway carrying information via the splanchnic nerves is not well understood. There is evidence that there is a relay at the T5–T13 level of the spinal cord (Lautt, 1980), but not much can be said about higher projections from this level.

Much more is known about afferents traveling with the vagus nerves. The first relay nucleus for afferents in this system is in the posterior portion of the NTS. A curious fact is that input from the liver goes almost exclusively to the left NTS in the rat (Adachi, 1981). The significance, if any, of this asymmetry and whether other organs share this peculiarity is unknown at the moment.

There is clear evidence that there are a variety of receptors for signals, all of which might be expected to play a role in the control of feeding. Afferent vagal fibers have been recorded which responded to changes in glucose, amino acids, osmolarity, sodium ion, temperature, and mechanical stimulation (Sawchenko & Friedman, 1979). In some cases, there is evidence for this information relaying in the NTS. In the caudal NTS, where visceral input is relayed, the same cells that respond to hepatic-portal glucose infusions are affected by direct ionto-phoretic application of glucose, suggesting that there are central glucoreceptors here (Adachi, Shimizu, Oomura, & Kobashi, 1984) as well as in the hypothal-amus (see below).

In general, the upward projection of visceral information as far as has been determined parallels, and to some extent overlaps with, and therefore is presum-ably integrated with, gustatory information. Thus, the next major relay nucleus for visceral information is in the PBN. Here portions of the nucleus receive discrete taste and visceral inputs, but there is a caudal portion where both inputs converge (Hermann, Kohlerman, & Rogers, 1983). The PBN and the NTS project to a variety of forebrain structures, most important among them are the ventro-basal complex of the thalamus, sometimes called the thalamic taste area, the hypothalamic paraventricular nucleus (now considered to be the chief hypotha-lamic nucleus involved in the modulation of feeding), and the central nucleus of the amygdala and cortical areas, known from other studies to be receiving areas for visceral and gustatory inputs. In addition, many of these brain areas not only receive inputs from relay nuclei lower in the neuraxis, but they send efferents back to these same nuclei.

In the lateral hypothalamic area, there is another case of convergence of inputs important in the control of feeding. Cells here are inhibited by iontophoretic application of glucose, identifying them as central glucose sensitive cells, and are also inhibited by the hepatic infusion of a glucose solution (Shimizu, Oomura, Novin, Grijalva, & Cooper, 1983). This area, which also probably receives taste information, appears to be a major point of convergence and possibly integration of signals known to be involved in food intake control.

Why is so much of the central nervous system involved in the control of feeding and at so many different levels, from the peripheral nervous system, through the brainstem up to the neo-cortex? The intake of complex energy-yielding substances is among the most primitive and basic behaviors in the entire animal kingdom. It is not likely, then, that even in higher organisms feeding behavior would be the province primarily of higher centers of the brain. Since it exists in even the lowest organisms, it must be represented at the lowest levels of the nervous system. There is now substantial behavioral evidence for this proposition, as it has been shown that a quite sophisticated degree of feeding regulation exists in the decerebrate rat (Norgren, Grill, & Pfaffman, 1977). This indicates that phylogenetically old structures of the pons and brainstem receiving peripheral inputs from viscera and gustatory sense provide much of the information and processing capacity for feeding.

Are higher portions of the brain really involved then in feeding and, if so, how? All the evidence so far indicates that higher centers are involved and importantly so. Whereas there is regulation to a degree at the pontine level demonstrated by the decerebrate rat, there is much that this preparation cannot do. Its general motor behavior is severely impaired so that it cannot search for food but must have food brought to it. However, this is a general impairment not specifically related to the feeding system, that is, decerebration greatly limits its entire behavioral repertoire. More specifically related to feeding is the inability of the decerebrate rat, deprived of connections to the forebrain, to learn a taste aversion (Norgren & Grill, 1982). This is a paradigm designed to show the associations that the rat makes between taste and the visceral and central effects of ingested and other material internalized by the organism. Thus, the higher parts of the brain are probably not necessary for what might be called the basic feeding reflex, which suggests its primitive nature. Rather the forebrain allows for the increasingly complex and flexible behaviors that are part of the feeding behaviors of animals possessed of such neural structures.

It should then come as no surprise that human feeding behavior is difficult to understand and control. The primitive neural structures that subserve feeding reflexes in the rat are identifiable and homologous in humans. However, sitting on top of these basic control mechanisms both literally and figuratively is the massively elaborated cerebral cortex, subject to complex inputs and producing at least as equally complex outputs of which we still have little understanding. Knowing something about the neural substrates of feeding, even if it comes largely from relatively primitive mammals, is at least a beginning to unraveling the mystery of normal and abnormal regulation of hunger and satiety in the human.

ACKNOWLEDGMENTS

This work was supported by grant USPHS NS07687 The author thanks Dr. Paula Geiselman for helpful suggestions in preparing this manuscript, and Julie Lee for her secretarial services.

REFERENCES

Adachi, A. (1981). Electrophysiological study of hepatic vagal projection to the medulla. *Neuroscience Letters, 24*, 19–23.

Adachi, A., Shimizu, N., Oomura, Y., and Kobashi, M. (1984). Convergence of hepatoportal glucose-sensitive afferent signals to glucose-sensitive units within the nucleus of the solitary tract. *Neuroscience Letters, 46*, 215–218.

Booth, D. A. (1977). Appetite and satiety as metabolic expectancies. In Y. Katsuki, M. Sato, S. F. Takagi, and Y. Oomura (Eds.), *Food intake and chemical senses* (pp. 317–330). Tokyo: University of Tokyo Press.

Cannon, V. B. (1963). *Bodily changes in pain, hunger, fear and rage* (2nd ed.). New York: Harper & Row.

Carlson, N. R. (1980). *Physiology of behavior* (2nd ed.). Boston: Allyn and Bacon.

Frohman, L. A., Goldman, J. K., and Bernardis, L. L. (1972). Metabolism of intravenously injected C^{14}-glucose in weaning rats with hypothalamic obesity. *Metabolism, 21*, 799–805.

Hermann, G. E., Kohlerman, N. J., and Rogers, R. C. (1983). Hepatic-vagal and gustatory afferent interactions in the brainstem of the rat. *Journal of the Autonomic Nervous System, 9*, 477–495.

Lasiter, P. S., Glanzman, D. L., & Mensah, P. A. (1982). Direct connectivity between pontine taste areas and gustatory neocortex in rat. *Brain Research, 234*, 111–121.

Lautt, W. W. (1980). Hepatic nerves: A review of their functions and effects. *Canadian Journal of Physiology and Pharmacology, 58*, 105–123.

Liebowitz, S. F. (1980). Neurochemical systems of the hypothalamus. In P. J. Morgane and J. Panksepp (Eds.), *Handbook of the hypothalmus* (Volume 3, Part A; pp. 299–437) New York: Marcel Dekker.

Louis-Sylvestre, J., & LeMagnen, J. (1980). A fall in glucose level precedes meal onset in free-feeding rats. *Neuroscience and Biobehavioral Reviews, 4* (Supp. 1), 13–16.

Mayer, J. (1955). Regulation of energy intake and the body weight: The glucostatic theory and the lipostatic hypothesis. *Annals of the New York Academy of Science, 63*, 15–43.

Morley, S. E., and Levine, A. S. (1982). Opiates, dopamine and feeding. In B. G. Hoebel and D. Novin (Eds.), *The neural basis of feeding and reward* (pp. 499–506). Brunswick, ME: Haer Institute.

Mrosovsky, N., and Powley, T. L. (1977). Set points for body weight and fat. *Behavioral Biology, 20*, 205–223.

Norgren, R., and Grill, H. J. (1982). Brain stem control of ingestive behavior. In W. D. Pfaff (Ed.), *Physiological mechanisms of motivation* (pp. 99–131). Berlin: Springer-Verlag.

Norgren, R., Grill, H. J., and Pfaffman, C. (1977). CNS projections of taste to the dorsal pons and limbic system with correlated studies of behavior. In Y. Katsuki, M. Sato, S. F. Takagi, and Y. Oomura (Eds.), *Food intake and chemical senses* (pp. 233–246). Tokyo: University of Tokyo Press.

Novin, D. (1983). The integration of visceral information in the control of feeding. *Journal of the Autonomic Nervous System, 9*, 233–246.

Novin, D., and VanderWeele, D. A. (1976). Visceral mechanisms in feeding: There is more to regulation than the hypothalamus. In J. Sprague and A. Epstein (Eds.), *Progress in psychobiology and physiological psychology* (pp. 193–241). New York: Academic Press.

Peck, J. W. (1976). Situational determinants of body weights defended by normal rats and rats with hypothalamic lesions. In D. Novin, W. Wyrwicka, G. A. & Bray (Eds.) *Hunger: Basic mechanisms and clinical implications* (pp. 297–312). New York: Raven Press.

Powley, T. L., and Keesey, R. E. (1970). Relationship of body weight to the lateral hypothalamic syndrome. *Journal of Comparative and Physiological Psychology, 70*, 25–36.

Rusiniak, K. W., Hankins, W. G., Garcia, J., and Brett, L. P. (1979). Flavor-illness aversions: Potentiation of odor by taste in rats. *Behavioral and Neural Biology, 25*, 1–15.

Sawchenko, P. E., and Friedman, M. I. (1979). Sensory functions of the liver—A review. *American Journal of Physiology, 236*, R5–R20.

Shimizu, N., Oomura, Y., Novin, D., Grijalva, C. V., and Cooper, P. H. (1983). Functional correlations between lateral hypothalamic glucose-sensitive neurons and hepatic portal glucose sensitive neurons in the rat. *Brain Research, 265*, 49–54.

Smith, G. P., Gibbs, J., and Kulkosky, P. J. (1982). Relationships between brain-gut peptides and neurons in the control of food intake. In B. G. Hoebel and D. Novin (Eds.), *The neural basis of feeding and reward* (pp. 149–166). Brunswick, ME: Haer Institute.

Stevenson, J. A. F. (1969). Neural control of food and water intake. In W. Haymaker, E. Anderson, and W. J. H. Nauta (Eds.), *The hypothalmus* (pp. 524–621). Springfield, IL: C. C. Thomas.

Toates, F. M. (1981). The control of ingestive behavior by internal and external stimuli—a theoretical review. *Appetite, 2*, 35–50.

Woods, S. C., Stein, L. S., McKay, L. D., & Porte, D., Jr. (1984). Suppression of food intake by intravenous nutrients and insulin in the baboon. *American Journal of Physiology, 247*, R393–R401.

4

HUMORAL MECHANISMS IN THE CONTROL OF EATING AND BODY WEIGHT

Gerard P. Smith
The Eating Disorders Institute
Cornell University Medical College

It seems certain that humoral mechanisms are involved in the control of eating behavior and in the maintenance of body weight, but not one humoral mechanism is supported by the necessary experimental evidence to be accepted as fact. In addition to the lack of scientific closure, there has been a marked change in the kind of humoral mechanisms that are receiving experimental attention. Ten years ago, nutrients were the candidate mechanisms (Smith, 1976). They have been replaced by peptide hormones released from endocrine cells in the gut (Gibbs & Smith, 1984).

The most active area of investigation has been guided by the gut hormone hypothesis of satiety (Gibbs, Young, & Smith, 1973a; Smith, 1984). This hypothesis states that gut hormones released by ingested food form at least part of the negative feedback mechanisms that terminate eating and elicit the behaviors and experiences characteristic of the initial phase of postprandial satiety. Although numerous peptides can inhibit food intake under some conditions (Gibbs & Smith, 1984), four peptides currently have sufficient experimental evidence of behavioral and structural specificity to emerge as candidate humoral mechanisms for satiety (Table 4.1).

All of these peptides inhibit food intake at doses that do not inhibit water intake. This behavioral specificity eliminates the possibility that the satiating effect of these peptides is a trivial result of a general behavioral depressant effect. This also demonstrates the important psychobiological principle that the behavioral context and neural state are critical determinants of the behavioral effect of peptides.

The structural-activity relationships have been worked out best for cholecystokinin (CCK). Three structural rules characterize the activity of CCK in classic visceral assays such as pancreatic acinar cells or gut smooth muscle. First, removal of the sulfated group on the tyrosyl residue in the seventh position from the C-terminal markedly reduces or abolishes the activity of CCK. Second, the closely related gut peptide gastrin is much less active. Third, the amphibian decapeptide ceruletide mimics the activity of CCK and is usually more potent on a molar basis. These three rules have also been demonstrated to characterize the satiety effect of CCK (Gibbs, Young, & Smith, 1973a, 1973b).

Although evidence of this kind is not available for the other three peptides, two structural analogues of bombesin share its satiating effect. These are gastrin-releasing peptide, the mammalian form of bombesin, and litorin (the amphibian form; Gibbs, Kulkosky, & Smith, 1981).

In considering the site of action for behavioral effects of circulating peptides, investigators frequently invoke Sutton's Law (Smith, 1982). That law states that since the brain is the organ of behavior, the site of behavioral action of peptides must be the brain. But the lipophobic structure and size of these four peptides make it very unlikely that they penetrate the blood-brain barrier and, in fact, there is no evidence for such penetration at this time (Oldendorf, 1981). In considering alternative indirect paths, we proposed that the satiety effect was based on smooth muscle effects of these peptides that could be detected by receptors of afferent axons traveling in the vagus and sympathetic nerves (Smith, Jerome, Cushin, Eterno & Simansky, 1981a).

This proposal has been heuristic. Abdominal vagotomy abolishes or markedly reduces the satiety effect of CCK (Smith, et al., 1981a), glucagon (Geary & Smith, 1983), and somatostatin (Levine & Morley, 1982) (Table 4.1). The effect of selective vagotomies on the satiety effect of CCK and glucagon has yielded evidence for double dissociation: Hepatic vagotomy abolishes the effect of glucagon, but not that of CCK (Geary & Smith, 1983; Smith et al., 1981a). Gastric vagotomy abolishes the effect of CCK, but not that of glucagon (Smith et al., 1981a; Geary & Smith, 1983). The effect of such selective vagotomies on the satiating potency of somatostatin has not been reported.

The loss of satiating potency after abdominal vagotomy does not prove the visceral afferent hypothesis because the abdominal vagal branches are a mixture of afferent and efferent fibers. The fact that the effect of vagotomy on the satiety effect of these peptides is not reproduced by peripheral anticholinergic blockade suggests that the loss of efferent fibers is not critical, but this pharmacological evidence is indirect (Smith et al., 1981a; Geary & Smith, 1983).

Recently, we obtained more critical evidence for the visceral afferent hypothesis (Smith, Jerome, & Norgren, 1983). Using a surgical approach to the ventral surface of the hindbrain, we were able to cut the afferent rootlets or the efferent rootlets of the vagus separately under microscopic control because the afferent rootlets enter the lateral surface of the medulla dorsal to the site where the efferent rootlets emerge. Bilateral lesion of vagal abdominal afferent fibers abolished the satiety effect of CCK, but bilateral lesion of vagal abdominal efferent

TABLE 4.1
Characteristics of Four Gut Peptides

Peptide	Inhibition of Feeding	Inhibition of Sham Feeding	Satiety Effect Blocked by	Synergistic Interaction with	Satiety Effect in Human
Cholecystokinin	Yes	Yes	Gastric vagotomy	—Pregastric food —Gastric load —Exogenous BBS	Yes
Bombesin	Yes	Yes	Visceral disconnection	Exogenous CCK	Yes
Pancreatic glucagon	Yes	No	Hepatic vagotomy	——	Yes
Somatostatin	Yes	——	Subdiaphragmatic vagotomy	——	——

Note: Dashes indicate no study has been published.

fibers did not (Smith et al., 1983). This procedure has not been used to analyze the satiating effect of glucagon or somatostatin.

In contrast to the significant effect of abdominal vagotomy on CCK, glucagon, and somatostatin, abdominal vagotomy did not change the satiety effect of bombesin (Smith, Jerome & Gibbs, 1981b). Stuckey, Gibbs, and Smith (1985) have recently reported, however, that when vagotomy is combined with lesion of the other visceral afferents that have cell bodies in the dorsal root ganglions and project into the spinal cord, the inhibitory effect of bombesin on meal size is abolished. But in addition to its inhibitory effect on meal size, bombesin also prolongs the postprandial intermeal interval. This effect, however, is not changed by lesion of the vagal and spinal visceral afferents. This suggests that the intermeal interval effect of bombesin must be mediated by another humoral mechanism that has access to the brain and/or is mediated by an action of bombesin on one of the circumventricular organs.

In addition to these effects of gut peptides on eating behavior, Woods and Porte (1983) have proposed that pancreatic insulin is a humoral mechanism for the control of body weight. Their proposal is based on the strong positive correlation between the basal concentration of plasma insulin and the size of the fat mass in the body of adult animals and humans. (This correlation may not necessarily apply to periods of metabolic adaptation such as growth, reproduction, hibernation or migration.) The pivot of the proposal is that the critical parameter is the concentration of insulin in the cerebrospinal fluid (CSF), not in the blood. They argue that the fluctuations of insulin in the blood as a result of food ingestion and acute metabolic alterations are too large and too transient to serve as a useful signal for adiposity. But the kinetics of entry of insulin into the CSF across the blood-CSF barrier is such that the plasma fluctuations are smoothed out and, thus, could provide a cumulative signal.

The experimental evidence for this proposal is mounting. Infusions of small doses of insulin into the baboon and rat decrease body weight (Woods, Lotter, McKay, & Porte, 1979; Brief & Davis, 1981; Nicolaidis, 1981). This decrease in body weight is apparently accounted for by the decrease in food intake. Woods, Ikeda, Stein, Figlewicz, West, & Porte, (1983) recently extended this idea by demonstrating that increased CSF insulin increases the satiating potency of peripherally administered CCK. This is the first suggestion of how alterations in a peptide signal for the control of fat mass can make functional contact with a peptide signal for the control of meal size. And this is the first experimental demonstration that fulfills the axiom that changes in the "long-term" control system for body weight in the adult (fat mass) must be expressed through the mechanisms of the "short-term" control system for meal size and meal frequency.

THERAPEUTIC IMPLICATIONS

Although there is no compelling evidence that the satiating effect of the four peptides is a physiological effect of the endogenous hormones released during a meal, this does not prevent us from considering their possible therapeutic usefulness. Bombesin (Muurhainen, Kissileff, Thornton, & Pi-Sunyer, 1983), CCK (Kissileff, Pi-Sunyer, Thornton, & Smith, 1981; Pi-Sunyer, Kissileff, Thornton, & Smith, 1982; Stacher, Steinringer, Schmierer, Schneider, & Winklehner, 1982), and pancreatic glucagon (Schulman, Carleton, Whitney, & Whitehorn, 1957; Penick & Hinkle, 1961) decrease meal size in humans. Bombesin and CCK do not have significant side effects, but repetitive injections of glucagon produced glycosuria and other metabolic abnormalities (Penick & Hinkle, 1961).

The results with CCK are most interesting. CCK did not change the rate of eating; CCK simply made subjects stop sooner. When lean or obese subjects ate less after CCK, they reported that the meal was as satisfying as the larger control meals (Kissileff et al., 1981; Pi-Sunyer et al., 1982). Videotape observations of the behavioral sequence that characterized satiety under these experimental conditions also did not reveal any differences between control meals and those eaten after CCK. Finally, the food diaries of these subjects did not show that they snacked more or advanced the time of the next meal after a CCK treatment. These results converge to suggest that the subjects treated the infused CCK as if it were food. This is what the gut hormone hypothesis predicts. But these human results do not prove the hypothesis because it is likely that the dose of CCK infused produced levels of circulating CCK that were larger than the normal circulating concentration of endogenous CCK released during a meal. This is only a guess, however, because plasma levels have not been measured under these conditions.

Can the satiating effect of CCK, bombesin, and glucagon be exploited to reduce body weight? There are four major impediments to such a therapeutic application. First, they are inactive orally. Second, the safety of *repetitive* administration of CCK and bombesin is not known. The metabolic effects of glucagon after repetitive administration appear to prohibit glucagon's therapeutic application, but it is possible that a glucagon analogue can be found that has a preferential satiating effect and fewer metabolic effects. Third, the satiating potency of these peptides may be diminished by individual and cultural food preferences. Fourth, the satiating effect of the peptides may be diminished by the regulatory mechanisms initiated by body weight loss.

Recent experiments concerned with the effect of food preferences, such as sweet taste, are encouraging—CCK retained (Gosnell & Hsiao, 1984; Bernz, Smith, & Gibbs, 1983) or increased (Waldbillig and Bartness, 1982) its satiating potency across a wide range of sucrose concentrations. And most relevant to these issues is the preliminary report that CCK administered prior to each of three meals for three weeks produced significant weight loss in genetically obese (fa/fa) rats without obvious side effects (Campbell & Smith, 1983). Despite these promising results, much more work is necessary to evaluate these therapeutic issues.

SUMMARY

Gut peptides released in response to ingested food have replaced circulating nutrients as the leading candidates for humoral mechanisms controlling eating and body weight. Bombesin, cholecystokinin, glucagon, and somatostatin have been proposed for the termination of eating and the elicitation of postprandial satiety. Insulin in the cerebrospinal fluid has been proposed as the signal by which the brain monitors the adipose mass and controls body weight. The effects of these peptides on meal size and body weight have been obtained by administration of exogenous peptides. There is no critical evidence for the hypothesis that these effects are physiological functions of the endogenous hormones. Finally, it is too early to tell if these peptides form a new type of therapy for disorders of eating and body weight in humans.

ACKNOWLEDGMENTS

I wish to thank Mrs. Marion Jacobson and Mrs. Jane Magnetti for typing this manuscript. The writing of the manuscript and the work from my laboratory cited in it were supported by Research Scientist Award MH00149 and Research Award MH15455 from the National Institute of Mental Health.

REFERENCES

Bernz, J. A., Smith, G. P., & Gibbs, J. (1983). A comparison of the effectiveness of intraperitoneal injections of bombesin (BBS) and cholecystokinin (CCK-8) to reduce sham feeding of different sucrose solutions. *Proceedings of the Eastern Psychological Association*, p. 95.

Brief, D., & Davis, J. D. (1981). Chronic intraventricular insulin infusions reduce food intake and body weight in rats. *Society for Neuroscience Abstracts, 7*, 655.

Campbell, R. G., & Smith, G. P. (1983). CCK-8 decreases body weight in Zucker rats. *Society for Neuroscience Abstracts, 9*, 902.

Geary, N., & Smith, G. P. (1983). Selective hepatic vagotomy blocks pancreatic glucagon's satiety effect. *Physiology & Behavior, 31*, 391–394.

Gibbs, J., Kulkosky, P. J., & Smith, G. P. (1981). Effects of peripheral and central bombesin on feeding behavior of rats. *Peptides, 2* (Supplement 2), 179–183.

Gibbs, J., & Smith, G. P. (1984). The neuroendocrinology of postprandial satiety. In L. Martini and W. F. Ganong, (Eds.) *Frontiers in neuroendocrinology* (Vol. 8, pp.223–245). New York: Raven Press.

Gibbs, J., Young, R. C., & Smith, G. P. (1973a). Cholecystokinin decreases food intake in rats. *Journal of Comparative & Physiological Psychology, 84*, 488–495.

Gibbs, J., Young, R. C., & Smith, G. P. (1973b). Cholecystokinin elicits satiety in rats with open gastric fistulas. *Nature, 245*, 323–325.

Gosnell, B. A., & Hsiao, S. (1984). Effects of cholecystokinin on taste preference and sensitivity in rats. *Behavioral Neuroscience, 98*, 452–460.

Kissileff, H. R., Pi-Sunyer, F. X., Thornton, J., & Smith, G. P. (1981). Cholecystokinin-octapeptide (CCK-8) decreases food intake in man. *American Journal of Clinical Nutrition, 34*, 154–160.

Levine, A. S., & Morley, J. E. (1982). Peripherally administered somatostatin reduces feeding by a vagal mediated mechanism. *Pharmacology, Biochemistry & Behavior, 16*, 897–902.

Muurhainen, N. E., Kissileff, H. R., Thornton, J., & Pi-Sunyer, F. X. (1983). Bombesin: Another peptide that inhibits feeding in man. *Society for Neuroscience Abstracts, 9*, 182.

Nicolaidis, S. (1981). Lateral hypothalamic control of metabolic factors related to feeding. *Diabetologia, 20*, 426–434.

Oldendorf, W. H. (1981). Blood-brain barrier permeability to peptides: Pitfalls in measurement. *Peptides, 2* (Supplement 2), 109–111.

Penick, S. B., & Hinkle, L. E., Jr. (1961). Depression of food intake induced in healthy subjects by glucagon. *New England Journal of Medicine, 264*, 893–897.

Pi-Sunyer, X., Kissileff, H. R., Thornton, J., & Smith, G. P. (1982). C-terminal octapeptide of cholecystokinin decreases food intake in obese men. *Physiology & Behavior, 29*, 627–630.

Schulman, J. L., Carleton, J. L., Whitney, G., & Whitehorn, J. C. (1957). Effect of glucagon on food intake and body weight in man. *Journal of Applied Physiology, 11*, 419–421.

Smith, G. P. (1976). Humoral hypotheses for the control of food intake. In G. Bray (Ed.), *Obesity in perspective*, (Vol. 2, pp. 19–29). Bethesda, MD: National Institute of Health.

Smith, G. P. (1982). Satiety and the problem of motivation. In D. W. Pfaff (Ed.), *The physiological mechanisms of motivation* (pp. 133–143). New York: Springer-Verlag.

Smith, G. P. (1984). Gut hormone hypothesis of postprandial satiety. In A. J. Stunkard & E. Stellar (Eds.), *Eating and its disorders* (pp. 67–75). New York: Raven Press.

Smith, G. P., Jerome, C., Cushin, B. J., Eterno, R., & Simansky, K. J. (1981a). Abdominal vagotomy blocks the satiety effect of cholecystokinin in the rat. *Science, 213*, 1036–1037.

Smith, G. P., Jerome, C., & Gibbs, J. (1981b). Abdominal vagotomy does not block the satiety effect of bombesin in the rat. *Peptides 2*, 409–411.

Smith, G. P., Jerome, C., & Norgren R. (1983). Vagal afferent axons mediate the satiety effect of CCK-8. *Society for Neuroscience Abstracts, 9*, 902.

Stacher, G., Steinringer, H., Schmierer, G., Schneider, C., & Winklehner, S. (1982). Cholecystokinin octapeptide decreases intake of solid food in man. *Peptides, 3*, 133–136.

Stuckey, J. A., Gibbs, J., & Smith, G. P. (1985). Neural disconnection of gut from brain blocks bombesin-induced satiety. *Peptides, 6*, 1249–1252.

Waldbillig, R. J., & Bartness, T. J. (1982). The suppression of sucrose intake by cholecystokinin is scaled according to the magnitude of the orosensory control over feeding. *Physiology & Behavior, 28*, 591–595.

Woods, S. C., Ikeda, H., Stein, L. J., Figlewicz, D. P., West, D. B., & Porte, D., Jr. (1983). Intraventricular insulin enhances the satiating effect of cholecystokinin. *Eighth International Conference on the Physiology of Food and Fluid Intake.*

Woods, S. C., Lotter, E. C., McKay, L. D., & Porte, D., Jr. (1979). Chronic intracerebroventricular infusion of insulin reduces food intake and body weight of baboons. *Nature, 282*, 503–505.

Woods, S. C., & Porte, D. Jr. (1983). The role of insulin as a satiety factor in the central nervous system. In A. J. Szabo (Ed.), *Advances in metabolic disorders, CNS regulation of carbohydrate metabolism* (Vol. 10, pp. 457–468). New York: Academic Press.

5

FUNCTION OF OPIOID PEPTIDES IN THE BRAIN AND GUT

Allen S. Levine
VA Medical Center

John E. Morley
University of Minnesota

DISTRIBUTION OF OPIOID PEPTIDES

Since the original identification of the opioid receptor and the isolation of the two opioid pentapeptides, methionine- and leucine-enkephalin, it has become clear that there are a number of endogenous opioid peptides. Three major gene families of opioid peptides have been identified viz. the enkephalin family, the proopiomelanocortin family, and the dynorphin/α-neo-endorphin family (Figures 5.1–5.3). Each of the opioid peptides appears to have its own endogenous receptor (Table 5.1). At pharmacological doses, the opioid peptides generalize to the other receptors, partially explaining the multiplicity of effects attributed to each of the opioids.

With our current knowledge of the three families of opioid peptides, it has become somwhat simpler to attempt to classify the distribution of opioid peptides (see Cuello, 1983, for review). The peptides belonging to the proopiomelanocortin family are distributed in the pituitary (Bloom et al., 1977; Pelletier et al., 1977) and hypothalamus (Krieger, Liotta, & Brownstein, 1977; Pelletier, 1980; Watson, Akil, Richard, & Barchas, 1978a; Watson, Barchas, & Li, 1977; Watson, Richard, & Barchas, 1978b). Within the pituitary these peptides seem to be produced in the anterior lobe and intermediate lobe cells. In the brain, the main group of neurons containing POMC peptides is found in the arcuate nucleus of the medial basal hypothalamus (Bloom et al., 1978). The fibers originating in this area are distributed in the area of the anterior commissure and extend in the lateral septum and nucleus accumbens. These fibers terminate in various areas of the brainstem, particularly in the periaqueductal gray matter, the nucleus

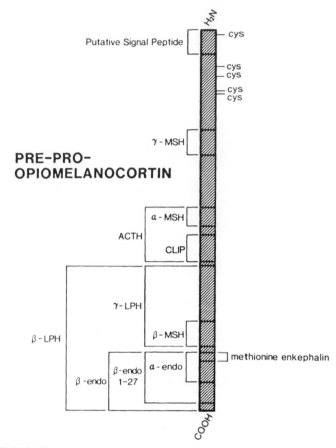

FIGURE 5.1   A schematic diagram of the structure of pre-pro-opiomelanocortin.

TABLE 5.1

Opioid Receptors and Their Putative Endogenous and Exogenous Agonists

Receptor	Endogenous Agonist	Exogenous Agonist
Mu	Morphiceptin	Morphine
Delta	Leucine-enkephalin	?
Iota	Methionine-enkephalin	?
Kappa	Dynorphin/α-neo-endorphin	Ketocyclazocine
		Tifluadom
		UH 50, 488
Sigma	?	Normetazocine
		? Phencyclidine
Epsilon	β-endorphin	?

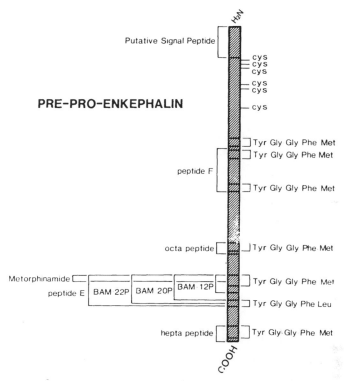

FIGURE 5.2   A schematic diagram of the structure of pre-pro-enkephalin.

tractus solitarii, and the locus ceruleus (Bloom et al., 1978). Immunoreactive fibers have also been identified in the olfactory cortex and hippocampus and in ventral portions of the brainstem.

Peptides from the pro-enkephalin family are widely distributed both periph-erally and centrally. Centrally, enkephalin-immunoreactive neurons are found in the telencephalon, the diencephalon, the brainstem, the cerebellum, and the spinal cord (see Cuello, 1983). Many of these neurons are distributed in areas related to pain and analgesia and tend to parallel the known distribution of opioid receptors (Hokfelt, Ljungdahl, Terenius, Elde, & Nilsson, 1977). The highest concentration of enkephalin fibers appears to be located in the globus pallidus and the caudate putamen. Also, many cell bodies are present in the nucleus caudate putamen, nucleus accumbens, and nucleus interstitialis of the stria ter-minalis (see Cuello, 1983). Enkephalins are also found peripherally in the adrenal medulla and the gastrointestinal tract (Elde, Hokfelt, Johansson, & Terenius, 1976; see Akil et al., 1984).

The distribution of the pro-dynorphin peptides is not well described (see Cuello, 1983; Khachaturian, Watson, Lewis, Coy, & Goldstein, 1982b; May-singer et al., 1982; Vincent, Hokfelt, Christensson, & Terenius, 1982; Watson,

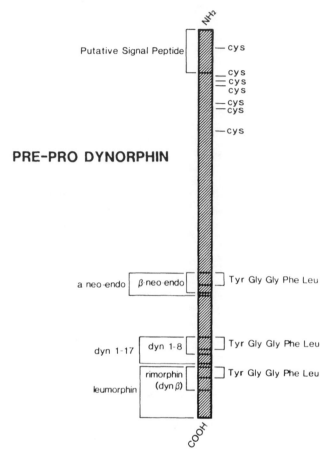

FIGURE 5.3   A schematic diagram of the structure of pre-pro-dynorphin.

Akil, Ghazarossian, & Goldstein, 1981; Watson et al., 1982a; Watson, Khachaturian, Akil, Coy, & Goldstein, 1982b). The posterior lobes of the pituitary
seem to be a major storage area for these peptides. Immunohistochemical studies
have indicated that leu-enkephalin, alpha-neo endorphin, and dynorphin are
associated with vasopressin in the nerve terminals of the posterior pituitary.
Prodynorphin is associated with vasopressin-producing cells in the magnocellular
nuclei of the hypothalamus. Pro-dynorphin peptides have also been identified in
regions of the gastrointestinal tract. The wide distribution of opioid peptides
suggests that these relatively small molecular weight compounds might have a
wide variety of effects on most organ systems. This review will emphasize only
a few of the regulatory roles the endogenous opioids play in maintaining homeostasis in many species. An overview of the major effects of the opioid peptides
is given in Table 5.2.

TABLE 5.2
Some of the Postulated Effects of Endogenous Opioids

1. Analgesia
2. Modulation of seizure activity
3. Modulation of body temperature
4. Respiratory depression
5. Production of hypotension (shock)
6. Modulation of sexual drive and reproductive function
7. Inhibition of gastrointestinal motility and secretions
8. Enhancement of feeding and drinking
9. Modulation of central reward mechanisms
10. Modulation of memory
11. Facilitation of social behavior
12. Modulation of hormonal release

THERMOREGULATION

The effects of opioids on body temperature are complex and depend on the species examined, the age of the animal, the injection site, the type of opioid, and the ambient temperature (see Martin, 1984, and Clark, 1981). Morphine given peripherally to a rat will result in hyperthermia when given in low doses and hypothermia in higher doses (Gunne, 1960; Herrman, 1942; Sloan, Brooks, Eisenman, & Martin, 1962). Several investigators have found that centrally injected morphine into rabbits results in hyperthermia (Banerjee, Burks, Feldberg, & Goodrich, 1968; Kandasamy & Williams, 1983); however, Lin and Su (1979) reported that injection of morphine into rats resulted in hypothermia. In mice, morphine will result in hypothermia when the mice are housed at 20°C, whereas at 30°C, these mice are hyperthermic following administration of morphine (Rosow, Miller, Pelikan, & Cochin, 1980). In cats (Cowan, Doxey, & Metcalf, 1976) and in rabbits (Kandasamy & Williams, 1983), central administration of kappa-receptor agonists induces hyperthermia. The sigma agonist SKF 10,047 will result in hyperthermia in the rabbit (Kandasamy & Williams, 1983), but not in the rat (Ward, Metcalf, & Rees, 1977). In rabbits, beta endorphin administered intrahypothalamically has been reported to result in both hypothermia and hyperthermia. Centrally administered DAMME results in hypothermia in chickens (Nistico, Rotiroti, Naccari, De Sarro, & Marino, 1980) and mice (Huidobro-Toro & Way, 1979), but hyperthermia in rabbits (Kandasamy & Williams, 1983). The thermic responsivity of rats to morphine is also dependent on age. The hyperthermic dose of morphine in rats results in the greatest increase in rectal temperature in senescent rats, whereas the hypothermic doses of morphine cause the greatest decrease in rectal temperature in young rats (McDougal, Marques, & Burks, 1980).

Many of the thermoregulatory effects of opioids can be reversed by naloxone. However, it should be noted that the hyperthermic response caused by morphine was not antagonized by naloxone. Naloxone has been shown to have moderate hypothermic and hyperthermic effects in rats (Cowan & McFarlane, 1976; Goldstein & Lowery, 1975). Thyrotropin-releasing hormone can reverse the hypothermic effects of naloxone and naloxone in combination with bombesin in a greater hypothermic response than when each of the latter agents are given individually (Morley, Levine, Oken, Grace, & Kneip, 1982e). Based on the above results, it is clear that our understanding of how opioids modulate temperature remains equivocal.

RESPIRATION

The depressive effects of opiates on respiration is well known, and clinically naloxone is commonly used to reverse respiratory suppression in patients. Narcotic analgesics appear to decrease the response of the "respiratory center" to carbon dioxide (Gen & Valdman, 1963). Opiates may selectively depress the CNS regulation of the respiratory center. Regions of the brainstem are sensitive to opiates, and also opioid receptors have been reported to be present in such areas of the brainstem involved in respiratory control (see McQueen, 1983). Also opioid-containing neurons have been shown to be present in the brainstem, particularly in the nucleus tractus solitarii (NTS) of the medulla oblongata. Iontophoretic application of morphine and met-enkephalin suppresses the peak discharge frequency of respiration units in the NTS of the brain of the cat (Denavit-Saubie, Champagnat, & Zieglgansberger, 1978). In general, it appears that opioids are probably involved in respiratory control during stressful conditions including pain, hypoxia, shock, and surgery, but not necessarily during normal respiratory regulation (McQueen, 1983).

As in other studies related to opioid regulation, many investigators have invoked the utilization of the opiate antagonist, naloxone, to evaluate the involvement of opioids in regulation of respiration. Naloxone increases ventilation in newborn rabbits, prevents ventilatory depression due to hyoxemia in newborn rabbits (Chernick, Madansky, & Lawson, 1980), and increases the ventilatory response following hypercapnia in fetal sheep (Moss & Scarpelli, 1979). Santiago, Remolina, Scoles, and Edelman (1981) demonstrated that intravenous naloxone (2 mg) did not affect respiratory sensitivity to carbon dioxide and restored flow-sensitive load compensation in adult humans with chronic obstructive pulmonary disease. Butland, Woodcock, Gross, and Geddes (1981), however, could not demonstrate any ventilatory effects in humans given 0.4–4 mg naloxone. As McQueen (1983) stressed, meaningful data from respiratory experiments in awake humans is extremely difficult to obtain. Naloxone has also been shown to increase phrenic nerve output in decerebrate and anesthetized cats (Lawson, Waldorp, & Eldridge, 1979) and to increase respiration in rats stimulated by carbon dioxide in both rats (Sowell, Bowen, & Carpenter, 1979) and humans (Santiago et al., 1981). Recently, it has been reported that tidal volume, respiratory frequency, and minute ventilation to steady-state hypoxia and steady-state hypercapnia in awake and unrestrained adult rats was unaffected by naloxone in doses up to 5.0 mg/kg (Steinbrook et al., 1984). Isom and Elshowihy (1982) did find a response of rats to naloxone as reflected by changes in tidal volume and frequency following inhalation of 10% CO_2 in O_2. Their time course did not conform to the known pharmacokinetics of naloxone. The increase in tidal volume occurred 5 minutes after injection and persisted for 25 minutes, whereas naloxone reached a peak serum concentration only after 15 minutes and has a half life of 40 minutes. Steinbrook et al. (1984) suggested that this response may also be due to the painful subcutaneous injection of 3.5 pH naloxone versus normal saline.

Zobrist, Allerton, and Isom (1981) studied the effects of intraventricular administration of D-ala[2]-methionine-enkephalinamide on respiration in unanesthetized rats. This long-acting met-enkephalin analogue resulted in a dose-dependent depression of respiratory rate and tidal volume which was naloxone-reversible. The enkephalin-induced respiratory depression was stimulated by an increased CO_2 concentration in the environment. Chronic administration of DAME resulted in tolerance to the respiratory depression, which paralleled the morphine response. The enkephalins seem to produce their respiratory effects by specific interactions with opioid receptors on the bulbar-pontine respiratory neurons present on the ventral surface of the brainstem.

OPIOID EFFECTS OF THE CARDIOVASCULAR SYSTEM

The neuroanatomical nuclei of the central nervous system known to play a role in autonomic regulation of the cardiovascular system contain opioid receptors and neurons which release opioids. For example, the nucleus of the solitary tract, a region known to be involved in regulating cardiac activity and feedback from the heart (Palkovits & Zaborszky, 1977), contains cell bodies for all three families of opioid peptides (Atweh & Kuhar, 1977). Many of these areas correspond with the areas containing high levels of norepinephrine. The anterior lobe of the pituitary releases beta-endorphin and ACTH, which results in the synthesis and release of adrenocorticoids which have potent pressor effects (see Akil et al., 1984). The posterior lobe of the pituitary contains the pre-pro-dynorphin family of peptides, which are co-released with vasopressin (Watson et al., 1982a). Administration of dynorphin and kappa agonists results in increased urination, which might affect blood pressure. Opioid peptides are also widely distributed in the peripheral autonomic nervous system. Enkephalins are present in sympathetic ganglia, in the vagus and the splanchnic nerves (Hokfelt, Johansson, Ljungdahl, Lundberg, & Schultzberg, 1980; Lundberg et al., 1979; Schultzberg et al., 1978a; Schultzberg et al., 1978b; Schultzberg et al., 1979). Recently,

Lang et al. (1983) have reported that distinct peaks for leu-enkephalin and met-enkephalin were found following extraction of guinea pig hearts which were then analyzed via HPLC. These peptides appear to be present in the noradrenergic nerve endings since chemical sympathectomy using 6-hydroxydopamine resulted in a 70% reduction in leu-enkephalin (Lang et al., 1983). Thus, the distribution of the opioid peptides suggests a possible role of these substances in cardiovascular physiology.

The known cardiovascular effects of opioid compounds are extremely complex and vary depending on the species examined, the type of preparation used, and the area into which the drug is injected. It has generally been reported that morphine has slight depressant effects on blood pressure and heart rate in humans (see Cohen & Coffman, 1979; Zelis, Mansour, Capone, & Mason, 1974). Systemic and pulmonary resistance decrease following administration of morphine, and this vascular resistance is reversed by naloxone (Cohen & Coffman, 1980). Clinically, this effect of morphine has been utilized to help treat patients with pulmonary edema even when they are anuric. Various opioid peptides have been reported to affect blood pressure, heart rate, and respiration following injection either peripherally or centrally. In the rat, intravenous administration of morphine results in a marked fall in heart rate and blood pressure which is short lived (Kiang & Wei, 1983). This effect is blocked by atropine or by transection of the vagus and therefore appears to be vagally mediated. Opioid receptors have been reported to be present on the vagal C-fiber afferents of the cardiopulmonary tree of rats (Fennessy & Rattray, 1971; Sapru, Willette, & Krieger, 1981; Wei, Lee, & Chang, 1980). Stimulation of such opioid receptors results in a vagal reflex with a fall in blood pressure, heart rate, and respiratory frequency.

The cardiovascular changes which occur following the injection of opioid peptides include depressor and pressor responses depending on the type of opioid agonist and the area of injection. It has been reported that pressor responses and tachycardia occur after lateral ventricular administration (Feldberg & Wei, 1978; Schaz et al., 1980; Yukimura, Stock, Stumpf, Unger, & Ganten, 1981), whereas hypotension and bradycardia occur after intracisternal injections or injections into the fourth ventricle (Bolme, Fuxe, Agnati, Bradley, & Smythies, 1978; Laubie, Schmitt, Vincent, & Remond, 1977). Based on such evidence, it has been suggested that forebrain delta receptors mediate the cardioexcitatory effects, and mu receptors in the brainstem mediate cardiodepressor effects (Feuerstein & Faden, 1982). The delta agonist D-ala^2-D-leu^5-enkephalin (DADLE) resulted in a dose-dependent depression of blood pressure, and the depressor effects of DADLE were reversed by low doses of naloxone (Hassen, Feuerstein, & Faden, 1982). The mu-agonist morphiceptin caused tachycardia which could be reversed by naloxone. These substances were administered to cats in the area of the nucleus of the tractus solitarius. Although the delta agonists were more effective than mu agonists in modifying cardiovascular function, the nucleus of tractus solitarius, a hindbrain region known to mediate cardiovascular activity, Hassen et al. (1982) found a predominance of mu-receptor sites in the nucleus of the solitary tract.

In the latter studies, anesthetized animals were utilized. Since anesthesia is known to interfere with the effects of opioids, Pfeiffer, Feuerstein, Zerbe, Faden, and Kopin, (1983) evaluated the effect of opioids in awake rats. The mu agonist (D-ala^2,MePhe^4,Gly^5-ol) enkephalin resulted in a prolonged increase in blood pressure, a decrease followed by an increase in heart rate. The selective mu antagonist, β-funaltrexamine (β-FNA) antagonized this effect. In contrast, a selective delta agonist had no effect on cardiovascular function. A kappa opioid agonist caused a pressor response which was not reversed by β-FNA. Feuerstein and Faden (1982) injected D-ala^2,D-leu^5-enkephalin and DAGO into anesthetized rats (anterior hypothalamic injections) and demonstrated tachycardia and hypertension. At higher doses, bradycardia also occurred while the pressor response was retained. The mu agonists were about 10 times more active than the delta compound. Pfeiffer et al. (1983) also found that with the increased heart rate and blood pressure observed with low doses of enkephalin were elevations of plasma norepinephrine and epinephrine, which indicates a stimulation of the sympathoadrenomedullary pathways. At high doses, an increased vagal outflow seemed to counteract the sympathetic activation.

A large amount of evidence has accumulated suggesting that endogenous opioids are involved in various types of shock, including endotoxic, hemorrhagic, and traumatic shock (see Holaday, 1984). Noting the similarities of opiate overdose effects to those of circulatory shock (depressed awareness, changes in endocrine function, decreased pain perception, and alterations in thermoregulation), Holaday and Faden (1978) demonstrated that naloxone antagonized the hypotensive effects of endotoxin-induced shock in rats. These investigators found that the therapeutic responses to naloxone generalized across species. The effect of naloxone was also shown to be stereospecific, providing evidence that this effect was dependent on opioid receptors. Reynolds et al. (1980) showed that naloxone's effects on shock occur due to an improvement in contractility rather than by changing heart rate or vascular resistance. Not only does naloxone reverse endotoxic shock in a number of species, it also increases circulating levels of β-endorphin and β-lipotropin. Besides affecting the cardiovascular system, naloxone also lowers body temperature and circulating white blood cells and platelets in the endotoxic model in the mouse (Wright & Weller, 1980). The action of naloxone on shock appears to be mediated within the brain and to involve the sympathomedullary system. The iodomethylate analogue of naloxone does not cross the blood-brain barrier and was reported to have no effect of endotoxic hypotension in rats. Adrenalectomy and adrenal demedullation enhances endotoxic shock susceptibility, and these surgical procedures block the pressor response to naloxone (Holaday, D'Amato, Ruvio, & Faden, 1982).

Other forms of shock are also sensitive to the actions of naloxone. Hemorrhagic and spinal shock also appear to be mediated via a central mechanism;

however, spinal shock appears to involve opiate receptors at central parasympathetic centers (see Holaday, 1984). Vargish et al. (1980) have indicated that burn shock in guinea pigs is reversed by naloxone. Recently, Rubin and colleagues (Rubin, Blaschke, & Guilleminault, 1981) have indicated that the blood pressure drop which occurs during non-rapid eye movement in humans does not occur following administration of naloxone. Hypotension induced by propranolol, clonidine, and alpha methyl dopa is reversed by administration of naloxone (see Ramirez-Gonzalez, Farsang, Tchakarov, & Kunos, 1982).

Holaday has suggested that delta agonists are involved in the control of shock (see Holaday, 1984). Whereas DADLE produced a pattern resembling shock after injection into the third ventricle, morphine had only minimal effects. When injected into the fourth ventricle, morphine produced bradycardia, but nothing resembling circulatory shock. Also, specific mu antagonists (β-FNA and naloxazone) did not reverse endotoxic shock hypotension (Holaday, Pasternak, D'Amato, Ruvio, & Faden, 1983; D'Amato & Holaday, 1984), whereas specific delta agonists (ICI M154,129) reversed endotoxic shock (D'Amato & Holaday, 1984; Holaday et al., 1983). However, the clinical use of opioid antagonists in shock remains problematic. Although naloxone clearly increases blood pressure in a variety of conditions, in humans there is little evidence that it improves survival. For example, in the case of hypotension and myocardial infarction, heightened awareness of pain could result in extension of the infarct. The ethical considerations of increasing awareness and pain in the critically ill patient while not improving survival suggest that use of naloxone in the clinical situation should await proof of its efficacy at improving survival in double-blind trials.

OPIOID EFFECTS ON IMMUNE FUNCTION

One of the most fascinating functions of the endogenous opiates is their putative involvement in immune function. In developing neural systems, opioids have been shown to alter both cell function and growth.

Opioid receptors are present on various cells which are part of the immune system, including granulocytes, monocytes, and lymphocytes (Lopkor, Abood, Hass, & Lionetti, 1980; Wybran, Appelboom, Famaey, & Gavaerts, 1979). Morphine and opioid peptides affect the reactivity of T cells to mitogenic stimulation, and they alter the number of T cells which participate in active rosettes (Plotnikoff & Miller, 1983; Wybran et al., 1979). Morphine decreased the percentage of active and total T-rosette-forming cells, whereas met-enkephalin increased the percentage of active T rosettes. These effects are naloxone reversible. There also appear to be some non-opioid effects of β-endorphin on immune function. Gilman, Schwartz, Milner, Bloom, and Feldman (1982) have reported that β-endorphin enhanced the proliferative response of spleen cells to the T-cell mitogens concanavilin A and phytohemagglutinin. Alpha-endorphin and D-Ala^2, met^5-enkephalin failed to produce the latter effect. In addition, naloxone failed to reverse the potentiating effect of β-endorphin. β-endorphin has been reported to bind specifically to transformed lymphocytes. This binding was not blocked by enkephalins or opiates, suggesting that there is a specific, non-opioid type of binding of β-endorphin. This compound may be a circulating hormone with peripheral effects which are non-opioid.

A subpopulation of lymphocytes referred to as natural killer cells are involved in the destruction of some tumor cells (Herberman & Ortaldo, 1981). Natural killer cell activity is reduced following exposure to a variety of stressors, including starvation and surgery (Herberman & Holden, 1978; Saxena, Saxena, & Adler, 1980). Shavit, Lewis, Terman, Gale, and Liebeskind (1984) recently reported that splenic natural killer cell activity is suppressed by an opioid form of inescapable foot shock and that this suppression was blocked by naltrexone. High doses of morphine also suppressed natural killer activity. This opioid stress paradigm reduces the response of T lymphocytes to mitogenic stimulation. Rats subjected to opioid-related foot shock before tumor implantation display a reduced survival time and percent survival. In contrast to the work of Shavit et al. (1984), several studies have shown that natural killer cell activity is increased by opioids, and this group of peptides has been reported by numerous investigators to stimulate the immune system (Kay, Allen, & Morley, 1984; Mathews, Froelich, Sibbitt, & Bankhurst, 1983). Natural killer cell activity was enhanced by β-endorphin and methionine enkephalin, whereas leucine enkephalin, alpha-endorphin, and morphine had no effect on cytotoxicity. The enhanced activity was inhibited by naloxone. Of particular interest was the finding that interferon-stimulated NK activity could be reversed by naloxone (Kay et al., 1984).

Tumor growth and survival time in mice with transplanted neuroblastoma is inhibited by chronic administration of heroin (Zagon & McLaughlin, 1981). The effects of heroin on tumor growth in these studies is reversed by the administration of naloxone. However, it has been shown that naloxone has antitumor effects of its own. Zagon and McLaughlin (1983) have recently reported that naltrexone markedly alters the course of murine neuroblastoma. Depending on the dose of naltrexone used, this opiate antagonist has both stimulatory and inhibitory effects on the growth of S20Y neuroblastoma in A/Jax mice. A low dose of naltrexone (.1 mg/kg) resulted in decreased tumor incidence, a delay in time of tumor appearance, and an increase in survival time. In contrast, 10 mg/kg naltrexone resulted in 100% tumor incidence, a reduction in the time before tumor appearance and a moderate decrease in survival time. Zagon and McLaughlin (1983) suggest that low naltrexone doses may result in more binding sites on the neuroblastoma cells producing a supersensitivity to basal concentrations of opioids. It is known that chronic treatment with narcotic antagonists increases the number of opioid receptor sites present and also causes opioid supersensitivity (Lahti & Collins, 1978). It has also been reported that leucine-enkephalin-treated mice demonstrated a significant increase in survival following inoculation with L1210 murine leukemia cells (Plotnikoff & Miller, 1983). At relatively high doses of methionine enkephalin (30 mg/kg), similar effects were found. Methionine and leucine enkephalin also were found to stimulate mouse lymphocyte blastogenesis following stimulation of phytohemagglutinin (PHA). Gilman et al. (1982) have shown stimulation of T-cell proliferation using β-endorphin. Dopamine also stimulated T cells, and methionine-enkephalin potentiates dopamine effects (Plotnikoff et al., 1976).

Blalock and Smith (1980) reported that human leukocyte interferon demonstrated structural and biological relatedness to ACTH and endorphins. Subsequently, these investigators reported that human leukocyte interferon binds to opioid receptors in vitro (Blalock & Smith, 1981). Interferon has been reported to alter discharge frequency in neurons of cortical explants (Calvet & Gresser, 1979). Dafny (1983) recently reported that interferon treatment one hour prior to naloxone injection in morphine-dependent animals markedly reduced abstinence behavior. Dafny (1983) also showed that when a single injection of interferon was given prior to chronic morphine treatment, a reduction in opiate addiction occurred. These data suggest that opioids may affect immunosuppression by their interrelationship with interferon. It should be noted, however, that Epstein, Rose, McManus, and Li (1982) failed to demonstrate any structural homology of natural and recombinant human leukocyte interferon (IFN-alpha) with either ACTH or β-endorphin.

SEXUAL AND REPRODUCTIVE FUNCTION

The endogenous opioids are involved in various aspects of sexual function ranging from sexual behavior to regulation of anterior pituitary gonadotropins. Opioids are well known to modulate a variety of other hormonal activities as well as sex hormones (see Morley, 1981, 1983). During sexual behavior, there is a concurrent activation of reward and analgesia (Kinsey, Pomeroy, Martin, & Gebhard, 1973; Whalen, 1961), two properties of endogenous opiates. Szechtman, Simantov, and Hershkowitz (1981) reported that there is reduced responsiveness to nociceptive stimuli during mating in rats, that opioid blockage with naloxone alters copulatory performance, and that prolonged copulation reduces opioid levels in the midbrain. Several investigators have reported that naloxone shortens the time to reach ejaculation (Myers & Baum, 1979; Quarantotti, Paglietti, Bonanni, Petta, & Gessa, 1979), whereas Szechtman et al. (1981) found an increase in the post-ejaculatory interval. In hamsters, plasma β-endorphin levels increase following repetitive ejaculations (Murphy, Bowie, & Pert, 1979). Opioids might also be involved in sexual drive. Sexual function is impaired in heroin addicts (Crowley & Simpson, 1978; Hollister, 1975), and during withdrawal premature ejaculation and spontaneous erections have been reported to occur in men (Parr, 1976). β-endorphin and D-ala^2-met-enkephalinamide when administered centrally will reduce the mounting behavior in male rats, and naloxone reverses this effect (Gessa, Paglietti, & Quarantotti, 1979; Meyerson & Terenius, 1977). Male Sprague-Dawley rats which show a reduced libido will increase mounting behavior and ejaculation following the injection of naloxone (4 mg/kg). Conflicting reports have been published indicating that naloxone either has no effect on sexual behavior in humans (Brady & Bianco, 1980) or that it will produce spontaneous penile erections and reduce the time from erection to ejaculation (Goldstein & Hansteen, 1977; Mendelson, Ellingboe, Keuhnle, & Mello, 1979). Henry (1982), in a recent review, has discussed the possible involvement of opioids in sadomasochistic behavior related to sexual activity. He suggests that pain, such as that inflicted in masochism, might increase opioid levels and result in heightened orgasm. Sadism, such as that which occurs when rats kill mice, is accompanied by analgesia, perhaps due to increased levels of opioids.

Opioids decrease the release of LH without affecting FSH release in the rat (Bruni, Van Vugt, Marshall, & Meites, 1977). Naloxone not only reverses such opioid agonist effects (Bruni et al., 1977; Rivier, Vale, Ling, Brown, & Guillemin, 1977; Shaar, Frederickson, Dininger, & Jackson, 1977) but also itself results in an elevation of LH and FSH in rats (Bruni et al., 1977). In the rat, morphine blocks ovulation, and naloxone reverses this antiovulatory effect of morphine (Barraclough & Sawyer, 1955; Packman & Rothchild, 1976). Opioids also suppress the preovulatory LH surge in proestrous rats, and naloxone antagonizes this effect. During proestrous, high doses of morphine suppress pituitary FSH secretion, which is also reversed by naloxone (Ieiri, Chen, Campbell, & Meites, 1980). Most investigators have assumed that the suppression of LH and FSH levels in the proestrous rat which occurs after opioid administration is due to the inhibition of GnRH release into pituitary portal blood. Ching (1983) has recently reported that rats treated with high-dose morphine (40 mg/kg) display reduced levels of GnRH by 50% in portal plasma. The naloxone reversal of opioid effects on LH and FSH occurred as a result of the restoration of GnRH secretion to levels which occur during proestrous. This is in agreement with the report that in the absence of GnRH, naloxone did not release LH from rat hemipituitary explants (Cicero, Schainker, & Meyer, 1979). However, Ching (1983) found that low doses of morphine (5–8 mg/kg) which decreased LH did so without affecting GnRH concentration.

A host of studies have evaluated the role of opioids on gonadotropins in humans (see Morley, 1983). In general, it appears that both LH and FSH activity are inhibited by opioid agents (Zanoboni, Zecca, Zanussi, & Zanoboni-Muciaccia, 1981). Naloxone causes an increase in LH levels and an increase in the number of LH pulses (Delitala et al., 1981; Ellingboe, Veldhuis, Mendelson, Kuehnle, & Mello, 1982; Grossman, et al., 1982; Morley et al., 1980a; Moult, Grossman,

Evans, Rees, & Besser, 1981; Ropert, Quigley, & Yen, 1981). In the early follicular phase of the menstrual cycle, naloxone has minimal effects on LH secretion, whereas in the late follicular phase, a marked effect occurs (Blankstein, Reyes, Winter, & Faiman, 1981; Quigley & Yen, 1980). The maximum effect of naloxone occurs during the midluteal phase (Quigley & Yen, 1980). Opioid agonists generally decrease LH and FSH secretion (see Tables I and II in Morley, 1983). In one study following the infusion of β-endorphin, an early rise in LH occurred at 15 minutes in women but not in men (Reid & Yen, 1981). The inhibitory opioid control of LH and FSH appears to occur at the hypothalamic level on the release of GnRH. Neither naloxone nor D-ala^{2}MetPhe^4,Met-(0)5-ol (DAMME) alter gonadotropin release following administration of GnRH. Also, intermittent hypothalamic release of GnRH seems to regulate the frequency modulation of pituitary gonadotropin pulsatile secretion (Santen & Ruby, 1979).

Prolactin is associated with amenorrhea, galactorrhea, and infertility in females and impotence in males. In mature male rats it has been reported that naloxone has a suppressive effect on basal prolactin (PRL) levels for a 30-minute period after injection. Lower doses of naloxone (0.1–0.4 mg/kg) seem to be more effective than higher doses (0.4–2.0 mg/kg) in reducing basal PRL secretion in rats (Ieiri et al., 1980). Muraki, Tokunaga, and Makino (1977) did not observe any effect of naloxone on PRL levels in proestrous rats, whereas Ieiri et al. (1980) found that a single injection of naloxone (0.2 mg/kg) at 1400 h completely inhibited the surge of PRL, and this effect was reversed by simultaneous administration of morphine (10 mg/kg). In human males, prolactin secretion is unaffected by naloxone administration (Blankstein, Reyes, Winter, & Faiman, 1980; Delitala, Devilla, & Di Biaso, 1980; Mayer, Wessel, & Kobberling, 1980; Volavka et al., 1980), and in women under certain circumstances small changes in prolactin have been noted (Cetel, Quigley, & Yen, 1983; Steardo et al., 1981). In contrast, many opioid agonists produce a naloxone-reversible increase in prolactin secretion.

Reid (1983), in a letter to *Lancet*, recently proposed that endogenous opioid activity might be directly involved in premenstrual syndrome (PMS). He suggested that several of the effects observed in PMS are common in opiate withdrawal. A sharp fall in opioid levels before menstruation could result in tension, anxiety, irritability, and even psychotic behavior. Such a fall in opioid levels has been reported to occur at the onset of menstruation. The level of β-endorphin arriving in the pituitary stalk peaks during the luteal phase. Such an increase in opioid activity could result in the increased desire to eat and also depression and fatigue by affecting catecholamine neurons. Although some of these thoughts appear to be wild speculation, the involvement of opioids in the regulation of gonadotropins suggests that PMS could involve endogenous opioid peptides.

Several reports have suggested that endogenous opioids could act as natural analgesics during pregnancy, labor, and parturition. In rats, a gradual rise in the threshold to noxious stimuli occurs between 16 to 4 days prior to parturition, with an abrupt rise 1 to 2 days before parturition. This antinociceptive effect of pregnancy is abolished by administration of naltrexone (Gintzler, 1980). In pregnant women, β-endorphin levels have been shown to increase progressively throughout pregnancy with a peak occurring at delivery (Genazzani, Facchinetti, & Parrini, 1981; Goland, Wardlaw, Stark, & Frantz, 1981). Opioid peptides have also been shown to be present in the placenta and appear to be synthesized de novo by this tissue (Tan & Yu, 1981). The role of these peptides in the placenta are not known, however they may affect maternal or fetal systems and have paracrine effects.

OPIOID EFFECTS ON THE GASTROINTESTINAL TRACT

The distribution of opioids in the GI tract suggests that these substances play a role in various aspects of the physiology of the GI tract. Pre-pro-enkephalin and pre-pro-dynorphin have been identified in neurons of the submucosal and myenteric plexuses of the gut, whereas the beta-endorphin precursor is probably not present in the gut (Schultzberg et al., 1980). Enkephalins are present in the cell bodies and nerve endings supplying the gastric antral mucosa and antral muscle layers, as well as in the gastric mucosal endocrine cells. The enkephalin-containing fibers in the guinea pig ileum seem to be polarized from the oral to the anal direction (Furness, Costa, & Miller, 1983). The exact distribution of dynorphin-like peptides in the GI tract is not presently known.

Opioids have been used for centuries as anti-diarrheal compounds, and it is now well known that opiate-like compounds have major effects on gut motility. Opioids also affect intestinal fluid and electrolyte transport (Awouters, Niemegeers, & Janssen, 1983) and affect the secretion of gastric acid (Morley et al., 1982d). These effects are dependent on the specific receptor agonist used and the type of preparation used, as well as the species of animal examined. For example, in the pig, opioids do not affect the lower esophageal sphincter, whereas in the opossum, at least five opiate receptor types have been identified (Rattan & Goyal, 1983). The putative physiological effects of opioids on the gastrointestinal tract are listed in Table 5.3.

Opioids and Gut Motility

Morphine and opioid-like peptides have been reported by many investigators to decrease the propulsive motility of the intestine (Awouters et al., 1983; Daniel, 1982; Daniel et al., 1959). Wood (1980) demonstrated that morphine suppresses the excitability of myenteric ganglion neurons on inhibition of transmitter release,

TABLE 5.3
Effects of Opioids on the Gastrointestinal Tract

1. *Gut Motility*
   —decreases propulsive intestinal motility
   —inhibits relaxation of lower esophageal sphincter
   —inhibits gastric emptying
2. *Intenstinal Fluid and Electrolyte Transport*
   —decreases chloride ion secretion
   —increases fluid and intestinal ion absorption
3. *Gastric Acid Secretion*
   —stimulation of acid secretion in humans
   —decreases acid secretion after central administration in rats

suggesting that the effect of morphine on motility is mediated by the enteric nervous system. Also, isolated cells prepared from jejunal or gastric circular muscle from the guinea pig contract in response to morphine, the enkephalins, and dynorphin (Bitar & Makhlouf, 1983). Thus, opiates may have direct effects on enteric nerves, as well as effects on intestinal smooth muscle.

The gastrocolonic response is due to an increase in distal colonic motor activity which occurs after eating. In humans this effect has been reported to involve efferent cholinergic neurons and opioid receptors in the GI tract (Sun, Snape, Cohen, & Renny, 1982). In humans, the long-acting synthetic enkephalin analogue DAMME inhibits the relaxation of the lower esophageal sphincter while having no effect on any other indices of esophageal motility (Howard, Belsheim, & Sullivan, 1982). In the opossum, intra-arterial injections of met-enkephalin and leu-enkephalin increase lower esophageal sphincter pressure, while injection of alpha-endorphin and beta-endorphin decrease pressure (Rattan & Goyal, 1980).

Other studies have indicated the direct involvement of the central nervous system in gastrointestinal motor function. Intracerebroventricular (i.c.v.) administration of morphine blocks intestinal transit more potently than does systemic administration (Galligan & Burks, 1983). Quarternary naloxone, which does not cross the blood-brain barrier, does not block the central effects of morphine on transit time (Schulz, Wuster, & Herz, 1979). In sheep, intravenous injections of small doses of E. coli endotoxin inhibited phasic contractions of the forestomach and altered the myoelectrical activity of the antrum, duodenal bulb, and jejunum. Prior administration of naloxone into the ventricle, but not when given intravenously, antagonized the endotoxin-induced alteration of the GI myoelectrical activity (Duranton & Bueno, 1984). This suggests an involvement of a central opioid mechanism for such effects of endotoxin. Margolin and associates have suggested that central administration of morphine releases an unidentified circulating neurohumoral substance which could alter GI motility (Margolin, 1963; Margolin & Plekss, 1965). A new opioid peptide, derived from the skin of South American amphibians, namely dermorphin, has been shown to delay gastric emptying (Broccardo, Improta, Nargi, & Melchiorri, 1982). The dose of i.c.v. dermorphin, which delays gastric emptying by 50%, is 1,000 times lower than the active subcutaneous dose.

More recently, Porreca and Burks (1983) have demonstrated a role for the spinal cord as a site for some of the opioid effects on GI transit in the mouse. Opioid receptors are present in the dorsal horn of the spinal cord (Atweh & Kuhar, 1977; Hokfelt et al., 1977; Pert, Kuhar, & Snyder, 1975). Also, the stomach and small bowel are innervated through the celiac ganglion originating from the thoracic region of the spinal cord (Roman & Gonella, 1981). Transection of the spinal cord failed to antagonize the anti-transit effects of intrathecally administered morphine, suggesting a direct effect within the spinal cord.

Aside from the location of action of opioids on gastrointestinal motility, the type of opiate agonist used also appears to be an important consideration. For example, both morphine and ketocyclazocine antagonized transit of the opaque marker through the small intestines of mice and rats when administered subcutaneously. Morphine was also effective when given intraventricularly, whereas ketocyclazocine was not (Porreca & Burks, 1983). This suggests that anatomically distinct distributions of receptors for kappa agonists may exist in the rat and the mouse, with these receptors being distant from the lateral cerebral ventricles. In another study, it has been reported that intrathecal administration of kappa agonists (ketocyclazocine or dynorphin) failed to affect transit time (Porreca, Filla, & Burks, 1983). Intrathecal administration of both mu (morphine) and delta agonists (DADLE, DSLET, DPLCE) in mice consistently inhibited gastrointestinal transit (Porreca & Burks, 1983). To further complicate the situation, DADLE and DSLET inhibited GI transit after i.c.v. administration, whereas DPLCE was ineffective (Porreca & Burks, 1983). The variation in distribution of different opioid peptides and the variable effects in different species indicates the importance of noting the tissue and species being evaluated. Contraction of the dog intestine is least affected by dynorphin (Burks, Hirning, Galligan, & Davis, 1982), whereas in the guinea pig, contraction of the intestine is highly sensitive to dynorphin (Goldstein, Tachibana, Lowney, Hunkapiller, & Hood, 1979).

In humans, administration of an enkephalin analogue delays gastric emptying (Sullivan, Lamki, & Corcoran, 1981). Since stressful stimuli modify gastroduodenal activity and release β-endorphin into the peripheral circulation (Stanghellini, Malagelada, Zinsmeister, Go, & Kao, 1983), Stanghellini and colleagues (Stanghellini, Malagelada, Zinsmeister, Go, & Kao, 1984) postulated that opioids are involved in the mediation of the disruptive effects induced by centrally acting stressful stimuli on postprandial motor activity in the proximal human gut. They found that opioid blockade with naloxone inhibited antral feeding. Thus their hypothesis was confirmed.

Opioids: Effects on Intestinal Fluid and Electrolyte Transport

Opiates not only act as antidiarrheal drugs by slowing motility, they also have major effects on electrolyte transport and intestinal fluid. Antisecretory effects of opiates have been demonstrated in isolated intestinal loops and in segments of intestinal mucosa in vitro (see Miller & Brown, 1984). For example, morphine increases the absorption of fluids and sodium and chloride ions from the dog intestine in situ and from isolated intestinal loops in the rat (Awouters et al., 1983). Some of the effects of opiates on electrolyte transport appear to be independent of blood flow (Powell, 1981). Rather, opioids reduce the short-circuit current and potential difference across isolated segments of ileal mucosa from guinea pigs and rabbits. This results in an inhibition of active chloride secretion. The opioid receptors which effect intestinal secretion appear to be localized in the intestinal mucosa. The mucosa contains a predominance of delta-type receptors, whereas the longitudinal muscle-myenteric plexus contains mu or kappa receptors (see Miller & Brown, 1984). This is concordant with the finding that delta agonists are more effective antisecretory agents than other opioid agonists. Brown and Miller (1983) have reported that intraventricular injection of the stable enkephalin, D-ala^2-met^5-enkephalinamide (DAMA), dose dependently increased basal fluid absorption in the medial ileum and decreased jejunal and proximal ileal fluid secretion following pretreatment with cholera toxin. This antisecretory effect of DAMA was blocked by subcutaneous administration of naltrexone, suggesting a specific opiate effect. Pretreatment of animals with phentolamine (an alpha-adrenergic antagonist) and guanethidine (a catecholamine-depleting agent) blocks the antisecretory effects of enkephalins, suggesting a sympathetic component to the antisecretory effect of opiates. Brown and Miller (1984) have recently suggested that the antisecretory effects of opiates are, in part, mediated by the CNS, perhaps by an increased activity in sympathetic nerve fibers innervating the upper small intestine. A recent study by Beubler and colleagues (Beubler, Bukhave, & Rask-Madsen, 1984) have suggested that the diarrhea associated with morphine withdrawal is mediated by local release of both prostaglandin and serotonin in the colon.

Opioid Effects on Gastric Acid Secretion

Brodie, Lottie, and Bauer demonstrated in 1970 that intraventricular administration of morphine decreased gastric volume and acidity in pylorus-ligated rats. Central administration of beta-endorphin also has been reported to decrease gastric acid secretion and appears to be about 30 times more potent than morphine when compared on a molar basis (Roze, Dubrasquet, Chariot, & Valle, 1980). A long-acting methionine-enkephalin analogue (D-ala^2-met-enkephalinamide), beta-endorphin, and dynorphin all have been reported to decrease TRH-induced gastric acid secretion in the rat (Morley, Levine, & Silvis, 1981b), and the methionine-enkephalin analogue reduced insulin-induced gastric acid secretion (Morley et al., 1981b). Central administration of D-ala^2-met-enkephalinamide is cytoprotective against cold-restraint-induced stress ulcers, apparently by decreasing gastric acid secretion (Morley, Levine, & Silvis, 1982e). In contrast, peripheral administration of the long-acting met-enkephalin analogue enhances stress ulcer formation, perhaps by decreasing blood flow to the gastric mucosa. Naltrexone, however, had a cytoprotective effect against stress-induced ulceration. This effect was independent of gastric acid secretion and appeared to involve an increase in mucosal blood flow.

In humans, it has been demonstrated that met-enkephalin stimulates gastric acid secretion without affecting serum gastrin levels, while naloxone inhibits basal and meal-stimulated acid secretion without lowering food-stimulated serum gastrin concentrations (Olsen, Kirkegaard, Petersen, & Christiansen, 1982; Olsen, Kirkegaard, Petersen, Lendorf, & Christiansen, 1981). Naloxone (40 µg/kg/h) was reported to decrease gastric acid secretion stimulated by sham feeding, intravenous pentagastrin, and intravenous histamine (Feldman & Cowley, 1982). However, Olsen et al. (1982) reported that although naloxone (10 µg/kg/h) suppressed met-enkephalin-stimulated acid secretion, naloxone had no effect on pentagastrin-stimulated acid secretion. Feldman, Walsh, and Taylor (1980) have reported that both naloxone and morphine reduced meal-stimulated acid secretion in humans. In dogs, met-enkephalin also enhanced pentagastrin- and histamine-stimulated acid secretion (Konturek, Pawlik, Walus, Coy, & Schally, 1978; Konturek et al., 1980). In contrast to humans and dogs, met-enkephalin has a potent inhibitory effect on hydrogen ion output in rhesus monkeys (Shea-Donohue, Adams, Arnold, & Dubois, 1983). The confusion in the literature concerning the effects of opioids on gastric acid secretion could be due to species diversity. It should also be noted that opioids affect a variety of systems which influence gastric acid secretion. For example, opiates reduce acetylcholine release, which would result in a suppression of acid secretion (Konishi, Tsunoo, & Osaka, 1981). In contrast, opiates increase gastric blood flow (Konturek et al., 1978) and stimulate the release of gastrin (Yamaguchi, Fuke, & Tusjta, 1978), both of which would increase acid output.

OPIOIDS AND FEEDING

A variety of opioid agonists have been reported to induce feeding, and blockade of the opioid receptor has been demonstrated to depress food intake. In 1929, Flowers, Dunham, and Barbour found that morphine increased water intake secondary to diuresis in rats. Martin, Wikler, Eades, and Pescor (1963) were the first to report that morphine could enhance food intake in rats. Grandison and Guidotti (1977) showed that the injection of beta-endorphin into the ventromedial hypothalamus increased feeding in rats.

The opioid antagonists, naloxone and naltrexone, are known to suppress food intake in many species under a variety of conditions. These conditions include spontaneous (Jaloweic, Panksepp, Zolovick, Najam, & Herman, 1981), starvation induced (Brands, Thornhill, Hirst, & Gowdey, 1979), norepinephrine induced (Morley, Levine, Murray, & Kneip, 1982b), muscimol induced (Morley, Levine, & Kneip, 1981a), 2-deoxyglucose induced (Lowy, Maickel, & Yim, 1980), and stress-induced feeding (Morley & Levine, 1980). However, naloxone poorly antagonized feeding induced by chronic starvation for three weeks (Morley, Levine, Gosnell, & Billington, 1984a), schedule feeding (Sanger & McCarthy, 1981), and insulin hypoglycemia (Levine & Morley, 1981), suggesting that the opioid feeding system is not the only inducer of feeding. Chronic administration of naloxone or naltrexone produced only small decreases in food intake and body weight in non-obese rats and mice (Mandenoff, Fumeron, Appelbaum, & Margules, 1982; Shimonura, Oku, Glick, & Bray, 1982). Also, a variety of hormones modulate the effectiveness of naloxone as a suppressor of food intake (Levine & Morley, 1983; Levine, Morley, Brown, & Handwerger, 1982; Morley, Levine, Grace, Kneip, & Gosnell, 1984b).

An important consideration is which opioid receptor modulates feeding. The current evidence suggests that several receptors and opioid peptides are involved, each producing its effect in a specific anatomical locus. Much evidence has now accumulated suggesting that the kappa opioid receptor and its endogenous ligands, dynorphin/α-neo-endorphin, are one of the major opioid systems involved in the regulation of feeding. Of the endogenous opioid ligands, dynorphin (kappa; Morley & Levine, 1981, 1983), beta-endorphin (epsilon; Leibowitz & Hor, 1982), and enkephalins (delta; Tepperman & Hirst, 1983) have been shown to enhance food intake in rats. However, peripheral infusions of beta endorphin appear to inhibit food intake (Morley & Levine, 1985). The mixed kappa opiate agonists/antagonists such as ketocyclazocine and butorphanol are more potent stimulators of feeding than the mu agonists (Morley, Levine, Grace, & Kneip, 1982a). The endogenous ligand dynorphin apparently stimulates feeding by involving two portions of the molecule. The non-opioid segment of the peptide may alter the conformation of the receptor and allow for the binding of the opioid segment of the peptide (Morley & Levine, 1983). This "double-lock" theory is similar to a model suggested by Chavkin and Goldstein (1981). Further evidence for a role for dynorphin in feeding comes from the studies showing that its levels alter in the CNS under conditions which modulate the feeding drive (Morley, Elson, Levine, & Shafer, 1983a).

It is of interest to speculate, from a teleological point of view, that opioids were originally the stimulus for feeding. This stimulus forced the animal to hunt for food, during which time pain may have occurred due to fighting. Survival might have been improved if a gene mutation caused a similar peptide to subserve the function of analgesia as well as feeding.

MEMORY

Much interest has been occasioned by the possible role of endogenous opioids in learning and memory. Opioid antagonism in animals has rather consistently been shown to facilitate retention of aversively-motivated and food-rewarded tasks (Olson, Olson, & Kastin, 1984). Opioid antagonism has been reported to either facilitate or inhibit memory acquisition.

Recently, much excitement was occasioned by a report that repeated naloxone administration could improve memory in patients with Alzheimer's disease (Reisberg et al., 1983). The changes seen, however, were minor, and pooling of the results from different naloxone doses could have resulted in positive results being due to the well-recognized practice effect seen with human memory testing. Low levels of β-endorphin have been reported in the CSF of patients with Alzheimer's disease, and levels of this peptide in the CSF correlated with the psychological ratings of dementia (Kaiya et al., 1983). In normal humans, naloxone has been shown either to have no effect on memory or to impair memory retention (Cohen, Cohen, Weingartner, Pickar, & Murphy, 1983; Grevert, Albert, Inturrisi, & Goldstein, 1983). Further studies are clearly indicated before attributing a role of opioids in human memory and in dementia.

EXORPHINS

A number of peptide hormone-like substances have been isolated from food (Fukushima, Watanabe, & Kushima, 1976; Jackson, 1981; Morley et al., 1980b; Zioudrou, Streaty, & Klee, 1979). It has been suggested that these food hormones (formones) may act on gut luminal receptors as exogenous regulators of gastrointestinal motility and hormone release (Morley, 1982). It has been shown that peptic digestion of some dietary proteins, such as casein and wheat gluten, results in the production of substances that have opiate-like activity in both receptor and bioassays (Zioudrou et al., 1979). These compounds were named exorphins in analogy with the endogenously derived opioid-like peptides (i.e., endorphins). The peptides responsible for the opioid properties of β-casein hydrolysates (β-casomorphins) have been isolated and sequenced (Brantl & Teschemacher, 1979; Brantl, Teschemacher, Henschen, & Lottspeich, 1979) and shown to produce naloxone-reversible analgesia after i.c.v. administration in rats (Brantl, Teschemacher, Blasig, Henschen, & Lottspeich, 1981).

Schusdziarra, Henrichs, Holland, Klier, and Pfeiffer (1981) have shown that oral administration of these exorphins to the dog leads to a more rapid and notably greater rise in postprandial peripheral vein insulin and glucagon. In humans, we could not reproduce the effects of exorphins on insulin and glucagon (Morley et al., 1983b). Exorphins do, however, appear to slow gastrointestinal somatostatin. Recently, β-casomorphin-like peptides have been identified in human cerebrospinal fluid and have been linked to the pathogenesis of post-partum psychosis (Lindstrom et al., 1984).

REFERENCES

Akil, H., Watson, S. J., Young, E., Lewis, M. E., Khachaturian, H., & Walker, J. M. (1984). Endogenous opioids: Biology and function. *Annual Review of Neuroscience, 7*, 223–255.

Atweh, S. F., & Kuhar, M. J. (1977). Autoradiographic localization of opiate receptors in rat brain. I. Spinal cord and lower medulla. *Brain Research, 124*, 53–67.

Awouters, F., Niemegeers, C. J. E., & Janssen, P. A. J. (1983). Pharmacology of anti-diarrheal drugs. *Annual Review of Pharmacology, 23*, 279–301.

Banerjee, U., Burks, T. F., Feldberg, W., & Goodrich, C. A. (1968). Temperature effects and catalepsy produced by morphine injection into the cerebral ventricles of rabbits. *British Journal of Pharmacology and Chemotherapy, 33*, 544–551.

Barraclough, C. A., & Sawyer, C. H. (1955). Inhibition of the release of pituitary ovulatory hormone in the rat by morphine. *Endocrinology, 57*, 329–337.

Beubler, E., Bukhave, K., & Rask-Madsen, J. (1984). Colonic secretion mediated by prostaglandin E_2 and 5-hydroxytryptamine may contribute to diarrhea due to morphine withdrawal in the rat. *Gastroenterology, 87*, 1042–1048.

Bitar, K. N., & Makhlouf, G. M. (1983). Specific opiate receptors on isolated mammalian gastric smooth muscle cells. *Nature, 297*, 72–74.

Blalock, J. E., & Smith, E. M. (1980). Human leukocyte interferon: Structural and biological relatedness to adrenocroticotropic hormone and endorphins. *Cell Biology, 77*, 5972–5974.

Blalock, J. E., & Smith, E. M. (1981). Human leukocyte interferon (HUIFN-alpha): Potent endorphin-like activity. *Biochemical & Biophysical Research Communications, 101*, 472–478.

Blankstein, J., Reyes, F. I., Winter, J. S. D., & Faiman, C. (1980). Effects of naloxone on prolactin and cortisol in normal women. *Proceedings of the Society for Experimental and Biological Medicine, 164*, 363–365.

Blankstein, J., Reyes, F. I., Winter, J. S., & Faiman, C. (1981). Endorphins and the regulation of the human menstrual cycle. *Clinical Endocrinology, 14*, 287–294.

Bloom, F. E., Battenberg, E., Rossier, J., Ling, N., Leppaluoto, J., Vargo, T. M., & Guillemin, R. (1977). Endorphins are located in the intermediate and anterior lobes of the pituitary gland, not in the neuropophysis. *Life Science, 20*, 43–48.

Bloom, F. E., Rossier, J., Battenberg, E., Bayon, A., French, E., Henricksen, S. J., Siggins, G. R., Segal, D., Browne, R., Ling, N., & Guillemin, R. (1978). Beta-endorphin: Cellular localization, electrophysiological and behavioral effects. *Advances in Biochemistry and Psychopharmacology: The Endorphins, 18*, 89–109.

Bolme, P., Fuxe, K. F., Agnati, L. F., Bradley, R., & Smythies, J. (1978). Cardiovascular effects of morphine and opioid peptides following intracisternal administration in chloralose-anesthetized rats. *European Journal of Pharmacology, 48*, 319–324.

Brady, J. P., & Bianco, F. C. (1980). Endorphins: Naloxone failure to increase sexual arousal in sexually unresponsive women: A preliminary report. *Biological Psychiatry, 15*, 627–631.

Brands, B., Thornhill, J. A., Hirst, M., & Gowdey, C. W. (1979). Suppression of food intake and body weight gain by naloxone in rats. *Life Science, 24*, 1773–1778.

Brantl, V., & Teschemacher, H. (1979). A material with opioid activity in bovine milk and milk products. *Naunyn-Schmeideberg's Archives of Pharmacology, 306*, 301–304.

Brantl, V., Teschemacher, H., Blasig, J., Henschen, A., & Lottspeich, F. (1981). Opioid activities of β-casomorphins. *Life Science, 28*, 1903–1909.

Brantl, V., Teschemacher, H., Henschen, A., & Lottspeich, F. (1979). Novel opioid peptides derived from casein (β-casomorphin). *Hoppe-Seyler's Journal of Physiological Chemistry, 360*, 1211–1216.

Broccardo, M., Improta, G., Nargi, M., & Melchiorri, P. (1982). Effects of dermorphin on gastrointestinal transit in rats. *Regulatory Peptides, 4*, 91–96.

Brodie, D. A., Lotti, V. J., & Bauer, B. G. (1970). Drug effects on gastric secretion and stress gastric hemorrhage in the rat. *American Journal of Digestive Diseases, 15*, 111–120.

Brown, D. R., & Miller, R. J. (1983). CNS involvement in the antisecretory action of [Met⁵]enkephalinamide on the rat intestine. *European Journal of Pharmacology, 90*, 441–444.

Brown, D. R., & Miller, R. J. (1984). Adrenergic mediation of the intestinal antisecretory action of opiates administered into the central nervous system. *Journal of Pharmacology and Experimental Therapeutics*, 231: 114–119, 1984.

Bruni, J. F., Van Vugt, D. A., Marshall, S., & Meites, J. (1977). Effects of naloxone, morphine and methionine enkephalin on serum prolactin, luteinizing hormone, follicle stimulating hormone, thyroid stimulating hormone and growth hormone. *Life Science, 21*, 461–466.

Burks, T. F., Hirning, L. D., Galligan, J. J., & Davis, T. P. (1982). Motility effects of opioid peptides in dog intestine. *Life Science, 31*, 2237–2240.

Butland, R. J., Woodcock, A. A., Gross, E. R., & Geddes, D. M. (1981). Endogenous opioids (endorphins) and the control of breathing (letter). *New England Journal of Medicine, 305*, 1096.

Calvet, M. C., & Gresser, I. (1979). Interferon enhances the excitability of cultural neurons. *Nature, 278*, 558–560.

Cetel, N. S., Quigley, M. E., & Yen, S. S. C. (1983). The control of prolactin secretion by endogenous opioids in man: Gonadal steroid dependent paradoxical response to naloxone. *Endocrinology, 110*, 964A.

Chavkin, C., & Goldstein, A. (1981). Specific receptor for the opioid peptide dynorphin: Structure-activity relationships. *Proceedings of the National Academy of Science, USA, 78*, 6543–6547.

Chernick, V., Madansky, D. L., & Lawson, E. E. (1980). Naloxone decreases the duration of primary apnea with neonatal asphyxia? *Pediatric Research, 14*, 357–359.

Ching, M. (1983). Morphine suppresses the proestrous surge of GnRh in pituitary portal plasma of rats. *Endocrinology, 112*, 2209–2211.

Cicero, T. J., Schainker, B. A., & Meyer, E. R. (1979). Endogenous opioids participate in the regulation of the hypothalamic-pituitary-luteinizing hormone axis and testosterone's negative feedback control of luteinizing hormone. *Endocrinology, 104*, 1286–1291.

Clark, W. G. (1981). Effects of opioid peptides on thermoregulation. *Federal Proceedings, 40*, 2754–2759.

Cohen, R. A., & Coffman, J. D. (1979). The effects of morphine on cutaneous capacitance and resistance vessels. *Circulation, 60*, (Part II), 80.

Cohen, R. A., & Coffman, J. D. (1980). Naloxone reversal of morphine-induced peripheral vasodilation. *Clinical Pharmacology and Therapeutics, 28*, 541–544.

Cohen, R. M., Cohen, M. R., Weingartner, H., Pickar, D., & Murphy, D. L. (1983). High dose naloxone affects task performance in normal subjects. *Psychiatry Research, 8*, 127–136.

Cowan, A., & MacFarland, I. R. (1976). Effect of morphine antagonists on drug induced hypothermia in mice and rats. *Psychopharmacology, 45*, 277–282.

Cowan, A., Doxey, J. C., & Metcalf, G. (1976). A comparison of pharmacological effects produced by leucine-enkephalin, methionine-enkephaline, morphine and ketocyclazocine. In H. W. Kosterlitz (Ed.), *Opiates and endogenous opioid peptides* (pp. 95–102). Amsterdam: Elsevier/North Holland.

Crowley, T. J., & Simpson, R. (1978). Methadone dose and human sexual behavior. *International Journal of Addiction, 13*, 285–295.

Cuello, A. C. (1983). Central distribution of opioid peptides. *British Medical Bulletin, 39*, 11–16.

Dafny, N. (1983). Modification of morphine withdrawal by interferon. *Life Science, 32*, 303–305.

D'Amato, R. J., & Holaday, J. W. (1984). Multiple opiate receptors in endotoxic shock: Evidence for delta involvement and mu-delta interactions in vivo. *Proceedings of the National Academy of Science, USA, 81*, 2898–2901.

Daniel, E. E. (1982). Pharmacology of adrenergic, cholinergic and drugs acting on other receptors in gastrointestinal muscle. In G. Bertaccini (Ed.), *Handbook of Experimental Pharmacology, Vol. 59: Mediators and drugs in gastrointestinal motility* (pp. 249–322). Berlin: Springer-Verlag.

Daniel, E. E., Sutherland, W. H., Bogoch, A. (1959). Effects of morphine and other drugs on motility of the terminal ileum. *Gastroenterology, 36*, 510–523.

Delitala, G., Devilla, L., & Di Biaso, D. (1980). Dopamine inhibits the naloxone induced gonadotropin rise in man. *Clinical Endocrinology, 13*, 515–518.

Delitala, G., Giusti, M., Devilla, L., Mazzocchi, G., Lotti, G., & Giordano, G. (1981). Effect of a met-enkephalin analogue and naloxone infusion on gonadotropin secretion in man. *Acta Europaea Fertilitatis (Roma), 12*, 287–288.

Denavit-Saubie, M., Champagnat, J., & Zieglgansberger, W. (1978). Effects of opiates and methionine-enkephalin on pontine and bulbar respiratory neurons of the cat. *Brain Research, 155*, 55–67.

Duranton, A., & Bueno, L. (1984). Central opiate mechanism involved in gastro-intestinal motor disturbances induced by E. coli endotoxin in sheep. *Life Science, 34*, 1795–1799.

Elde, R., Hokfelt, T., Johansson, O., & Terenius, L. (1976). Immunohistochemical studies using antibodies to leucine enkephalin: Initial observations on the nervous system of the rat. *Neuroscience, 1*, 349–351.

Ellingboe, J., Veldhuis, J. D., Mendelson, J. H., Kuehnle, J. C., & Mello, N. K. (1982). Effect of endogenous opioid blockade on the amplitude and frequency of pulsatile luteinizing hormone secretion in normal man. *Journal of Clinical Endocrinology and Metabolism, 54*, 854–857.

Epstein, L. B., Rose, M. E., McManus, N. H., & Li, C. H. (1982). Absence of functional and structural homology of natural and recombinant human leukocyte interferon (IFN-α) with human α-ACTH and β-endorphin. *Biochemical and Biophysical Research Communications., 104*, 341–346.

Feldberg, W., & Wei, E. (1978). Central cardiovascular effects of enkephalin and C-fragment of lipotropin. *Journal of Physiology, 280*, 18P.

Feldman, M., & Cowley, Y. M. (1982). Effect of an opiate antagonist (naloxone) on the gastric acid secretory response to sham feeding, pentagastrin, and histamine in man. *Digestive Disease Science, 27*, 308–310.

Feldman, M., Walsh, J. H., & Taylor, I. L. (1980). Effect of naloxone and morphine on gastric acid secretion and on serum gastrin and pancreatic polypeptide concentrations in humans. *Gastroenterology, 79*, 294–298.

Fennessy, M. R., & Rattray, J. F. (1971). Cardiovascular effects of intravenous morphine in the anesthetized rat. *European Journal of Pharmacology, 14*, 1–8.

Feuerstein, G., & Faden, A. I. (1982). Differential cardiovascular effects of μ, γ, and κ opiate agonists at discrete hypothalamic sites in the anesthetized rat. *Life Science, 31*, 2197–2200.

Flowers, S. H., Dunham, E. S., & Barbour, H. G. (1929). Addiction edema and withdrawal edema in morphinized rats. *Proceedings of the Society for Experimental and Biological Medicine, 26*, 572–574.

Fukushima, M., Watanabe, S., & Kushima, K. (1976). Extraction and purification of a substance with luteinizing hormone-release activity from leaves of *Avena sativa*. *Tohoku Journal of Experimental and Clinical Medicine, 119*, 115–119.

Furness, J. B., Costa, M., & Miller, R. J. (1983). Distribution and projections of nerves with enkephalin like immunoreactivity in the guinea-pig small intestine. *Neuroscience, 8*, 653–664.

Galligan, J. J., & Burks, T. F. (1983). Centrally mediated inhibition of small intestinal transit and motility by morphine in the rat. *Journal of Pharmacology and Experimental Therapy, 226*, 356–361.

Gen, M. C. & Valdman, A. V. (1963). Experimental data in the pharmacology of bulbar respiratory centre. In A. V. Valdman (Ed.), *Problems of pharmacology of reticular formation and synaptic transmission* (pp. 190–215). Leningrad: Leningrad Medical Institute.

Genazzani, A. R., Facchinetti, F., & Parrini, D. (1981). β-lipotropin and β-endorphin plasma levels during pregnancy. *Clinical Endocrinology, 14*, 409–418.

Gessa, G. L., Paglietti, E., & Quarantotti, B. P. (1979). Induction of copulatory behavior in sexually inactive rats by naloxone. *Science, 204*, 203–205.

Gilman, S. C., Schwartz, J. M., Milner, R. J., Bloom, F. E., & Feldman, J. D. (1982). β-endorphin enhances lymphocyte proliferative responses. *Proceedings of the National Academy of Science, USA, 79*, 4226–4230.

Gintzler, A. R. (1980). Endorphin-mediated increases in pain threshold during pregnancy. *Science, 210*, 193–195.

Goland, R. S., Wardlaw, S. L., Stark, R. I., & Frantz, A. G. (1981). Human plasma β-endorphin during pregnancy, labor, and delivery. *Journal of Clinical Endocrinology and Metabolism, 52*, 74–78.

Goldstein, A., & Hansteen, R. W. (1977). Evidence against involvement of endorphins in sexual arousal and orgasm in man. *Archives of General Psychiatry, 34*, 1179–1180.

Goldstein, A., & Lowery, P. J. (1975). Effect of the opiate antagonist naloxone on body temperature in rats. *Life Science, 17*, 927–932.

Goldstein, A., Tachibana, S., Lowney, L. I., Hunkapiller, M., & Hood, L. (1979). Dynorphin-(1–13), an extraordinarily potent opioid peptide. *Proceedings of the National Academy of Science, USA, 76*, 6666–6670.

Grandison, L., & Guidotti, A. (1977). Stimulation of food intake by muscimol and beta-endorphin. *Neuropharmacology, 16*, 533–536.

Grevert, P., Albert, L. H., Inturrisi, C. E., & Goldstein, A. (1983). Effects of eight-hour naloxone infusions on human subjects. *Biological Psychiatry, 18*, 1375–1392.

Gunne, L. M. (1960). The temperature response in rats during acute and chronic morphine administration. A study of morphine tolerance. *Archives of International Pharmacodynamic Therapy, 129*, 416–428.

Hassen, A. H., Feuerstein, G. Z., & Faden, A. I. (1982). Cardiovascular responses to opioid agonists injected into the nucleus of tractus solitarius of anesthetized cats. *Life Science, 31*, 2193–2196.

Henry, J. L. (1982). Circulating opioids: Possible psychological roles in central nervous function. *Neuroscience Biobehavior Review, 6*, 229–245.

Herberman, R. B., & Holden, H. T. (1978). Natural cell-mediated immunity. *Advances in Cancer Research, 27*, 305–377.

Herberman, R. B., & Ortaldo, J. R. (1981). Natural killer cells: Their roles in defenses against disease. *Science, 214*, 24–30.

Herrman, J. B. (1942). The pyretic action of small doses of morphine. *Journal of Pharmacology and Experimental Therapeutics, 76*, 309–315.

Hokfelt, T., Johansson, O., Ljungdahl, A., Lundberg, J. M., & Schultzberg, M. (1980). Peptidergic neurones. *Nature, 284*, 515–521.

Hokfelt, T., Ljungdahl, A., Terenius, L., Elde, R., & Nilsson, G. (1977). Immunohistochemical analysis of peptide pathways possibly related to pain and analgesia: Enkephalin and substance P. *Proceedings of the National Academy of Science, USA, 74*, 3081–3085.

Holaday, J. W. (1984). Neuropeptides in shock and traumatic injury: Sites and mechanisms of action. In E. E. Muller & R. M. MacLeod (Eds.), *Neuroendocrine perspectives* (Vol. 3, pp. 161–199). Elsevier Science Publishers.

Holaday, J. W., D'Amato, R. J., Ruvio, B. A., & Faden, A. I. (1982). Action of naloxone and TRH on the autonomic regulation of circulation. *Advances in Biochemistry and Psychopharmacology, 33*, 353–361.

Holaday, J. W., & Faden, A. I. (1978). Naloxone reversal of endotoxin hypotension suggests role of endorphins in shock. *Nature (London), 275*, 450–451.

Holaday, J. W., Pasternak, G. W., D'Amato, R. J., Ruvio, B. A., & Faden, A. I. (1983). Naloxazone lacks therapeutic effects in endotoxic shock yet blocks the effects of naloxone. *European Journal of Pharmacology, 89*, 293–296.

Hollister, L. E. (1975). The mystique of social drugs and sex. In M. Sandler & G. L. Gessa (Eds.), *Sexual behavior: Pharmacology and biochemistry* (pp. 85–92). New York: Raven Press.

Howard, J. M., Belsheim, M. R., & Sullivan, S. N. (1982). Enkephalin inhibits relaxation of the lower oesophageal sphincter. *British Medical Journal, 285*, 1605–1606.

Huidobro-Toro, J. P., & Way, E. L. (1979). Studies on the hyperthermic response of β-endorphin in mice. *Journal of Pharmacology and Experimental Therapeutics, 211*, 50–58.

Ieiri, T., Chen, H. T., Campbell, G. A., & Meites, J. (1980). Effects of naloxone and morphine on the proestrous surge of prolactin and gonadotropins in the rat. *Endocrinology, 106*, 1568–1570.

Isom, G. E., & Elshowihy, R. M. (1982). Naloxone-induced enhancement of carbon dioxide stimulated respiration. *Life Science, 31*, 113–118.

Jackson, I. M. D. (1981). Abundance of immunoreactive thyrotropin releasing hormone-like material in the alfalfa plant. *Endocrinology, 108*, 344–346.

Jaloweic, J. E., Panksepp, J., Zolovick, A. J., Najam, N., & Herman, B. (1981). Opioid modulation of ingestive behavior. *Pharmacology, Biochemistry, and Behavior, 15*, 477–484.

Kaiya, H., Tanaka, T., Takeuchi, K., Morita, K., Adachi, S., Shirakawa, H., Ueki, H., & Namba, M. (1983). Decreased level of β-endorphin like immunoreactivity in cerebrospinal fluid of patients with senile dementia of Alzheimer type. *Life Science, 33*, 1039–1043.

Kandasamy, S. B., & Williams, B. A. (1983). Peptide and non-peptide opioid-induced hyperthermia in rabbits. *Brain Research, 265*, 63–71.

Kay, N., Allen, J., & Morley, J. E. (1984). Endorphins stimulate normal human peripheral blood lymphocyte natural killer activity. *Life Science, 35*, 53–59.

Khachaturian, H., Watson, S. J., Lewis, M. E., Coy, D., & Goldstein, A. (1982). Dynorphin immunocytochemistry in the rat central nervous system. *Peptides, 3*, 941–945.

Kiang, J. G., & Wei, E. T. (1983). Inhibition of an opioid-evoked vagal reflex in rats by naloxone, SMS 201-995 and ICI 154,129. *Regulatory Peptides, 6*, 255–262.

Kinsey, A. C., Pomeroy, W. B., Martin, C. E., & Gebhard, P. H. (1973). *Sexual behavior in the human female*. New York: Pocket Books.

Konishi, S., Tsunoo, A., & Osaka, M. (1981). Enkephalins as transmitter for presynaptic inhibition in sympathetic ganglia. *Nature (London), 294*, 80–82.

Konturek, S. J., Pawlik, W., Walus, K. M., Coy, D. H., & Schally, A. V. (1978). Methionine-enkephalin stimulates gastric secretion and gastric mucosal blood flow. *Proceedings of the Society for Experimental and Biological Medicine, 158*, 156–160.

Konturek, S. J., Tasler, J., Cheszkowski, M., Mikos, E., Coy, D. H., & Schally, A. V. (1980). Comparison of methionine-enkephalin and morphine in the stimulation of gastric acid secretion in the dog. *Gastroenterology, 78*, 294–300.

Krieger, D. T., Liotta, A., & Brownstein, M. J. (1977). Presence of corticotropin in brain of normal and hypophysectomized rats. *Proceedings of the National Academy of Science, USA, 74*, 648–652.

Lahti, R., & Collins, R. J. (1978). Chronic naloxone results in prolonged increases in opiate binding by an endogenous material from the brain. *European Journal of Pharmacology, 51*, 185–186.

Lang, R. E., Hermann, K., Dietz, R., Gaida, W., Ganten, D., Kraft, K., & Unger, T. (1983). Evidence for the presence of enkephalins in the heart. *Life Science, 32*, 399–406.

Laubie, M., Schmitt, H., Vincent, M., & Remond, G. (1977). Central cardiovascular effects of morphinomimetic peptides in dogs. *European Journal of Pharmacology, 46*, 67–71.

Lawson, E. E., Waldorp, T. G., & Eldridge, F. L. (1979). Naloxone enhances respiratory outputs in cats. *Journal of Applied Physiology: Respiratory, Environmental and Exercise Physiology, 47*, 1105–1111.

Leibowitz, S. F., & Hor, L. (1982). Endorphinergic and α-noradrenergic systems in the paraventricular nucleus: Effects on eating behavior. *Peptides, 3*, 421–428.

Levine, A. S., & Morley, J. E. (1981). Peptidergic control of insulin-induced feeding. *Peptides, 2*, 261–264.

Levine, A. S., & Morley, J. E. (1983). Adrenal modulation of opiate induced feeding. *Pharmacology, Biochemistry and Behavior, 19*, 403–406.

Levine, A. S., Morley, J. E., Brown, D. M., & Handwerger, B. A. (1982). Extreme sensitivity of diabetic mice to naloxone-induced suppression of food intake. *Physiological Behavior, 28*, 987–989.

Lin, M. T., & Su, C. Y. (1979). Metabolic, respiratory, vasomotor and body temperature responses to beta-endorphin and morphine in rabbits. *Journal of Physiology (London), 296*, 179–189.

Lindstrom, L. H., Nyberg, F., Terenius, L., Bauer, K., Besev, G., Gunne, L. M., Lyrenas, S., Willdecklund, G., & Lindberg, B. (1984). CSF and plasma beta-casomorphin-like opioid-peptides in postpartum psychosis. *American Journal of Psychiatry, 141*, 1059–1066.

Lopkor, A., Abood, L. G., Hass, W., & Lionetti, F. J. (1980). Stereoselective muscarinic acetylcholine and opiate receptors on human pahagocytic leukocytes. *Biochemical Pharmacology, 29*, 1361–1365.

Lowy, M. T., Maickel, R. P., & Yim, G. K. W. (1980). Naloxone reduction of stress-related feeding. *Life Science, 26*, 2113–2118.

Lundberg, J. M., Hokfelt, T., Kewenter, J., Petterson, G., Ahlman, H., Edin, R., Dahlstrom, A., Nilsson, G., Terenius, L., Vvnas-Wallenstein, K., & Said, S. (1979). Substance P-, VIP- and enkephaline-like immunoreactivity in the human vagus nerve. *Gastroenterology, 77*, 468–471.

Mandenoff, A., Fumeron, F., Appelbaum, M., & Margules, D. L. (1982). Endogenous opiates and energy balance. *Science, 215*, 1536–1538.

Margolin, S. (1963). Centrally mediated inhibition of gastrointestinal propulsive motility by morphine over a non-neural pathway. *Proceedings of the Society for Experimental and Biological Medicine, 112*, 311–315.

Margolin, S., & Plekss, O. J. (1965). A neurohumoral substance discharged into blood perfusate from isolated rabbit heads by intracerebral morphine. *Med. Pharmacol. Exp., 12*, 1–7.

Martin, W. R. (1984). Pharmacology of opioids. *Pharmacological Reviews, 35*, 283–323.

Martin, W. R., Wikler, A., Eades, C. G., & Pescor, F. T. (1963). Tolerance to and physical dependence on morphine in rats. *Psychopharmacologia (Berlin), 4*, 247–260.

Mathews, P. M., Froelich, C. J., Sibbitt, W. L., & Bankhurst, A. D. (1983). Enhancement of natural cytotoxicity by β-endorphin. *Journal of Immunology, 130*, 1658–1662.

Mayer, G., Wessel, J., & Kobberling, J. (1980). Failure of naloxone to alter exercise-induced growth hormone and prolactin release in normal man. *Clinical Endocrinology, 13*, 413–416.

Maysinger, D., Hollt, V., Seizinger, B. R., Mehraein, P., Pasi, A., & Herz, A. (1982). Parallel distribution of immunoreactive alpha-neo-endorphin and dynorphin in rat and human tissue. *Neuropeptides, 2*, 211–225.

McDougal, J. N., Marques, P. R., & Burks, T. F. (1980). Thermic responses to morphine in old and young rats. *Proceedings of the Western Pharmacological Society, 23*, 235–238.

McQueen, D. S. (1983). Opioid peptide interactions with reparatory and circulatory systems. *British Medical Bulletin, 39*, 77–82.

Mendelson, J., Ellingboe, J., Keuhnle, J., & Mello, N. (1979). Effects of naltrexone on mood and neuroendocrine function in normal adult males. *Psychoneuroendocrinology, 3*, 231–236.

Meyerson, B. J., & Terenius, L. (1977). β-endorphin and male sexual behavior. *European Journal of Pharmacology, 42*, 191–192.

Miller, R. J., & Brown, D. R. (1984). Opiates and the gut. *Viewpoints on Digestive Disease, 16*(2), 5–8.

Morley, J. E. (1981). The endocrinology of the opiates and opioid peptides. *Metabolism, 30*, 195–209.

Morley, J. E. (1982). Food peptides: A new class of hormones? *Journal of the American Medical Association, 247*, 2379–2380.

Morley, J. E. (1983). Neuroendocrine effects of endogenous opioid peptides in humans. A review. *Psychoneuroendocrinology, 8*, 361–379.

Morley, J. E., Baranetsky, N. G., Wingert, T. D., Carlson, H. E., Hershman, J. M., Melmed, S., Levin, S. R., Jamison, K. R., Weitzman, R., Chang, R. J., & Varner, A. A. (1980a). Endocrine effects of naloxone-induced opiate receptor blockade. *Journal of Clinical Endocrinology and Metabolism, 50*, 251–257.

Morley, J. E., Elson, M. K., Levine, A. S., & Shafer, R. B. (1983a). The effects of stress on central nervous system concentrations of the opioid peptide, dynorphin. *Peptides, 3*, 901–906.

Morley, J. E., & Levine, A. S. (1980). Stress induced eating is mediated through endogenous opiates. *Science, 209*, 1259–1261.

Morley, J. E., & Levine, A. S. (1981). Dynorphin-(1–13) induces spontaneous feeding in rats. *Life Science, 29*, 1901–1903.

Morley, J. E., & Levine, A. S. (1983). Involvement of dynorphin and the kappa opioid receptor in feeding. *Peptides, 4*, 797–800.

Morley, J. E., & Levine, A. S.(1985). Pharmacology of eating behavior. In R. George & R. Okun (Eds.), *Annual review of pharmacology and toxicology* Palo Alta, CA: Annual Reviews Inc., 25, 127–146.

Morley, J. E., Levine, A. S., Gosnell, B. A., & Billington, C. J. (1984a). Which opioid receptor mechanism modulates feeding? *Appetite, 5*, 61–68.

Morley, J. E., Levine, A. S., Grace, M. & Kneip, J. (1982a). An investigation of the role of kappa opiate receptor agonists in the initiation of feeding. *Life Science, 31*, 2617–2626.

Morley, J. E., Levine, A. S., Grace, M., Kneip, J., & Gosnell, B. A. (1984b). The effect of ovariectomy, estradiol and progesterone on opioid modulation of feeding. *Physiological Behavior, 33*, 237–241.

Morley, J. E., Levine, A. S., & Kneip, J. (1981a). Muscimol induced feeding: A model to study the hypothalamic regulation of appetite. *Life Science, 29*, 1213–1218.

Morley, J. E., Levine, A. S., Murray, S., & Kneip, J. (1982b). Peptidergic regulation of norepinephrine induced feeding. *Pharmacology, Biochemistry and Behavior, 16*, 225–228.

Morley, J. E., Levine, A. S., Oken, M. M., Grace, M., & Kneip, J. (1982c). Neuropeptides and thermoregulation: The interactions of bombesin, neurotensin, TRH, somatostatin, naloxone and prostaglandins. *Peptides, 3*, 1–6.

Morley, J. E., Levine, A. S., & Silvis, S. E. (1982d). Central regulation of gastric acid secretion: The role of neuropeptides. *Life Science, 31*, 399–410.

Morley, J. E., Levine, A. S., & Silvis, S. E. (1981b). Endogenous opiates inhibit gastric acid secretion induced by central administration of thyrotropin releasing hormone (TRH). *Life Science, 29*, 293–297.

Morley, J. E., Levine, A. S., & Silvis, S. E. (1982e). Endogenous opiates and stress ulceration. *Life Science, 31*, 693–699.

Morley, J. E., Levine, A. S., Yamada, T., Gebhard, R. L., Prigge, W. F., Shafer, R. B., Goetz, F. C., & Silvis, S. E. (1983b). Effect of exorphins on gastrointestinal function, hormonal release and appetite. *Gastroenterology, 84*, 1517–1523.

Morley, J. E., Mayer, N., Pekary, A. E., Melmed, S., Carlson, H. E., Briggs, J. E., & Hershman, J. M. (1980b). A prolactin inhibitory factor with immunocharacteristics similar to thyrotropin releasing factor (TRH) is present in rat pituitary tumors (GH3 and W%), testicular tissue and a plant material, alfalfa. *Biochemical and Biophysical Research Communications, 96,* 47–53.

Moss, I. R., & Scarpelli, E. M. (1979). Generation and regulation of breathing in utero: Fetal CO_2 response test. *Journal of Applied Physiology: Respiratory, Environmental and Exercise Physiology, 47,* 527–531.

Moult, P. J., Grossman, A., Evans, J. M., Rees, L. H., & Besser, G. M. (1981). The effect of naloxone on pulsatile gonadotropin release in normal subjects. *Clinical Endocrinology, 14,* 321–324.

Muraki, T., Tokunaga, Y., & Makino, T. (1977). Effects of morphine and naloxone on serum LH, FSH, and prolactin levels on hypothalamic content of LH-RF in proestrous rats. *Endocrinology (Japan), 24,* 313–315.

Murphy, M. R., Bowie, D. L., & Pert, C. B. (1979). Copulation elevates plasma β-endorphin in the male hamster. *Society for Neuroscience Abstracts, 5,* 470.

Myers, B. M., & Baum, M. J. (1979). Facilitation by opiate antagonists of sexual performance in the male rat. *Pharmacology, Biochemistry and Behavior, 10,* 615–618.

Nistico, G., Rotiroti, D., Naccari, F., De Sarro, G. B., & Marino, E. (1980). Effects of intra-ventricular β-endorphin and D-Ala²-methionine-enkephalinamide on behaviour, spectrum power of electro-cortical activity and body temperature in chicks. *Research Communications in Chemical Pathology and Pharmacology, 28,* 295–308.

Olsen, P. S., Kirkegaard, P., Petersen, B., & Christiansen, J. (1982). Effect of naloxone on met-enkephalin-induced gastric acid secretion and serum gastrin in man. *Gut, 23,* 63–65.

Olsen, P. S., Kirkegaard, P., Petersen, B., Lendorf, A., & Christiansen, J. (1981). The effect of a synthetic met-enkephalin analogue (FK 33-824) on gastric acid secretion and serum gastrin in man. *Scandinavian Journal of Gastroenterology, 16,* 531–533.

Olson, G. A., Olson, R. D., & Kastin, A. J. (1984). Endogenous opiates: 1983. *Peptides, 5,* 975–992.

Packman, P. M., & Rothchild, J. A. (1976). Morphine inhibition of ovulation: Reversal by naloxone. *Endocrinology, 99,* 7–10.

Palkovits, M., & Zaborszky, L. (1977). Neuroanatomy of central cardiovascular control. Nucleus tractus solitarii: Afferent and efferent neuronal connections in relation to the baroreceptor reflex arc. *Progress in Brain Research, 47,* 9–34.

Parr, D. (1976). Sexual aspects of drug abuse in narcotic addicts. *British Journal of Addiction, 71,* 261–268.

Pelletier, G. (1980). Ultrastructural localization of a fragment (16K) of the common precursor for adrenocorticotropin and beta-LPH in the rat hypothalamus. *Neuroscience Letters, 16,* 85–90.

Pelletier, G., Leclerc, R., LaBrie, F., Cote, J., Chretien, M., & Lis, M. (1977). Immunohisto-chemical localization of beta-LPH hormone in the pituitary gland. *Endocrinology, 100,* 770–776.

Pert, C. B., Kuhar, M. J., & Snyder, S. H. (1975). Autoradiographic localization of the opiate receptor in rat brain. *Life Science, 16,* 1849–1854.

Pfeiffer, A., Feuerstein, G., Zerbe, R. L., Faden, A. I., & Kopin, K. J. (1983). μ-receptor mediated opioid cardiovascular effects at anterior hypothalamic sites through sympatho-adrenomedullary and parasympathetic pathways. *Endocrinology, 113,* 929–938.

Plotnikoff, N. P., Kastin, A. J., Coy, D. H., Christensen, C. W., Schally, A. V., & Spirtes, M. A. (1976). Neuropharmacological actions of enkephalin after systemic administration. *Life Science, 19,* 1283–1288.

Plotnikoff, N. P., & Miller, G. C. (1983). Enkephalins as immunomodulators. *International Journal of Immunopharmacology, 5,* 437–441.

Porreca, F., & Burks, T. F. (1983). The spinal cord as a site of opioid effects on gastrointestinal transit in the mouse. *Journal of Pharmacological and Experimental Therapeutics, 227,* 22–27.

Porreca, R., Filla, A., & Burks, T. F. (1983). Studies in vivo with dynorphin-(1–9): Analgesia but not gastrointestinal effects following intrathecal administration to mice. *European Journal of Pharmacology, 91*, 291–294.

Powell, D. W. (1981). Muscle or mucosa: The site of action of antidiarrheal opiates? *Gastroenterology, 80*, 406–408.

Quarantotti, B. P., Paglietti, E., Bonanni, A., Petta, M., & Gessa, G. L. (1979). Naloxone shortens ejaculation latency in male rats. *Experientia, 35*, 524–525.

Quigley, M. E., & Yen, S. S. C. (1980). The role of endogenous opiates in LH secretion during the menstrual cycle. *Journal of Clinical Endocrinology and Metabolism, 51*, 179–181.

Ramirez-Gonzalez, M. D., Farsang, C., Tchakarov, L., & Kunos, G. (1982). Opiate antagonists reverse the centrally mediated antihypertensive action of propranolol in spontaneously hypertensive rats. *European Journal of Pharmacology, 81*, 167–170.

Rattan, S., & Goyal, R. K. (1980). Effect of morphine and endogenous opiates on the opossum lower esophageal sphincter. *Gastroenterology, 78*, 1241.

Rattan, S., & Goyal, R. K. (1983). Identification and localization of opioid receptors in the opossum lower esophageal sphincter. *Journal of Pharmacology and Experimental Therapeutics, 224*, 391–398.

Reid, R. (1983). Endogenous opioid activity and the premenstrual syndrome (letter). *Lancet, ii*, 786.

Reid, R. L., & Yen, S. S. C. (1981). Beta-endorphin stimulates the secretion of insulin and glucagon in humans. *Journal of Clinical Endocrinology and Metabolism, 52*, 592–594.

Reisberg, B., Ferris, S. H., Anand, R., Mir, P., Geibel, V., & DeLeon, M. J. (1983). Effects of naloxone in senile dementia: A double-blind trial. *New England Journal of Medicine, 308*, 721–722.

Reynolds, D. G., Gurll, N. J., Vargish, T., Lechner, R., Faden, A. I., & Holaday, J. W. (1980). Blockade of opiate receptors with naloxone improves survival and cardiac performance in canine endotoxic shock. *Circulatory Shock, 7*, 39–48.

Rivier, C., Vale, W., Ling, N., Brown, M., & Guillemin, R. (1977). Stimulation in vivo of the secretion of prolactin and growth hormone by β-endorphin. *Endocrinology, 100*, 238–241.

Roman, C., & Gonella, J. (1981). Extrinsic control of digestive tract motility. In L. R. Johnson (Ed.), *Physiology of the gastrointestinal tract* (pp. 289–333). New York: Raven Press.

Ropert, J. F., Quigley, M. E., & Yen, S. S. C. (1981). Endogenous opiates modulate pulsatile luteinizing hormone release in humans. *Journal of Clinical Endocrinology and Metabolism, 52*, 583–585.

Rosow, C. E., Miller, J. M., Pelikan, E. W., & Cochin, J. (1980). Opiates and thermoregulation in mice. I. Agonists. *Journal of Pharmacology and Experimental Therapeutics, 213*, 273–283.

Roze, C., Dubrasquet,M., Chariot, J., & Vaille, C. (1980). Central inhibition of basal pancreatic and gastric secretions by β-endorphin in rats. *Gastroenterology, 79*, 659–664.

Rubin, P., Blaschke, T. F., & Guilleminault, C. (1981). Effect of naloxone, a specific opioid inhibitor, on blood pressure fall during sleep. *Circulation, 63*, 117–121.

Sanger, D. J., & McCarthy, P. S. (1981). The anorectic effect of naloxone is attenuated by adaptation to a food-deprivation schedule. *Psychopharmacology, 74*, 217–220.

Santen, R. J., & Ruby, E. B. (1979). Enhanced frequency and magnitude of episodic luteinizing hormone discharge as a hypothalamic mechanism for increased luteinizing hormone secretion. *Journal of Clinical Endocrinology and Metabolism, 48*, 315–319.

Santiago, T. V., Remolina, C., Scoles, V., & Edelman, N. H. Endorphins and the control of breathing. Ability of naloxone to restore flow-resistive load compensation in chronic obstructive pulmonary disease. *New England Journal of Medicine, 304*, 1190–1195.

Saxena, R. K., Saxena, Q. B., Adler, W. H. Regulation of natural killer activity in vivo: Part I— Loss of natural killer activity during starvation. *Indian Journal of Experimental Biology, 18*, 1383–1386.

Schaz, K., Stock, G., Simon, W., Schlor, K.-H., Unger, T., Rockhold, R., & Ganten, D. (1980). Enkephalin effects on blood pressure, heart rate and baroreceptor reflex. *Hypertension, 2*, 395–407.

Schultzberg, M., Hokfelt, T., Lundberg, J. M., Terenius, L., Elfvin, L.-G., & Elde, R. (1978a). Enkephalin-like immunoreactivity in nerve terminals in sympathetic ganglia and adrenal medulla and in adrenal medullary gland cells. *Acta Physiologica Scandinavica, 103*, 475–477.

Schultzberg, M., Hokfelt, T., Nilsson, G., Terenius, L., Rehfeld, J. F., Brown, M., Elde, R., Goldstein, M., & Said, S. (1980). Distribution of peptide and catecholamine containing neurons in the gastrointestinal tract of rat and guinea-pig: Immunohistochemical studies with antisera to Substance P, vasoactive intestinal polypeptide, enkephalins, somatostatin, gastrin/cholecystokinin, neurotensin and dopamine beta-hydroxylase. *Neuroscience, 5*, 689–744.

Schultzberg, M., Hokfelt, T., Terenius, L., Elfvin, L.-G., Lundberg, J. M., Brandt, J., Elde, R. P., & Goldstein, M. (1979). Enkephalin immunoreactive nerve fibers and cell bodies in sympathetic ganglia of the guinea pig and rat. *Neuroscience, 4*, 249–279.

Schultzberg, M., Lundberg, J. M., Hokfelt, T., Terenius, L., Brandt, J., Elde, R. P., & Goldstein, M. (1978b). Enkephalin-like immunoreactivity in gland cells and nerve terminals of the adrenal medulla. *Neuroscience, 3*, 1169–1186.

Schulz, R., Wuster, M., & Herz, A. (1979). Centrally and peripherally mediated inhibition of intestinal motility by opioids. *Naunyn-Schmiedeberg's Archives of Pharmacology, 308*, 255–260.

Schusdziarra, V., Henrichs, I., Holland, A., Klier, M., & Pfeiffer, E. F. (1981). Evidence for an effect of exorphins on plasma insulin and glucagon levels in dogs. *Diabetes, 30*, 362–364.

Shaar, C. J., Frederickson, R. C. A., Dininger, N. B., & Jackson, L. (1977). Enkephalin analogues and naloxone modulate the release of growth hormone and prolactin—evidence for regulation by an endogenous opioid peptide in brain. *Life Science, 21*, 853–860.

Shavit, Y., Lewis, J. W., Terman, G. W., Gale, R. P., & Liebeskind, J. C. (1984). Opioid peptides mediate the suppressive effect of stress on natural killer cell cytotoxicity. *Science, 223*, 188–190.

Shea-Donohue, P. T., Adams, N., Arnold, J., & Dubois, A. (1983). Effects of met-enkephalin and naloxone on gastric emptying and secretion in rhesus monkeys. *American Journal of Physiology, 245*, G196–G200.

Shimonura, Y., Oku, J., Glick, Z., & Bray, G. A. (1982). Opiate receptors, food intake and obesity. *Physiological Behavior, 28*, 441–443.

Sloan, J. W., Brooks, J. W., Eisenman, A. J., & Martin, W. R. (1962). Comparison of the effects of single doses of morphine and thebaine on body temperature, activity and brain and heart levels of catecholamines and serotonin. *Psychopharmacologia, 3*, 291–301.

Sowell, J. G., Bowen, S. R., & Carpenter, F. G. (1979). Hyperventilation in rats treated with morphine and naloxone. *Federal Proceedings, 38*, 681.

Stanghellini, V., Malagelada, J-R., Zinsmeister, A. R., Go, V. L. W., & Kao, P. C. (1983). Stress-induced gastroduodenal motor disturbances in humans: Possible humoral mechanisms. *Gastroenterology, 85*, 83–91.

Stanghellini, V., Malagelada, J-R., Zinsmeister, A. R., Go. V. L. W., & Kao, P. C. (1984). Effect of opiate and adrenergic blockers on the gut motor response to centrally acting stimuli. *Gastroenterology, 87*, 1104–1113.

Steardo, L., Maj, M., Monteleone, P., Zizolfi, S., Buscino, G. A., & Kemali, D. (1981). Naloxone-induced decrease of plasma prolactin in healthy women. *Acta Neurologica, 36*, 379–383.

Steinbrook, R. A., Feldman, H. A., Fencl, V., Forte, V. A., Jr., Gabel, R. A., Leith, D. E., & Weinberger, S. E. (1984). Naloxone dose not affect ventilatory responses to hypoxia and hypercapnia in rats. *Life Science, 34*, 881–887.

Sullivan, S. N., Lamki, L., & Corcoran, P. (1981). Inhibition of gastric emptying by enkephalin analogue. *Lancet, ii*, 86–87.

Sun, E. A., Snape, W. J., Jr., Cohen, S., & Renny, A. (1982). The role of opiate receptors and cholinergic neurons in the gastrocolonic response. *Gastroenterology, 82*, 689–693.

Szechtman, H., Simantov, R., & Hershkowitz, M. (1981). Sexual behavior decreases pain sensitivity and stimulates endogenous opioids in male rats. *European Journal of Pharmacology, 70*, 279–285.

Tan, L., & Yu, P. H. (1981). De novo biosynthesis of enkephalins and the homologues in the human placenta. *Biochemical and Biophysical Research Communications, 98*, 752–760.

Tepperman, F. S., & Hirst, M. (1983). Effects of intrahypothalamic injection of D-ala^2,D-Leu^5-enkephalin on feeding and temperature in the rat. *European Journal of Pharmacology, 96*, 243–249.

Vargish, T., Reynolds, D. G., Gurll, N. J., Lechner, R. J., Holaday, J. W., & Faden, A. I. (1980). Naloxone reversal of hypovolemic shock in dogs. *Circulatory Shock, 7*, 31–38.

Vincent, S. R., Hokfelt, T., Christensson, I., & Terenius, L. (1982). Dynorphin-immunoreactive neurons in the central neurons system of the rat. *Neuroscience Letters, 35*, 185–190.

Volavka, J., Bauman, J., Pevnick, J., Reker, D., James, B., & Cho, D. (1980). Short-term hormonal effects of naloxone in man. *Psychoneurendocrinology, 5*, 225–234.

Ward, S. J., Metcalf, G., & Rees, J. M. H. (1977). The comparative pharmacology of morphine, ketocyclazocine and 2-hydroxy-5,9-dimethyl-2-allyl-6,7-benzomorphan in rodents. *Journal of Pharmacy and Pharmacology, 29*, 54P.

Watson, S. J., Akil, H., Fischli, A., Goldstein, A., Zimmerman, E., Nilaver, G., & van Wimersma Greidanus, T. B. (1982a). Dynorphin and vasopressin: Common localization in magnocellular neurons. *Science, 216*, 85–87.

Watson, S. J., Akil, H., Ghazarossian, V. E., & Goldstein, A. (1981). Dynorphin immunocytochemical localization in brain and peripheral nervous system: Preliminary studies. *Proceedings of the National Academy of Science, USA, 78*, 1260–1263.

Watson, S. J., Akil, H., Richard, C. W., & Barchas, J. D. (1978a). Evidence for two separate opiate peptide neuronal systems and the coexistence of beta-LPH, beta-endorphin and ACTH immunoreactivities in the same hypothalamic neurons. *Nature, 275*, 226–228.

Watson, S. J., Barchas, J. D., & Li, C. H. (1977). Beta-LPH: Localization of cells and axons in rat brain by immunocytochemistry. *Proceedings of the National Academy of Science, USA, 74*, 5155–5158.

Watson, S. J., Khachaturian, H., Akil, H., Coy, D., & Goldstein, A. (1982b). Comparison of the distribution of dynorphin systems and enkephalin systems in brain. *Science, 218*, 1134–1136.

Watson, S. J., Richard, C. W., & Barchas, J. D. (1978b). Adrenocorticotropin in rat brain: Immunocytochemical localization in cells and axons. *Science, 200*, 1180–1182.

Wei, E. T., Lee, A., & Chang, J. K. (1980). Cardiovascular effects of peptides related to enkephalins and beta-casomorphin. *Life Science, 26*, 1517–1522.

Whalen, R. E. (1961). Effects of mounting without intromission and intromission without ejaculation on sexual behavior and maze learning. *Journal of Comparative Physiology and Psychology, 4*, 405–415.

Wood, J. D. (1980). Intracellular study of effects of morphine on electrical activity of myenteric neurones in cat small intestine. *Gastroenterology, 79*, 1222–1230.

Wright, D. J. M., & Weller, M. D. I. (1980). Inhibition of naloxone by endotoxin-induced reactions in mice. *British Journal of Pharmacology, 70*, 99P.

Wybran, J., Appelboom, T., Famaey, J. P., & Gavaerts, A. (1979). Suggestive evidence of receptors for morphine and methionine-enkephalin on normal human blood lymphocytes. *Journal of Immunology, 123*, 1068–1070.

Yamaguchi, I., Fuke, H., & Tusjta, M. (1978). Relationship between gastric secretion and serum gastrin levels in dogs anesthetized with morphine and urethane. *Japanese Journal of Pharmacology, 28*, 521–526.

Yukimura, T., Stock, G., Stumpf, H., Unger, T., & Ganten, D. (1981). Effects of (D-ala^2)-methionine enkephalin on blood pressure, heart rate and baroreceptor sensitivity in conscious cats. *Hypertension, 3*, 528–533.

Zagon, I. S., & McLaughlin, P. J. (1981). Heroin prolongs survival time and retards tumor growth in mice with neuroblastoma. *Brain Research Bulletin, 7*, 25–32.

Zagon, I. S., & McLaughlin, P. J. (1983). Naltrexone modulates tumor response in mice with neuroblastoma. *Science, 221*, 671–673.

Zanoboni, A., Zecca, L., Zanussi, C., & Zanoboni-Muciaccia, W. (1981). Naloxone and anterior pituitary hormone effect on TRH stimulation test. *Neuroendocrinology, 33*, 140–143.

Zelis, R., Mansour, E. J., Capone, R. J. & Mason, D. T. (1974). The cardiovascular effects of morphine. *Journal of Clinical Investigation, 54*, 1247–1258.

Zioudrou, C., Streaty, R. A., & Klee, W. A. (1979). Opioid peptides derived from food proteins: The exorphins. *Journal of Biological Chemistry, 254*, 2446–2449.

Zobrist, R. H., Allerton, H. W., & Isom, G. E. (1981). Characterization of the respiratory activity of (D-Ala^2)methionine-enkephalinamide. *European Journal of Pharmacology, 70*, 121–128.

6

CENTRAL NERVOUS SYSTEM ACTION OF NEUROPEPTIDES TO INDUCE OR PREVENT EXPERIMENTAL GASTRODUODENAL ULCERATIONS

Yvette Taché
School of Medicine
University of California

BRAIN DAMAGE AND GASTRIC PATHOGENESIS

The existence of a relationship between the central nervous system (CNS) and gastric pathology has been suspected since the end of the last century (Brown-Sequard, 1876). In 1932, Cushing described ulcerations and perforations of the stomach and duodenum in patients with intracranial disease. During the last decades, through the advancement of stereotaxic procedures and the use of electrical stimulations or lesions, several neuroanatomic sites have been implicated as playing a role in the development of gastroduodenal ulcerations (Grijalva, Lindholm, & Novin, 1980). Table 1 lists the reported influence of electrolytic brain damage on the production of gastric pathology in various animal species. Cortical lesions in the entorhinal or posterior cingulate cortex or in the hippocampus induced the formation of gastric pathology in unrestrained rats. Lesions of the anterior cingulate cortex or complete ablation of the neocortex produced negligible amounts of gastric mucosal alterations (Henke & Savoie, 1982; Henke, Savoie, & Callahan, 1981; Schallert, Whishaw, & Flannigan, 1977). Lesions of the anterior hypothalamus or preoptic area produced acute gastric mucosal hemorrhages, while lesions placed in the posterior, lateral, and ventromedial hypothalamus are associated with gastric ulcers in rats, cats, or guinea pigs (French, Porter, von Amerongen, & Raney, 1952; Kim et al., 1976; Lindholm, Shumway, Grijalva, Schallert, & Ruppel, 1975; Long, Leonard, Chou, & French, 1962; Luparello, 1967; Maire & Patton, 1956; Schallert et al., 1977). Posterior lateral lesions of the amygdala increased the severity of gastric damage in stressed rats, whereas amygdala lesions placed anteromedially produced opposite effects (Henke, 1979). In the brain stem, median and dorsal raphé nuclei lesions elicited

TABLE 6.1
Electrolytic Brain Lesions and Gastric Pathology

| Brain Sites | Species | Gastric Pathology | | References |
		Hemorr-hages	Ulcers	
Cortex				
Neocortex	rat	0	0	Schallert et al., 1977
Entorhinal	rat	+	+	Henke et al., 1981
Anterior cingulate	rat	0	0	Henke & Savoie, 1982
Posterior cingulate	rat	+	+	Henke & Savoie, 1982
Limbic system				
Hippocampus	rat	+	+	Kim et al., 1976
Amygdala posterolateral	rat	+	+	Henke, 1979
Amygdala ventromedial	rat	0	0	Henke, 1979
Thalamus				
Lateral	rat	0	0	Lindholme et al., 1975
Hypothalamus				
Anterior	cat, guinea pig, rat	+	0	Grijalva et al., 1980
Preoptic area	cat, rat	+	0	Grijalva et al., 1980
Lateral	cat, rat	+	+	Grijalva et al., 1980
Ventromedial	cat, guinea pig	+	+	Grijalva et al., 1980
Brain stem				
Subtantia nigra	rat	0	0	Schallert et al., 1979
Raphé nuclei	rat	+	+	Hoshino et al., 1980

gastric ulcers similar to stress (Hoshino, Moura, Menezes, Capelari, & Valas Boas, 1980). Lesions placed in the substantia nigra have no effect (Schallert et al., 1977).

Whereas these studies revealed the relationships between specific brain structures and ulcer production, little was known regarding the biochemical signals acting on these brain sites to trigger gastric pathology or to influence experimental stress ulcerations (Osumi, Muramatsu, & Fujiwara, 1977).

BRAIN NEUROPEPTIDES

During the last decades, over 50 neuropeptides have been identified in the brain, mostly in the hypothalamus. They have been either structurally sequenced from purified brain extracts or immunologically detected based on peptides previously characterized elsewhere in vertebrate tissues (gastrointestinal tract, pituitary, or thyroid glands; Krieger, 1983). Table 6.2 lists the major categories of brain peptides described to date. Structurally sequenced peptides included hypothalamic-releasing hormones, neurohypophyseal hormones, opioid peptides, and a number of other peptides (bradykinin, angiotensin II, substance P, neurotensin, CCK 8, VIP, PHI, NPY, hydra head activator, and CGRP). Peptides demonstrated to be present using techniques of radioimmunoassay and immunohistochemistry included gastrointestinal and pituitary peptides and calcitonin. These

TABLE 6.2
Mammalian Brain Peptides

A. Sequenced Neuropeptides

Releasing Factors	*Others*
Thyrotropin-releasing hormone (TRH)	Bradykinin
Gonadotropin-releasing hormone (LHRH)	Carnosine
Somatostatin 14, 25, 28	Angiotensin II
Corticotropin-releasing factor (CRF)	Substance P
Growth hormone-releasing factor (GRF)	Substance K
Hypophyseal Hormones	Neurotensin
Vasopressin	Cholecystokinin 8 (CCK-8)
Oxytocin	Vasoactive Intestinal Peptide (VIP)
Neurophysins	PHI active
Melanocyte-stimulating hormones	Neuropeptide Y (NPY)
	Hydra Head Activator
Opioid Peptides	Calcitonin Gene-Related Peptide (CGRP)
β-endorphin	Neuromedin K
Enkephalins (leu or met)	Neuromedin L
Dynorphin	Cerebelline
Metorphamides	Galanin
FMRF amides	

B. Immunohistochemically Demonstrated Neuropeptides

Gastrointestinal Peptides	*Others*
Bombesin	Calcitonin
Motilin	Atrial Natriuretic Peptide
Secretin	Ranatensin
Gastrin	Insulin Growth Factor II (IGFII)
Gastric Inhibitory Peptide (GIP)	Epidermal Growth Factor (EGF)
Glucagon	
Insulin	
Pituitary Peptides	
Adrenocorticotropic Hormone (ACTH)	
Luteinizing Hormone (LH)	
Growth Hormone (GH)	
Thyrotropin (TSH)	
Prolactin	

TABLE 6.3
Brain Peptides Injected into the CSF: Influence on the
Development of Gastric Lesions in Stressed Rats

Protective Effects	*Aggravating Effects*
Bombesin (0.1-5 μg)	TRH (1-30 μg)
Calcitonin (0.4 μg)	VIP (30 μg)
Neurotensin (20–30 μg)	
Opioid Peptides (2–20 μg)	
No Effects	
CCK-8 (30 μg)	
Gastrin (30 μg)	
Bradykinin (30 μg)	
Substance P (5–30 μg)	
Somatostatin (5–30 μg)	

neuropeptides have emerged as a new class of brain chemical transmitters and have been demonstrated to produce marked effects on several homeostatic systems (Zadina, Banks & Kastin, 1986).

In 1979, two peptides, β-endorphin and bombesin, were found to prevent gastric lesions when injected into the cerebrospinal fluid (CSF) of rats exposed to cold-restraint stress (Taché, Simard, & Collu, 1979). Since then, growing evidence indicates that specific neuropeptides act within the brain to prevent or induce gastric pathology and to alter gastric secretory and motor functions (Table 6.3).

CNS ACTION OF NEUROPEPTIDES
TO PREVENT GASTRIC DUODENAL ULCERATIONS

Bombesin

The tetradecapeptide was originally isolated from the skin of the frog *Bombina bombina*. The mammalian counterpart, a 27-amino acid isolated from porcine gut, shares a C-terminal decapeptide homology with bombesin except that Glu-His are interchanged in position 7 (McDonald et al., 1979). The distribution of bombesin-like peptides and their specific receptors have been mapped in the brain and the spinal cord of various animal species (Moody, Thoa, O'Donohue, & Jacobowitz, 1981; Panula, Yang, & Costa, 1982; Pert, Moody, Pert, Dewald, & Rivier, 1980).

As mentioned previously, bombesin was the first peptide reported to act within the brain to influence the development of stress-induced gastric erosion in rats.

Intracerebreventricular or intracisternal injection of bombesin markedly suppressed both the incidence and the severity of hemorrhagic lesions elicited by one hour or three hours of restraint in the cold (Hernandez, Nemeroff, Orlando, & Prange, 1983; Taché et al., 1979). Bombesin given intravenously is much less potent, suggesting a central action (Figure 1). The protective effect of intracerebroventricular bombesin was shown to be dose related (0.1–5 μg) and independent of an interaction with opiate receptors or changes in core temperature (Taché et al., 1979). Bombesin also offered protection against experimental duodenal ulcers: The peptide given intracisternally (0.1–10 μg) but not intravenously (100 μg/kg) dose-dependently reduced the incidence of duodenal ulcerations induced by cysteamine in rats (Hernandez, Adcock, Nemeroff, & Prange, 1982).

The mechanisms through which bombesin instilled into the CSF prevented the formation of experimental gastric and duodenal lesions could involve changes in gastric secretions and motility. Intracisternal injection of bombesin in doses ranging from 10 ng to 1 μg dose-dependently suppressed gastric acid and pepsin secretion, increased gastric mucus and bicarbonate secretion, and delayed gastric emptying (Dubrasquet, Rozé, Ling, & Florencio, 1982; Hernandez et al., 1982; Porreca & Burks, 1983; Taché, 1982; Taché et al 1980b; Taché, Brown, & Collu, 1981;1982).

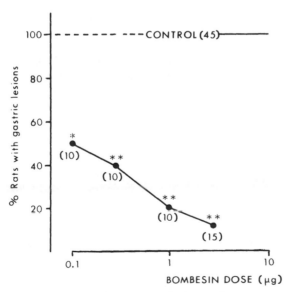

FIGURE 6.1 Dose-dependent inhibition of gastric hemorrhagic lesions induced by bombesin given intracerebroventricularly before exposing rats to cold (4° C) restraint stress for one hour.

Opioid Peptides

The brain contains at least three anatomically separated neuronal networks of opioid peptides: an enkephalin, a β-endorphin, and a dynorphin family which act on distinct types of receptors (δ, μ, k; Watson, Khachaturian, Akil, Coy, & Goldstein, 1982; Wood, 1982).

β-endorphin (0.5–5 μg) injected intracerebroventricularly dose-dependently reduced gastric lesions elicited by one-hour exposure to cold restraint stress (Taché et al., 1979). Higher doses (10–70 μg) exerted a protective effect against stress ulcers, but not in a dose-dependent manner (Hernandez et al., 1983).

Enkephalins (met or leu) given intracisternally (30 μg) did not modify gastric ulcers induced by three-hour cold-restraint stress (Hernandez et al., 1983). Stable enkephalin analogs such as [D-Ala^2,N-Met-Phe^4,-Met-(0)^5-ol])-enkephalin (1–2 μg) or [D-Ala^2]-Met-enkephalinamide (20 μg) injected intracerebroventricularly in rats significantly reduced the incidence of gastric lesions induced by two to three hours of cold-restraint stress. The protective effect was reversed by naloxone (Ferri et al., 1983; Morley, Levine, & Silvis, 1982).

Although the mechanisms of their protective action remain to be determined, opioid peptides injected into the CSF markedly inhibited gastric acid secretion (Ferri et al., 1983; Morley et al., 1982; Rozé, Dubrasquet, Chariot, & Vaille, 1980; Taché et al., 1980).

Calcitonin

Intracisternal injection of calcitonin (0.4 ug) prevented gastric erosions induced by cold-restraint stress. The lack of mucosal lesions in rats treated with calcitonin is correlated with an increase in gastric pH values (Morley, Levine, & Silvis, 1981).

High-affinity binding sites for calcitonin have been described and localized in various brain areas by autoradiography (Rizzo & Goltzman, 1981), and immunoreactive calcitonin has been found in the hypothalamus and CSF (Becker et al., 1983). However, a recent report indicates that immunoreactive calcitonin mRNA and calcitonin are not detected in rat brain and pituitary (Rosenfeld et al., 1983). Obviously more information on the characterization of endogenous ligand for calcitonin receptors in the brain is needed.

Neurotensin

This tridecapeptide was isolated from the mammalian hypothalamus and, like other neuropeptides, was shown to possess a characteristic regional distribution with a highly individual neuronal circuitry in hypothalamic and extrahypothalamic structures (Uhl, Kuhar, & Snyder, 1977; Yound & Kuhar, 1981).

Intracisternal (30 μg) but not intravenous (100 μg/kg) injection of the peptide prevented the formation of gastric ulcers elicited by three hours of cold-restraint stress in rats (Nemeroff, Hernandez, Orlando, & Prange, 1982). Peptide action was shown to be dose dependent in doses ranging from 10 to 30 μg, whereas lower doses were ineffective (Hernandez et al., 1983; Nemeroff et al., 1982; Taché et al., 1979). Unlike bombesin, neurotensin (1–30 μg) given intracisternally did not prevent duodenal ulceration induced by cisteamine (Hernandez et al., 1982). The mechanisms responsible for the protective action appear to be unrelated to the effects of the peptide on thermoregulation (Nemeroff et al., 1982). Neurotensin did not significantly change gastric pH in stressed animals, and intraperitoneal injection of the H_2-receptor blocker, cimetidine, which raised gastric pH in stressed rats, failed to decrease significantly the incidence of gastric pathology (Nemeroff et al., 1982). The protective effect of neurotensin was abolished by pretreatment with inhibitors of prostaglandin synthesis, aspirin, and indomethacin and by blocking of dopamine receptors with haloperidol. These data suggest that neurotensin protective action is not related to changes in gastric acid secretion and is dependent on functional gastrointestinal prostaglandin synthetic pathways, as well as brain dopaminergic systems (Adcock et al., 1983; Hernandez, Stanley, Melvin, & Prange, 1985).

CENTRAL NERVOUS SYSTEM ACTION OF NEUROPEPTIDES TO PRODUCE GASTRIC ULCERATION

Two neuropeptides, thyrotropin-releasing hormone (TRH) and vasointestinal peptide (VIP), have been reported to produce gastric lesions or to aggravate experimental gastric erosions.

TRH

Intracisternal injection of TRH (0.1–1 μg) or a stable TRH analog, RX 77368, (3,3-dimethyl-pro)-TRH (0.01–0.1 μg) induced gastric hemorrhagic lesions in 24-hour-fasted, conscious rats maintained at room temperature (Goto & Taché, 1985). Gastric erosions developed in the corpus and the antrum within four hours following peptide injection. TRH action is mediated by the central nervous system because the intravenous injection of the peptide at doses 25 times greater had no effect (Goto & Taché, 1985). Experiments on the effects of intracerebroventricularly administered TRH on various experimental gastric lesions indicate that TRH (3–10 μg) aggravated indomethacin-, serotonin-, and to a lesser degree, aspirin-induced gastric ulcers (Maeda-Hagiwara, Watanabe, & Watanabe, 1983). TRH given intracisternally in doses ranging from 10 to 30 μg enhanced cold-restraint-induced gastric erosions (Hernandez et al., 1983). Lower doses given intracerebroventricularly (5, 10 μg) did not alter the development of stress-induced ulcers (Maeda-Hagiwara et al., 1983; Taché et al., 1979).

The mechanisms by which injection of TRH or TRH analogues injected into the CSF promote gastric lesions could involve increases in the activity of the parasympathetic nervous system to alter gastric function. TRH or RX 77368 given intracisternally stimulated vagal efferent activity recorded by platinum electrodes attached to bundles of the cervical vagus (Taché et al., 1985) to produce cholinergic discharge and an increase in gastrointestinal motor activity and gastric acid and pepsin secretion (Lahann & Horita, 1982; Taché et al., 1980a; Taché, Goto, Lauffenburger, & Lesiege, 1984). Gastric lesions produced by TRH probably result from the integrated stimulatory effects of the peptide on both gastric secretory and motor function. This is suggested by the fact that neither bethanechol nor histamine given at secretory doses affect the gastric mucosa. Moreover, a low dose of atropine which suppressed TRH-stimulated gastric acid secretion did not prevent the potentiating effect of TRH on indomethacin ulcers (Maeda-Hagiwara et al., 1983).

Although the physiological significance of these findings remains to be established, it is tempting to speculate that TRH may play a role in the pathogenesis of certain types of experimentally induced gastric ulcers. In support of this possibility the facts are that high concentrations of TRH immunoreactivity and specific receptors are present in the hypothalamus and the nuclei of vagus complex (Kubek, Rea, Hodes, & Aprison, 1983; Sharif & Burt, 1983) and that the endogenous release of TRH in the brain elicited by cold (Arancibia, Tapia-Arancibia, Assenmacher, & Astier, 1983) is associated with rapid and enhanced formation of gastric hemorrhagic lesions in restrained rats (Senay & Levine, 1967).

VIP

Intracisternal injection of VIP (30 μg) has been reported to significantly increase the severity of gastric ulceration in cold-restrained rats (Hernandez et al., 1983). The mechanism of its action is unknown. The peptide injected intracisternally (1–10 μg) did not modify gastric acid secretion in pylorus-ligated rats (Taché, unpublished observation).

PEPTIDES FOUND INACTIVE TO INFLUENCE GASTRIC MUCOSA

Corticotropin-releasing factor (CRF) or growth hormone releasing factor (GRF) given intracisternally in a 10 μg dose did not affect the gastric mucosa in unstressed rats (Goto & Taché, 1984). Substance P, somatostatin, cholecystokinin (CCK-8), gastrin, or bradykinin administered intracisternally in 5–30 μg doses did not modify the severity of gastric erosions induced by restraint and cold (Hernandez et al., 1983; Nemeroff et al., 1982; Taché et al., 1979).

CONCLUSIONS

From the literature reviewed, it appears that the central nervous system action action of some neuropeptides in producing gastroduodenal lesions is a new subject of considerable interest. Several of these peptides injected into the brain have unique protective or aggravating effects on the development of gastric or duodenal ulceration (Table 3). The previous methods used so far for studying the influence of the brain on gastric mucosal integrity were based exlusively on electrical stimulation or lesions of various brain structures. Such approaches have generated some conflicting data without determining whether the variations were due to differences in species, stimulation parameters, lesion size, or a combination of these variables (Grijalva et al., 1980).

Neuropeptides are new standard probes for studying brain-gut relationships. Moreover, the facts that they produce gastroduodenal ulceration when injected into the CSF and that they are present in the brain, as are their receptors suggest their involvement in the regulation of gastric function in health and disease.

ACKNOWLEDGMENTS

This work was supported by the National Institutes of Health (NIADDK, Grants AM 30110-03, AM 33061-01, and AM 17328-01). S. Heil is gratefully acknowledged for helping in the preparation of the manuscript.

REFERENCES

Adcock, J., Hernandez, D., Nemeroff, C., & Prange, J. (1983). Effects of prostaglandin synthesis inhibition on neurotensin and sodium salicylates-induced gastric cytoprotection in rats. *Life Science, 32*, 2905–2910.

Arancibia, S., Tapia-Arancibia, L., Assenmacher, I., & Astier, H. (1983). Direct evidence of short-term cold-induced TRH release in the median eminence of unanesthetized rats. *Neuroendocrinology, 37*, 225–228.

Becker, K. L., Silva, O. L., Post, R. N., Ballenger, J. C., Carmen, J. S., Snider, R. H., Moore, D. F. (1980). Immunoreactive calcitonin in cerebrospinal fluid of man. *Brain Research, 194*, 598–602.

Brown-Sequard, C. E. (1876). Des alterations qui surviennent dans la muqueuse de l'estomac, consecutivement aux lesions cerebrales. *Progr. Med. Paris, 4*, 136–137.

Cushing, H. (1932). Peptic ulcers and the interbrain. *Surgery Gynecology & Obstetrics, 55*, 1–34.

Dubrasquet, M., Roze, C., Ling, N., & Florencio, H. (1982). Inhibition of gastric and pancreatic secretions by cerebroventricular injections of gastrin-releasing peptide and bombesin in rats. *Regulatory Peptides, 3,* 105–112.

Ferri, S., Arrigo-Reina, R., Candeletti, S., Costa, F., Murari, G., Speroni, E., & Scoto, G. (1983). Central and peripheral sites of action for the protective effect of opioids of the rat stomach. *Pharmacological Research Communication, 15,* 409–419.

French, J. D., Porter, R. W., von Amerongen, F. K., & Raney, R. B. (1952). Gastrointestinal hemorrhage and ulceration associated with intracranial lesions. A clinical and experimental study. *Surgery, 32,* 395–407.

Grijalva, C., Lindholm, E., & Novin, D. (1980). Physiological and morphological changes in the gastrointestinal tract induced by hypothalamic intervention: An overview. *Brain Research Bulletin, 5*(Suppl. 1), 19–31.

Henke, P. (1979). The hypothalamus-amygdala axis and experimental gastric ulcers. *Neuroscience Biobehavioral Review, 3,* 75–82.

Henke, P., & Savoie, R. (1982). The cingulate cortex and gastric pathology. *Brain Research Bulletin, 8,* 489–492.

Henke, P., Savoie, R. J., & Callahan, B. M. (1981). Hippocampal deafferentation and deefferentation and gastric pathology in rats. *Brain Research Bulletin, 7,* 395–398.

Hernandez, D., Adcock, J., Nemeroff, C., & Prange, A. (1982). The effect of intracisternally administered bombesin on cysteamine-induced duodenal ulcers in rats. *European Journal of Pharmacology, 84,* 205–209.

Hernandez, D., Nemeroff, C., Orlando, R., & Prange, A. (1983). The effect of centrally administered neuropeptides on the development of stress-induced gastric ulcers in rats. *Journal of Neuroscience Research, 9,* 145–157.

Hernandez, D. E., Stanley, D. A., & Melvin, J. A., Prange, A. J. (1985). Role of brain neurotransmitters on neurotensin-induced gastric cytoprotection. *Pharmacology Biochemistry and Behavior, 22,* 509–513.

Hoshino, K., Moura, J. L., Menezes, C. E., Capelari, J., & Valas Boas, M. (1980). Vagotomy and adrenalectomy effects on the gastric ulcers induced by the raphé nuclei lesion in the rat. *Rev Cienc Biomed, 1,* 79–88.

Kim, C. H., Choi, H., Kim, J. K., Kim, M. S., Parke, J., Ahn, B. T., & Kang, S. H. (1976). Influence of hippocampectomy on gastric ulcer in rats. *Brain Research, 109,* 245–254.

Krieger, D. T. (1983). Brain peptides: What, where and why? *Science, 222,* 975–984.

Kubek, M., Rea, M., Hodes, Z., Aprison, M. (1983). Quantitation and characterization of thyrotropin-releasing hormone in vagal nuclei and other regions of the medulla oblongata of the rat. *Journal of Neurochemistry, 40,* 1307–1313.

Lahann, T. R., & Horita. A. (1982). Thyrotropin releasing hormone; centrally mediated effects on gastrointestinal motor activity. *Journal Pharmacology Experimental Therapeutics, 222,* 66–70.

Lindholm, E., Shumway, G. S., Grijalva, C. V., Schallert, T., & Ruppel, M. (1975). Gastric pathology produced by hypothalamic lesions in rats. *Physiological Behavior, 14,* 165–169.

Long, D. M., Leonard, A. S., Chou, S. N., & French, L. A. (1962). Hypothalamus and gastric ulceration. Gastric effects of hypothalamic lesions. *Archives of Neurology, 7,* 13–21.

Luparello, T. J. (1967). Neurogenic gastroduodenal erosions in the guinea pig. *Journal of Psychosomatic Research, 11,* 299–306.

Maeda-Hagiwara, M., Watanabe, H., & Watanabe, K. (1983). Enhancement by intracerebroventricular thyrotropin-releasing hormone of indomethacin-induced gastric lesions in the rat. *British Journal of Pharmacology, 80,* 735–739.

Maire, F. W. & Patton, H. D. (1956). Neural structures involved in the genesis of preoptic pulmonary edema, gastric erosions and behavior changes. *American Journal of Physiology, 184,* 345–350.

McDonald, T. J. Jörnall, H., Nilsson, G., Vagne, M., Ghatei, M., Bloom, S. R., and Mutt, V. (1979). Characterization of a gastrin-releasing peptide from porcine non-antral gastric tissue. *Biochemical Biophysical Research Communications, 90,* 227–233.

Moody, T., Thoa, N., O'Donohue, T., & Jacobowitz, D. (1981). Bombesin-like peptides in rat spinal cord: Biochemical characterization, localization and mechanism of release. *Life Science, 29,* 2273–2279.

Morley, J., Levine, A., & Silvis, S. (1981). Intraventricular calcitonin inhibites gastric acid secretion. *Science, 214,* 671–673.

Morley, J., Levine, A., & Silvis, S. (1982). Endogenous opiates and stress ulceration. *Life Science, 31,* 693–699.

Nemeroff, C., Hernandez, D. E., Orlando, R. C., & Prange, A. (1982). Cytoprotective effect of centrally administered neurotensin on stress-induced gastric ulcers. *American Journal of Physiology, 242,* G342–G346.

Osumi, Y., Muramatsu, I., & Fujiwara, M. (1977). The effects of destruction of noradrenergic ascending ventral bundles and tetrabenazine on formation of stress induced gastric ulcer. *European Journal of Pharmacology, 41,* 47–51.

Panula, P., Yang, H., & Costa, E. (1982). Neuronal location of the bombesin-like immunoreactivity in the central nervous system of the rat. *Regulatory Peptides, 4,* 275–283.

Pert, A., Moody, T., Pert, C., Dewald, I., & Rivier, J. (1980). Bombesin: Receptor distribution in brain and effects on nociception and locomotor activity. *Brain Research, 193,* 209–220.

Porreca, F., & Burks, T. (1983). Centrally administered bombesin affects gastric emptying and small and large bowel transit in the rat. *Gastroenterology, 85,* 313–317.

Rizzo, A., & Goltzman, D. (1981). Calcitonin receptors in the central nervous system of the rat. *Endocrinology, 108,* 1672–1677.

Rosenfeld, M. G., Mermod, J. J., Amara, S. G., Swanson, L. W., Sawchenko, P. E., Rivier, J., Vale, W., & Evans, R. (1983). Production of a novel neuropeptide encoded by calcitonin gene via tissue-specific RNA processing. *Nature, 304,* 129–135.

Roze, C., Dubrasquet, M., Chariot, J., & Vaille, C. (1980). Central inhibition of basal pancreatic and gastric secretion by beta-endorphin in rats. *Gastroenterology, 79,* 659–664.

Schallert, T., Whishaw, I. Q., & Flannigan, K. P. (1977). Gastric pathology and feeding deficits induced by hypothalamic damage in rats: Effects of lesion type, size and placement. *Journal Comparative Physiology Psychology, 91,* 598–610.

Senay, E., & Levine, R. (1967). Synergism between cold and restraint for rapid production of stress ulcers in rats. *Proceedings Society Experimental Biology Medicine, 124,* 1221–1223.

Sharif, N. A., & Burt, D. R. (1983). Biochemical similarity of rat pituitary and CNS TRH receptors. *Neuroscience Letters, 39,* 57–64.

Taché, Y. (1982). Bombesin: Central nervous system action to increase gastric mucus in rats. *Gastroenterology, 83,* 75–80.

Taché, Y., Brown, M., Collu, R., (1981). Central nervous system actions of bombesin-like peptides. In R. Collu, J. R. Ducharme, A. Barbeau, & F. Tolis (Eds.), *Brain neurotransmitters and hormones* (pp. 183–196). New York: Raven Press.

Taché, Y., Goto, Y., Lauffenburger, M., & Lesiege, D. (1984). Potent central nervous system action of p-Glu-His-(3,3'-dimethyl)-Pro-NH₂, a stabilized analog of TRH, to stimulate gastric secretion in rats. *Regulatory Peptides, 8,* 71–78.

Taché, Y., Goto, Y., Hamel, D., Pekary, A., & Novin, D. (1985). Mechanisms underlying intracisternal thyrotropin-releasing hormone induced stimulation of gastric secretion in rats. *Regulatory Peptides 13:* 21–30.

Taché, Y., Simard, P., & Collu, R. (1979). Protection by bombesin of cold-restraint stress induced hemorrhagic lesions in rats. *Life Science, 24,* 1719–1726.

Taché, Y., & Vale, W., Brown, M. (1980a). Thyrotropin-releasing hormone: Central nervous system action to stimulate gastric acid secretion. *Nature, 287,* 149–151.

Taché, Y., Vale, W., Rivier, J., & Brown, M. (1980b). Brain regulation of gastric secretion influence of neuropeptides. *Proceedings National Academy Sciences USA, 77,* 5515–5519.

Uhl, B. R., Kuhar, M. J., & Snyder, S. H. (1977). Neurotensin: Immunohistochemical localization in rat central nervous system. *Proceedings National Academy Science USA, 74,* 4059–4063.

Watson, S., Khachaturian, H., Akil, H., Coy, D., & Goldstein, A. (1982). Comparison of the distribution of dynorphin systems and enkephalin system in brain. *Science, 218,* 1134–1136.

Wood, P. (1982). Multiple opiate receptors: Support for unique mu, delta and kappa sites. *Neuropharmacology, 21,* 487–498.

Yound, W. S., & Kuhar, M. J. (1981). Neurotensin receptor localization by light microscopic autoradiography in rat brain. *Brain Research, 206,* 273–285.

Zadina, J. E., Banks, W. A., & Kastin, A. J. (1986). Central Nervous system effects of peptides, 1980–1985: A cross-listing of peptides and their central actions from the first six years of the journal. *Peptides, 7,* 497–537.

7

OPIOID, α_2-NORADRENERGIC AND ADRENOCORTICOTROPIN SYSTEMS OF HYPOTHALAMIC PARAVENTRICULAR NUCLEUS

Sarah Fryer Leibowitz
The Rockefeller University

The discovery of endogenous opioid peptides has inspired extensive investigation into the function of these substances in the control of physiological and behavioral processes. Studies to date have demonstrated diverse effects, with opiate stimulants and antagonists, on a variety of autonomic-metabolic phenomena, including cardiovascular and respiratory responses, temperature control, and glucose metabolism; on basic consummatory behaviors, including eating, drinking, and sexual responses; on nociception; and on more complex emotional, social, and learning behaviors (Henry, 1982; Leibowitz, 1986; Margules, 1979a; Morley, Levine, Yim, & Lowy, 1983; Olson, Olson, & Kastin, 1984; Sanger, 1981). Although important questions still exist as to whether these effects have physiological significance, evidence is accumulating in support of the idea that endogenous opioids may have important functions as mediators of various physiological processes involved in the maintenance of bodily homeostasis, particularly under unstable and unpredictable environmental conditions. These opioid functions appear to manifest themselves, at least in part, through their interaction with the various monoamine neurotransmitters, as well as through other neuropeptide-neuroendocrine systems.

The focus of the present review is on hypothalamic endorphinergic systems, their role in the control of eating behavior, and their relation to α_2-noradrenergic and adrenocorticotropic systems of the hypothalamus. The nature of these systems' interaction in appetite control is also discussed in relation to other related phenomena, such as reward, stress, and nociception. The proposed hypotheses state that: (a) Endorphinergic receptor mechanisms within the hypothalamus in response to energy expenditure have a role in regulating certain behavioral and physiological responses that are adaptive in repleting energy stores; (b) One hypothalamic site specifically involved in this process is the paraventricular nucleus (PVN) in the anteromedial region of the hypothalamus; (c) The opioids, particularly in their control of eating behavior, may under certain conditions induce their effects in close conjunction with or through a PVN α_2-noradrenergic receptor system. However, under different circumstances, the opioids may also work independently of this α_2-noradrenergic circuit, acting through other hypothalamic and possibly extra-hypothalamic structures; (d) The full expression of these PVN opiate-α_2-noradrenergic effects depends, in part, on the functional integrity of the PVN-adrenocorticotropin (ACTH)-adrenal cortex axis; (e) The potentiating effect of opioids and norepinephrine (NE) on food intake involves homeostatic mechanisms controlling appetite for specific macronutrients and also possibly hedonic mechanisms determining the rewarding properties of food; and (f) Specific conditions during which the PVN neurochemical systems become activated include acute food deprivation, mild stress, and the active period of the diurnal cycle, specifically the early phase when food-seeking behavior and ingestion are most pronounced. For nocturnal animals, such as the rat, this would be during the first few hours of the dark period.

Each of these conditions has in common the fact that energy stores of the body are at risk of becoming depleted. In order to rapidly and homeostatically replete these energy stores, the brain and body must work together through the release of PVN opiates, NE, and the adrenal glucocorticoids to immediately increase gluconeogenesis and make available energy-rich nutrients. In addition to the metabolically adaptive responses, the animal must initiate physiologically and behaviorally adaptive responses which focus on the procurement of energy from the environment. Such responses may include food seeking and food ingestion; the enhancement of appetite for specific foods; an increase in the rewarding potential of food; and possibly an associated decrease in nociception, to permit greater focus on the process of food procurement. Additional autonomic responses, that may occur during this essential function and that have been associated with the opiates and NE within the hypothalamus, include changes in blood pressure, heart rate, respiration, body temperature, and metabolic rate.

This review will first describe evidence for the function of hypothalamic opiates in the stimulation of eating behavior. It will also summarize findings suggesting a similar function for an α_2-noradrenergic system of the hypothalamus and then examine the possibility that these neurotransmitter mechanisms are closely linked in their process of appetite control. Finally, these regulatory functions, relative to eating behavior, will be discussed in a broader framework to provide greater and more general understanding of how these neurochemical systems operate to meet the body's physiological requirements.

PVN OPIATE SYSTEM

The available evidence appears to be unequivocal in showing that brain opioid systems have a stimulatory effect on food ingestion (Leibowitz, 1986; Morley et al., 1983; Sanger, 1981). This function of the opioids contrasts with that demonstrated for most other neuropeptides (e.g., cholecystokinin, bombesin, and neurotensin), which are known to inhibit eating behavior (Gibbs & Smith, 1984; Leibowitz, 1986; Leibowitz & Stanley, 1986; Stanley, Hoebel, & Leibowitz, 1983). Systematically administered opiate agonists have been shown to enhance feeding in satiated animals, in contrast to systemic injections of the opiate antagonists naloxone and naltrexone which suppress feeding (Leibowitz & Stanley, 1986; Morley et al., 1983; Sanger, 1981). Recent studies have investigated the question of where in the body or brain these opiate drugs may be acting to alter behavior. Several laboratories have now determined that the mediating opiate receptors exist largely within the brain and that the hypothalamus, in particular, may play a key role. Whereas intraventricular administration of the opiate drugs in the rat is effective in modulating feeding (McKay, Kenney, Eden, Williams, & Woods, 1981; Morley & Levine, 1981), hypothalamic injection of these drugs has been shown to be more effective at lower doses (Gosnell, Morley & Levine, 1986; Grandison & Guidotti, 1977; Lanthier, Stanley, & Leibowitz, 1985; Leibowitz & Hor, 1982; McLean & Hoebel, 1983; Stanley, Lanthier, & Leibowitz, 1984; Tepperman, Hirst, & Gowdey, 1981; Woods & Leibowitz, 1985). Extra-hypothalamic sites, including the septum, amygdala, nucleus accumbens, and ventral tegmental are also found to be responsive to opiate stimulation (Lanthier et al., 1985; Mucha & Iversen, 1986; Stanley et al., 1984).

Within the hypothalamus, the PVN has consistently been demonstrated to be a particularly sensitive brain site to both the feeding-stimulatory effects of the opiate agonists and the feeding-suppressive effects of the opiate antagonists. In satiated animals, this nucleus activates food ingestion after local administration of the μ-receptor agonist morphine (Lanthier et al., 1985; McLean and Hoebel, 1983; Woods & Leibowitz, 1985), the κ-receptor agonists dynorphin and MR-2043 (Gosnell et al., 1986; Scott, Jawaharlal, & Hoebel, 1984), and the endogenous opioids β-endorphin (Leibowitz & Hor, 1980, 1982) and enkephalin (McLean & Hoebel, 1983; Stanley et al., 1984; Tepperman & Hirst, 1983). These reports suggest that several subtypes of opiate receptors in the PVN, in particular the μ, δ, κ and possibly ε receptors, may be essential to feeding stimulation. These effects of the opiate agonists are sensitive to blockade by locally administered opiate receptor antagonists (Leibowitz & Hor, 1980, 1982; McLean & Hoebel, 1983; Tepperman et al., 1981; Woods & Leibowitz, 1985), supporting the suggestion that the mediating opiate receptors exist within this region. Furthermore, naloxone injection into the PVN is itself effective in suppressing feeding induced by mild food deprivation (Gosnell et al., 1986; Woods & Leibowitz, 1985), and PVN lesions appear to significantly attenuate (but not abolish) the feeding-stimulatory effect of peripherally administered morphine (Shor-Posner, Azar, Filart, Tempel & Leibowitz, 1986a). Anatomical studies have indicated that the PVN is moderately to densely innervated by various opiate systems (Atweh & Kuhar, 1977; Duka, Schubert, Schubert, Stroiber, & Herz, 1981; Goodman, Snyder, Kuhar, & Young, 1980; Khachaturian et al.,

1982; Khachaturian, Lewis, & Watson, 1983; Pearson, Brandeis, Simon, & Hiller, 1980; Pert, Kuhar, & Snyder, 1975; Simon, 1975; Terenius, 1980). Terminals containing β-endorphin, enkephalins, and dynorphins have been identified, and autoradiographic studies have revealed the existence of μ, δ, and κ receptors. These investigations provide clear anatomical support for the proposed existence of PVN opiate receptor sites involved in energy homeostasis.

It is possible that other brain sites also play a role; however, systematic mapping and lesion studies have yet to be conducted to permit us to draw any firm conclusions. For example, the apparent sensitivity of the ventromedial hypothalamus to opiate stimulation (Gosnell et al., 1986; Grandison & Guidotti, 1977; Tepperman & Hirst, 1983; Tepperman et al., 1981) may be attributed to the spread of the opiate drugs to more sensitive sites, possibly dorsally into the PVN (Lanthier et al., 1985; Stanley et al., 1984; Woods & Leibowitz, 1985). While naloxone injected directly into this brain site was effective in inhibiting feeding (Thornhill & Saunders, 1984; Woods & Leibowitz, 1985), an additional study failed to observe any effect of ventromedial hypothalamic destruction on the anorectic effect of peripherally injected naloxone (King et al., 1979). A similarly ambiguous set of data exists for the dorsomedial nucleus of the hypothalamus, where locally administered naloxone is ineffective as an anorectic agent (Woods & Leibowitz, 1985), but where electrolytic lesions attenuate the anorexia induced by peripheral naloxone injection (Bellinger, Bernardis, & Williams, 1983). The perifornical region of the lateral hypothalamus, similar to the PVN, has recently been shown to produce quite dramatic changes in feeding after local morphine, met-enkephalin, and naloxone injection (Lanthier et al., 1985; Stanley et al., 1984; Woods & Leibowitz, 1985). This brain site, therefore, warrants further study with additional opiate drugs, as well as with electrolytic lesions. As mentioned earlier, a few extra-hypothalamic sites are also found to be sensitive to opiate stimulation and will similarly need to be investigated for their potential role in opiate control of feeding.

Morphine, a relatively selective μ-receptor agonist with ability to cross the blood-brain barrier, is effective in stimulating eating behavior in the rat after systemic administration, as well as after administration directly into the hypothalamus (see Morley et al., 1983, and Leibowitz, 1986, for review). As mentioned above, electrolytic PVN lesions significantly attenuate (but do not abolish) the feeding-stimulatory action of peripheral morphine. This finding suggests that opiate receptors in the PVN may have some role in the mediation of this eating response, whether induced through peripheral or central drug administration. Consistent with this suggestion is the additional finding that the rats' responsiveness to peripheral and PVN injection of morphine varies similarly as a function of the circadian cycle. That is, in both cases, the feeding response elicited by morphine in satiated animals is considerably greater just prior to the onset of the dark period than it is at the onset of the light period (Bhakthavatsalam & Leibowitz, 1986b). Based on this result and on similar evidence obtained with closely linked α_2-noradrenergic receptors of the PVN (Bhakthavatsalam & Leibowitz, 1986a; Jhanwar-Uniyal and Leibowitz, 1986; and see below), it is possible that PVN opiate receptors, presumably of the μ-subtype, increase in number or sensitivity as the circadian cycle moves toward the dark phase and that these receptors help to mediate the increase in feeding behavior that occurs naturally during the most active time in the rat's cycle.

Recent investigations, in which the animals were permitted to choose their nutrient intake from three separate sources of protein, carbohydrate, and fat, have revealed that peripherally injected morphine has specific effects on the animals' nutrient selection, depending on the state of the animal (Marks-Kaufman, 1982; Shor-Posner et al., 1986a). Under conditions of food deprivation, rats stimulated with morphine exhibit a selective increase in fat ingestion, the opposite to that observed after naloxone injection (Daniel, Stanley, & Leibowitz, 1985; Marks-Kaufman, 1982; Marks-Kaufman and Kanarek, 1981; Shor-Posner et al., 1986a). In satiated animals, however, this pattern changes. Under these conditions, PVN injection of opiate agonists, similar to peripheral morphine, potentiate protein ingestion to a significantly greater extent than fat selection (Shor-Posner et al., 1986a). Under both satiated and deprived conditions, carbohydrate ingestion is either unaffected or even suppressed. These findings argue for a more specific role of hypothalamic opiate receptors in feeding control, a role that involves a selective change in appetite for certain nutrients, rather than just a change in quantity of food ingested.

PVN α_2-NORADRENERGIC SYSTEM

α_2-Noradrenergic stimulation of the PVN, like opiate stimulation, is also known to potentiate feeding in the rat (Goldman, Marino, & Leibowitz, 1985; Leibowitz, 1978, 1980, 1986). Over the past decade, a wide variety of data have converged to support the idea that NE released within the PVN has a physiological function in the stimulation of eating (Jhanwar-Uniyal, Fleischer, Levin, & Leibowitz, 1982; Leibowitz, 1980, 1986; Martin & Myers, 1975). Briefly, the evidence demonstrates that exogenous NE, at near physiological doses, is effective in potentiating eating in satiated animals and that this phenomenon is mediated by α_2-noradrenergic receptors localized in the PVN (Goldman et al., 1985; Leibowitz, 1978). Discrete electrolytic lesions of the PVN abolish eating induced by central NE or peripheral clonidine (CLON) injection (Leibowitz, Hammer, & Chang, 1983; McCabe, DeBellis, & Leibowitz, 1984). Furthermore, PVN injection of α_2-noradrenergic receptor blockers, in contrast to antagonists of α_1-noradrenergic, β-adrenergic, dopaminergic, serotonergic, and opiate receptors, antagonize the action of PVN-injected NE and CLON (Goldman et al., 1985; Leibowitz, 1975; Slangen & Miller, 1969).

The importance of endogenous NE release in the eating process is indicated by the finding that PVN injections of antidepressant compounds also enhance eating, apparently through presynaptic release of endogenous NE (Leibowitz, Arcomano, & Hammer, 1978). It has also been found that chronic PVN NE and CLON infusions induce hyperphagia and body weight gain (Leibowitz, Roossin, & Rosenn, 1984c; Lichtenstein, Marinescu, & Leibowitz, 1984), consistent with the idea that total 24-hour food intake, in addition to one single meal, may ultimately be modulated by α_2-noradrenergic stimulation. The possibility that endogenous PVN NE and α_2 receptors are active in appetite regulation is strongly supported by the finding that NE turnover within the PVN or medial hypothalamus is significantly increased in food-deprived animals (Jhanwar-Uniyal et al., 1982) and that α_2 receptors in the PVN, in contrast to other hypothalamic or extra-hypothalamic areas, are profoundly down-regulated by food deprivation (Jhanwar-Uniyal et al., 1982; Jhanwar-Uniyal & Leibowitz, 1986a).

Although hypothalamic injection of NE has for some time been known to elicit eating (Grossman, 1962), only recently has light been shed on the specific nature of the appetite control exerted by endogeneous NE (Leibowitz, 1986). Detailed studies of the animals' meal patterns after NE administration have demonstrated that this neurotransmitter enhances eating by increasing meal size, rather than by altering meal frequency (Shor-Posner et al., 1985). The animals' rate of eating is also potentiated. In addition to changing the pattern of eating, PVN-injected NE is found to modulate the animals' appetite for specific foods. In particular, NE, as well as CLON and the antidepressant agents, have clearly been demonstrated to selectively enhance carbohydrate intake (Leibowitz, Brown, Tretter, & Kirschgessner, 1985a; Leibowitz, Weiss, Yee, & Tretter, 1985b), while a reduction in carbohydrate ingestion has been revealed by PVN injection of the catecholamine neurotoxin 6-hydroxydopamine (Shor-Posner, Azar, Jhanwar-Uniyal, Filart & Leibowitz, 1986b). This selective noradrenergic action relative to carbohydrate consumption is of particular interest in light of the finding that gastric loads of a carbohydrate meal significantly depress endogenous NE release, specifically within the PVN (Myers & McCaleb, 1980). This leads us to propose that, in the normal sequence of events, an increase in PVN noradrenergic activity is associated with eating onset, particularly of carbohydrate-rich foods, and at a critical time thereafter the ingested food feedbacks in a negative manner to inhibit further NE release in the PVN and further eating (Leibowitz, 1986).

For several reasons, these events are believed to occur most critically at the early stages of the rats' active (dark) period. It has been shown that exogenous NE is consistently more effective in potentiating eating at this particular time, in contrast to other times later in the dark or in the light period (Bhakthavatsalam & Leibowitz, 1986a). Furthermore, a sharp rise in PVN α_2-receptor density also occurs at the onset of the dark cycle (Jhanwar-Uniyal, Roland, & Leibowitz, 1986). This early dark period appears to be important in revealing the above-described alterations in PVN α_2 receptors as a result of food deprivation. As little as 3 hours without food during the early dark is sufficient to severely down-regulate these receptors, in contrast to 3–6 hours of food deprivation introduced later in the dark phase or during the day (Jhanwar-Uniyal & Leibowitz, 1986a).

PVN OPIATE AND α_2-NORADRENERGIC SYSTEMS IN RELATION TO GLUCOCORTICOSTEROIDS

It has been well established that, just prior to the onset of the dark period, a sharp rise occurs in the blood levels of the adrenal hormone, corticosterone (CORT; e.g., Krieger & Hauser, 1978; Wilkinson, Shinsako, & Dallman, 1979). This peak of CORT appears to be linked to eating onset, as opposed to other behaviors, which has led to the proposal that this glucocorticosteroid may be involved in appetite regulation. In our earlier work, we demonstrated that norad-renergically elicited feeding was abolished by hypophysectomy and adrenalec-tomy and significantly and selectively restored by CORT replacement (Leibowitz, 1980; Leibowitz, Chang, & Oppenheimer, 1976; Roland, Oppenheimer, Chang, & Leibowitz, 1985a). This evidence and more recent studies (Leibowitz, Roland, Hor, & Squillari, 1984b; Roland, Bhakthavatsalam, & Leibowitz, 1986b) clearly reveal that the size of the meal initiated by PVN NE in the rat is closely related to the level of circulating CORT and thus to the activity of corticotropin-releasing-factor neurons located in the PVN (Swanson, Sawchenko, Rivier, & Vale, 1983). As plasma CORT rises from 1 to 10 µg%, the potency of α_2-noradrenergic stimulation rises accordingly. As mentioned earlier, circulating CORT normally rises during the late afternoon, to peak just prior to the onset of the dark cycle. It is precisely at this time in the diurnal cycle when the animals are most responsive to NE and CLON stimulation (Bhakthavatsalam & Leibowitz, 1986a). It is believed, therefore, that at this key point, PVN NE and peripheral CORT collaborate closely in the physiological control of eating behavior. This proposal is consistent with recent data showing the dependence of genetic and lesion-induced overeating and obesity on CORT (for reviews see Bray, 1984; Leibowitz, Jhanwar-Uniyal, & Roland, 1984a; Roland et al., 1986).

Similar results to those of NE have recently been obtained with morphine stimulation. The feeding-stimulatory effect of peripherally administered mor-phine is found to be abolished by adrenalectomy (Bhakthavatsalam & Leibowitz, 1986b). Furthermore, this eating response, which is lost despite an enhanced uptake of morphine into the brain after adrenalectomy (Holaday, Law, Loh, & Li, 1979), is completely restored by peripheral CORT administration. This rela-tionship between morphine-induced feeding and circulating CORT, similar to that observed with opiate-induced hypothermia (Holaday, Law, Tseng, Loh, & Li, 1977) and with the opiate form of stress-induced analgesia (MacLennan et al., 1982), is apparently reflected in the diurnal studies of morphine respon-siveness, which have revealed the strongest morphine eating effect at the start of the dark period, precisely when endogenous CORT levels are at their highest (Bhakthavatsalam & Leibowitz, 1986b; Kavaliers & Hirst, 1985). This diurnal rhythm is similar to that observed with opiate-mediated analgesia (McGivern & Berntson, 1980), as well as for endogenous opiate activity (Kerdelhue et al., 1983).

Comparable results to these obtained with peripheral opiate manipulations have now been observed with PVN injections of morphine. With this form of opiate stimulation, the elicited eating response is significantly attenuated by adrenalectomy, restored by CORT, and is strongest when endogenous CORT levels are highest (Bhakthavatsalam & Leibowitz, 1986b). These findings strengthen the proposal that peripheral and PVN-injected morphine are acting via similar brain mechanisms and that this opiate receptor effect on eating behavior is CORT-dependent. It should be noted, however, that eating evoked by PVN morphine administration, although significantly attenuated by adrenalectomy, remains partially intact in the absence of CORT (Bhakthavatsalam & Leibowitz, 1986b). Further, the eating-stimulatory effects of intraventricular dynorphin (Morley et al., 1983) and PVN-injected enkephalin (McLean & Hoebel, 1982) are unaffected by adrenalectomy. These contrasting effects of adrenalectomy on opiate-induced eating are very possibly due to the different routes used for drug administration (and thus different brain areas affected) and/or to the different types of opiate receptors, μ, κ, δ, which are mediating the actions, respectively, of morphine, dynorphin, and met-enkephalin. From the results obtained to date, we conclude that opiate-induced eating depends to some degree on adrenal function but not to the same extent as NE and not in the case of all receptor subtypes. The PVN μ receptor, in contrast to the κ and δ receptors, appears to be most responsive to fluctuations in circulating CORT.

INTERACTION BETWEEN PVN
OPIATE-α_2-NORADRENERGIC RECEPTOR SYSTEMS

With the evidence just described, it has become clear that both opiate and α_2-noradrenergic stimulation are associated with a potentiation of eating behavior and that their behavioral action is mediated, in part, by receptors in the PVN. The issue we wish to address now is whether NE and the opiate peptides function independently to control food ingestion or whether they interact in a synergistic or serial fashion to produce their effect. Whereas a considerable amount of evidence supports the possibility of a close link between these potential neurotransmitters in appetite regulation, there are certain findings that argue for some degree of independence.

In favor of the argument for a close interaction are the findings that NE and the opiates are particularly effective within the same brain area, namely the PVN (Lanthier et al., 1985; McLean & Hoebel, 1983; Leibowitz, 1978; Stanley et al., 1984; Woods & Leibowitz, 1985), and that their eating stimulatory effect within the medial hypothalamus is positively correlated in magnitude and is similarly blocked by antagonists of α_2-noradrenergic receptor sites (Leibowitz & Hor, 1982; McLean & Hoebel, 1983; Tepperman & Hirst, 1983; Tepperman et al., 1981). Consistent with a variety of other data linking opiate and catecholaminergic systems in the brain (Bläsig & Herz, 1980; Palmer, Seiger, Hoffer, & Olson, 1983), these results suggest that the opiate and α_2-noradrenergic receptors function sequentially in feeding regulation, with the opiates apparently working through the NE synapse. Electrophysiological experiments have revealed inhibitory effects of morphine and enkephalin on PVN neuronal firing (Muehlethaler, Gaehwiler, & Dreifuss, 1980; Pittman, Hatton, & Bloom, 1980), similar to that observed with NE (Moss, Urban, & Cross, 1972). The possiblity that the opiates actually operate through NE release in the PVN is consistent with the observation that peripheral injections of morphine, at doses that potentiate eating behavior, significantly decrease NE concentration and increase NE turnover in the PVN (Jhanwar-Uniyal, Woods, Levin, & Leibowitz, 1984). Furthermore, as described above, the eating stimulatory effect of peripheral morphine, like PVN-injected NE and morphine, is abolished by adrenalectomy, restored by CORT replacement, and strongest when endogenous CORT levels are highest. A link between the opiate and α_2-noradrenergic receptor systems has also been established in experiments of peripheral autonomic (cholinergic) function. With both naloxone feeding suppression (Jones & Richter, 1981) and NE-elicited feeding (Sawchenko, Gold, & Leibowitz, 1981), peripheral injections of atropine methyl nitrate are found to abolish their respective effects on food intake. These results strengthen the proposal that the opiates and NE function via similar mechanisms controlled through the medial hypothalamus. These mechanisms involve the hypothalamic-pituitary-adrenal axis and possibly neurochemical systems of the peripheral nervous system.

The above pharmacological evidence, suggesting a sequentially organized, opiate-to-NE neurocircuit, leads to the proposal that opiate stimulation may modulate the action of NE at its PVN synapse. As just described, peripherally administered morphine enhances NE turnover in the PVN (Jhanwar-Uniyal et al., 1984). To examine further the impact of morphine on PVN noradrenergic function, rats with and without chronic subcutaneous morphine pellets were tested for their responsiveness to PVN NE injection (Leibowitz & Hor, 1982; Leibowitz, & Hor, 1980). These chronic morphine implants were found to greatly potentiate the animals' eating response to NE administration. The magnitude of this morphine-induced enhancement was greatest for animals exhibiting low to moderate baseline sensitivity to NE and actually reversed into a suppressive effect in animals already showing a strong NE response in the absence of morphine.

Thus, it appears that through their modulatory action on α_2-noradrenergic receptors and on presynaptic NE release, opiates in the PVN may have an important synergistic interaction with the NE system in the control of appetite.

This suggestion is consistent with the biochemical and anatomical evidence revealing moderate to dense populations of opiate and α_2-noradrenergic receptors in the PVN (Duka et al., 1981; Goodman et al., 1980; Kuhar, Pert, & Snyder, 1973; Leibowitz, Jhanwar-Uniyal, Dvorkin, & Makman, 1982; Pearson et al., 1980; Pert et al., 1975), and also with additional evidence, in other behavioral models, that has linked opiates and α_2-noradrenergic receptor systems (Unnerstall, Kopajtic, & Kuhar, 1984). While the synergistic effects of opiates on noradrenergic function may occur directly within the PVN itself, it may be noted that opiate agonists have a stimulatory effect on the release of ACTH and consequently of CORT (Van Vugt & Meites, 1980). In light of the finding that PVN NE function depends on circulating CORT (see above), opiate-induced CORT release may be predicted to serve as an intermediate link in the potentiation of NE eating. Direct evidence for this suggestion is provided by recent biochemical studies (Jhanwar-Uniyal & Leibowitz, 1986b) which have shown CORT to have a major impact on the density of α_2 receptors in the PVN.

This evidence is strongly suggestive of an important and close link between PVN opiate, α_2-noradrenergic, and pituitary-adrenal systems in the control of eating behavior. One needs to be cautious, however, in entirely accepting this hypothesis, since there is some other evidence which appears to dissociate these systems. As described above, the eating stimulatory effects of δ and κ agonists, in contrast to the μ agonist morphine (Bhakthavatsalam & Leibowitz, 1986b) and NE (Leibowitz et al., 1984b), are unaffected by adrenalectomy (McLean & Hoebel, 1982; Morley et al., 1983). Further, electrolytic PVN lesions, which abolish feeding induced by α_2-noradrenergic stimulation (Leibowitz et al., 1983; McCabe et al., 1984), leave partially intact the eating response elicited by peripheral morphine injection (Shor-Posner et al., 1986a). Finally, α_2-noradrenergic and opiate stimulation have differential effects on diet selection. Whereas NE and CLON selectively stimulate the animals' preference for carbohydrate (Leibowitz et al., 1985a), peripheral and central opiate stimulation increases fat and protein intake, while at the same time actually decreasing carbohydrate selection (Daniel et al., 1985; Marks-Kaufman, 1982; Marks-Kaufman & Kanarek, 1981; Shor-Posner et al., 1986a).

The extent to which these findings do, in fact, reflect a dissociation of the opiate and α_2-noradrenergic systems, rather than the additional involvement of multiple brain sites, cannot be determined until systematic studies of different brain areas are conducted. It is clear, from cannula mapping and lesion studies, that opiate receptor sites outside the PVN, and possibly outside the hypothalamus, may be involved in the feeding process. These sites, however, would not be expected to interact with α_2 receptor sites controlling feeding which are more concentrated in the medial hypothalamus, in particular the PVN (Leibowitz, 1978). Thus, in order to study the opiate-α_2-noradrenergic interaction, we need to focus our attention and manipulations directly on the PVN, to answer such questions as whether PVN opiate stimulation, in contrast to peripheral or intraventricular opiate drugs, is affected by adrenalectomy or PVN lesions and whether it has any specific effects on carbohydrate ingestion. Based on the available evidence, (Leibowitz, 1986), it is proposed that in the PVN, and perhaps only in this nucleus, the α_2 and opiate receptor systems, in conjunction with the PVN-pituitary-adrenal axis, interact closely to initiate and maintain adaptive feeding responses (Leibowitz & Hor, 1982; Woods & Leibowitz, 1985). Outside the PVN, the opiate receptors may function either independently or in conjunction with other monoamine systems to control feeding. One site in particular may be the lateral perifornical hypothalamus, where morphine has a potent, possibly adrenal-independent, stimulatory influence on food intake in the absence of any NE α_2-receptor sensitivity. At this site, dopamine and epinephrine (β-adrenergic) have been suggested to control protein ingestion (Leibowitz, 1980, 1986), and thus it may be through this mechanism that morphine similarly alters protein intake. Feeding induced by electrical stimulation of this lateral hypothalamic area can be blocked by naloxone administration (Carr & Simon, 1983).

PVN OPIATE α_2-NORADRENERGIC-ADRENOCORTICOTROPIN SYSTEM: ROLE IN NUTRITIONAL HOMEOSTASIS, UNDER NORMAL CONDITIONS AND AFTER ACUTE FOOD DEPRIVATION AND STRESS

The opiate and noradrenergic systems of the brain are widespread and are believed to serve an important role in the elaboration of a large number of physiological and behavioral respsonses. In many instances, the opiates and α_2-noradrenergic receptor mechanisms mediating specific adaptive behaviors are believed to exist in close proximity within a particular brain area and to interact closely to produce optimal control of the behavior (Bläsig & Herz, 1980; Unnerstall et al., 1984). With regard to feeding behavior, the rescarch described above leads us to propose the following hypotheses outlined in Figure 7.1. It is suggested that, under specific conditions involving energy expenditure (namely, food deprivation, stress,

HYPOTHALAMIC OPIATE - α2-NORADRENERGIC-ADRENOCORTICOTROPIN
SYSTEMS CONTROLLING FEEDING

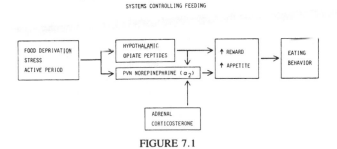

FIGURE 7.1

and in the active period of the diurnal cycle), the opiate receptor systems of the brain become activated and consequently potentiate eating behavior as part of their overall effort to rapidly restore body energy stores. This function is performed primarily through the hypothalamus. In the medial hypothalamus, in particular the PVN, the endogenous opiate pepetides act in close association with the local α_2-noradrenergic receptor system, which also enhances feeding; however, in other hypothalamic areas, such as the lateral perifornical site, the opiates work independently of this noradrenergic system, possibly interacting with other local catecholamine systems. The opiate and α_2-noradrenergic systems of the PVN operate in conjunction with the adrenal hormone, CORT, which enables the organism to adjust optimally to sudden environmental changes. In their effort to replenish energy stores, the endogenous opiates, NE and CORT, function, both homeostatically and nonhomeostatically, by increasing appetite for specific macronutrients and also by increasing the rewarding quality of food, possibly through alterations of taste. A well-coordinated interplay between these and other neurochemical-neuroendocrine systems is clearly required for the execution of such complex adaptive changes in sensory, motivational, and affective processes in the brain.

Brain endorphins and NE, as well as adrenal CORT, are known to be released particularly under such activating and/or unstable conditions as food deprivation, stress, and at the initiation of the active diurnal period. In response to food deprivation, β-endorphin levels, specifically in the hypothalamus, are significantly reduced (Gambert, Garthwaite, Pontzer, & Hagen, 1980) and NE turnover, specifically in the medial hypothalamus, is significantly increased (Jhanwar-Uniyal et al., 1982; Martin & Myers, 1975; Stachowiak, Bialowas, & Jurkowski, 1978; Van der Gugten & Slangen, 1977). Associated with these neurochemical events, in addition to enhanced food intake, is a naloxone-sensitive increase in analgesia (McGivern, Berka, Berntson, Walker, & Sandman, 1979). Similar events have been observed in situations involving acute stress (e.g., Amir & Amit, 1979; Amir, Brown, & Amit, 1980; Antelman, Szechtman, Chin, & Fisher, 1975; Bodnar, Kelly, Brutus, & Glusman, 1980; Morley & Levine, 1980; Rossier et al., 1977; Smythe, Bradshaw, & Vining, 1983; Tanaka et al., 1983), and the enhancing effect of stress on hypothalamic NE turnover can be reliably potentiated by blockade of opiate receptor function (Tanaka et al., 1982).

While this evidence is generally supportive of the hypothesis outlined in Figure 7.1, what are lacking, particularly relative to the opiate system, are systematic studies that involve more discrete brain sites and that provide a more direct and critical evaluation of specific predictions. A few such tests have been conducted so far on the PVN α_2-noradrenergic system, which responds in a rapid, dramatic, and highly site-specific fashion to food deprivation and refeeding. For example, food deprivation significantly increases NE turnover, specifically in the PVN (Jhanwar-Uniyal et al., 1982). This effect, after as little as three hours of food deprivation, is associated with a sharp down-regulation of

α_2 receptors only in this nucleus, and this down-regulation can be reversed by a few hours of refeeding (Jhanwar-Uniyal & Leibowitz, 1986a). Thus, in the case of NE, it appears that we may be dealing with an anatomically localized and relatively specific food-directed system of the brain. With regard to the opiate receptor system, we have, at present, little available evidence to draw any specific conclusions along these lines. Although the results described above support a close and site-specific association between the opiates and NE function in the PVN, the cannula mapping and PVN lesion studies indicate that the opiates act more diffusely throughout the hypothalamus and even in extra-hypothalamic structures. Thus, in biochemical studies of physiologically induced opiate activity, we will need to consider all these sites in our effort to determine whether the opiates, in certain brain areas, have a specific function relative to food intake, or whether these peptides perform a more general activating function, such as in response to stressful stimuli.

In addition to food deprivation and stress, the active period of the diurnal cycle, when feeding behavior sharply increases, has been associated with a significant increase in both opiate and NE activity within the hypothalamus. Diurnal rhythms of brain β-endorphin, met-enkephalin, and NE, as well as feeding and analgesia, have been described (Armstrong, 1981; Frederickson, Wesche, Edwards, Harrell, & Burgis, 1978; Manshardt & Wurtman, 1968; Mash, Soliman, & Walker, 1980; McGivern et al., 1979; Rosenfeld & Rice, 1979). Once again, these biochemical studies of brain endorphins and NE have been conducted on large brain areas, as well as under a wide range of experimental and behavioral conditions. Thus, their significance to our specific hypothesis for feeding behavior, outlined in Figure 7.1, remains in question.

Recent studies, conducted in more discrete brain areas, provide the first clear indication that diurnal rhythms of brain neurotransmitter activity may have a physiological consequence in the control of food intake. In one study, the response of the rats to opiate and α_2-noradrenergic receptor agonists, applied directly to the PVN, was found to be greatest at the start of the dark period, when feeding in the rat naturally occurs (Bhakthavatsalam & Leibowitz, 1986a, 1986b). In a second study, this diurnal pattern of drug responsiveness was shown to reflect a neurochemical change within the brain (Jhanwar-Uniyal et al., 1986). Through biochemical procedures, this report revealed a sharp increase in α_2-receptor binding sites, exclusively within the PVN, precisely at the start of the dark period when behavioral responsiveness also peaks. Similar biochemical studies on the opiate receptors are needed to determine whether the enhanced feeding response observed with opiate agonists at this time of the diurnal cycle, similar to that observed with NE, actually reflects a physiologically significant change in opiate receptor function.

The possibility of a surge of opiate receptor activity, as well as α_2-noradrenergic activity, at the onset of the dark phase receives further support from evidence linking the opiate and α_2-receptor systems of the PVN to the adrenal release of

CORT (Figure 7.1). As described above for brain NE and the opiate peptides, adrenal CORT is also known to be released by stress (Amir et al., 1980), food deprivation (Dallman, 1984), and during the initial phase of the active period (Krieger & Hauser, 1978). From the data just described, a specific consequence of this release in the dark cycle appears to be a dramatic increase in PVN α_2-receptor number, associated with an increased response to PVN NE and morphine stimulation. Further, the loss of circulating CORT after adrenalectomy rapidly down-regulates the α_2 receptors, again specifically within the PVN, and attenuates or abolishes the stimulating action of PVN NE and morphine and peripheral morphine on eating behavaior. It is known that adrenalectomy reduces food intake, particularly under unstable environmental conditions (Bhakthavatsalam & Leibowitz, 1986b; Dallman, 1984; Jhanwar-Uniyal et al., 1985a), and it is possible that this reduction in eating is attributed to a decrease in activity at the hypothalamic opiate and α_2-receptor sites. Consistent with this proposal is the finding that night-time feeding, specifically of carbohydrate (NE-mediated) and to a lesser extent protein (opiate-mediated), is particularly disturbed by removal of the adrenals (Jhanwar-Uniyal & Leibowitz, 1986b). While this evidence is certainly suggestive of a CORT interaction with PVN or opiate receptor function similar to that of NE, other available evidence precludes us from generalizing our conclusions to all opiate systems in other brain areas (McLean & Hoebel, 1983; Morley et al., 1983).

The question now is, through what efferent mechanisms in the brain do the opiates and NE act to potentiate feeding? Since these neurochemical systems are believed to respond to such conditions as stress, food deprivation, and in the active period, one may ask whether the drive triggered by these neurotransmitters in specific hypothalamic areas represents a general source of energy for all motivated behaviors or whether it is specific to feeding, perhaps a particular aspect of this behavior. Although our knowledge is limited, we may refer to at least two pieces of evidence which argue for relative specificity in the effects of hypothalamic opiates and NE on feeding. First, in both cases, food ingestion appears to be more selectively initiated, as compared to water ingestion which is either unaffected, suppressed, or only slightly enhanced (Leibowitz, 1980, 1986; Morley et al., 1983). Second, as described above, both the opiates and NE, in addition to enhancing total calorie intake, have highly selective effects on nutrient selection.

This and other evidence for behavioral specificity opens the door to questions concerning the particular aspects of feeding behavior that may be activated. Although we have insufficient information to determine whether these central neurochemical systems actually evoke sensations of hunger, we do know that they affect the ingestion of specific foods, and this change in appetite is believed to occur in response to a homeostatic imbalance. At the start of the night-time feeding period in the rat, energy stores are known to be very low, and hypoglycemia may occur just prior to a meal (LeMagnen, 1981). Recent evidence has shown that at this period of the diurnal cycle, rats permitted to select their macronutrients ingest first a meal of carbohydrate, followed shortly by a meal of protein (Leibowitz & Shor-Posner, 1986). In light of the evidence that NE selectively stimulates carbohydrate ingestion, whereas morphine (in ad lib-fed animals) preferentially increases protein ingestion (Shor-Posner et al., 1986a), it is proposed that the α_2-noradrenergic and opiate receptor systems in the hypothalamus induce, respectively, the carbohydrate and protein meals that naturally occur in the early hours of the dark. Consistent with this proposal is the evidence that ingestion or gastric loading of specific nutrients can affect the binding of radioligands to opiate and α_2-noradrenergic receptors in the hypothalamus, as well as the release of β-endorphin and NE (Dum, Gramsch, & Herz, 1983; Jhanwar-Uniyal et al., 1982; Myers & McCaleb, 1980). These neurochemical changes occur exclusively in the hypothalamus and, in the case of the α_2-noradrenergic system, specifically in the medial hypothalamus or in the PVN itself.

In addition to their proposed function in the homeostatic control of appetite for specific macronutrients, NE and the opiates may also potentiate eating in a nonhomeostatic fashion, through their action on reward systems in the brain. Both the catecholamines (Wise, 1978) and opiates (Stein & Belluzzi, 1979) have generally been associated with rewarding processes, and, thus, they may logically be expected to affect the reinforcing properties of food substances, possibly through their action on taste mechanisms. Morphine has been shown to have electrophysiological effects on parabrachial taste units, which can be blocked by naloxone (Hermann & Novin, 1980). Furthermore, the PVN, which projects to the parabrachial nucleus (Swanson & Sawchenko, 1983), is known to support self-stimulation reward (Atrens & von Vietinghoff-Riesch, 1972). In addition, NE in this nucleus, or just lateral to it, may act as a positive reinforcer for motivated behavior (Cytawa, Jurkowlaniec, & Bialowas, 1980; Wise & Stein, 1969); and food deprivation, which is known to broaden the acceptable range of food substances, has been associated with increased release of hypothalamic NE (Jhanwar-Uniyal et al., 1982; Martin & Myers, 1975) and endorphins (Gambert et al., 1980).

In studies of various sweet diets, morphine has been shown to broaden the range of acceptable saccharin solutions, whereas naloxone works in the opposite direction to narrow this range (Cooper, 1983; LeMagnen, Marfaing-Jallat, Miceli, & Devos, 1980; Lynch & Libby, 1983; Siviy & Reid, 1983). Stressful tail pinch, perhaps through brain opiates, induces sucrose hyperphagia unrelated to hunger (Bertierre, Mame Sy, Baigts, Mandenoff, & Apfelbaum, 1984). Hyperphagia induced by a highly palatable diet is also attenuated by naltrexone, at a dose which has no effect on ingestion of a less palatable, standard diet (Apfelbaum & Mandenoff, 1981). While an early report suggests that NE-induced eating may be particularly dependent on diet palatability (Booth & Quartermain, 1965), this has been disputed by a recent report (Sclafani & Toris, 1981). It appears that the stimulating effect of NE on food intake is largely specific to ingestion of carbohydrate, whether sweet or nonsweet; and, in contrast to morphine, does not readily extend to the ingestion of a saccharin-water solution (Leibowitz et al., 1985b). Stress, which releases opiate peptides in the hypothalamus (Henry, 1982; Olson et al., 1984), has recently been found to increase appetite for sucrose, an effect blocked by naltrexone (Bertierre et al., 1984). On the basis of these data, several investigators have postulated a role for endogenous opiates in mediating appetite for sweet or palatable foods, independent of homeostatic imbalance.

The importance of the hypothalamic, opiate, and α_2-noradrenergic systems in control of natural feeding is underscored by additional evidence showing disturbances in daily feeding patterns and even body weight consequent to chronic manipulations of these neurotransmitter systems. For example, chronic naloxone administration is effective in suppressing the hyperphagia and obesity induced by a highly palatable cafeteria diet (Mandenoff, Fumeron, Apfelbaum, & Margules, 1982). Furthermore, chronic PVN infusion of NE and CLON or chronic peripheral CLON administration reliably potentiates daily food intake, particularly carbohydrate ingestion, and body weight gain (Leibowitz et al., 1985a; Lichtenstein et al., 1984; Schlemmer, Casper, Narasimhachari, & Davis, 1979).

The possibility that endogenous NE and endorphins may be disturbed in animals with genetic obesity is suggested by a variety of evidence (Cruce, Thoa, & Jacobowitz, 1976; Ferguson-Segall, Flynn, Walker, & Margules, 1982; Gibson, Liotta, & Krieger, 1981; King et al., 1979; Levin & Sullivan, 1979; Margules, Moisset, Lewis, Shibuya, & Pert, 1978; Oltmans, 1983; Recant, Voyles, Luciano, & Pert, 1980). However, in contrast to the studies on brain NE, the studies of the opiates have, with the exception of Gibson et al. (1981), generally detected a change (increase) in peripheral rather than central neurotransmitters, and it has been proposed that this peripheral effect may actually develop subsequent to the obesity (Rossier, Rogers, Shibasaki, Guillemin, & Bloom, 1979). In other studies of nongenetic obesity models, no clear relationship between peripheral β-endorphin, naloxone sensitivity, and level of obesity was detected (Gunion & Peters, 1981). In obese humans, the opiate antagonists naloxone and naltrexone reliably suppress food ingestion to a greater extent than in normal-weight subjects (Atkinson, 1982; Sternbach, Annitto, Pottash, & Gold, 1982). This effect, however, is not always reliable (O'Brien, Stunkard, & Ternes, 1982) and generally requires particularly high doses of the antagonist (Atkinson, 1982).

Margules (1979a) has proposed that middle-aged obesity represents a mild form of Cushing's Disease, in which excess circulating β-endorphin and CORT cause gluconeogenesis, lipogenesis, and increased adiposity. His working hypothesis states that β-endorphin works through the autonomic nervous system, not only to control the influence of nutrients through food ingestion, but also to conserve the outflow of bodily resources by reducing energy expenditure (Margules, 1979b). This highly integrated system is not indispensable for food intake in a predictable environment, but is called into action when the reward system is disrupted and food is scarce. It is of interest that, in patients with anorexia nervosa, significantly higher levels of CSF β-endorphin have been observed in underweight subjects (Kaye, Pickar, Naber, & Ebert, 1982), and lower levels of CSF NE have been detected in weight-recovered subjects (Kaye, Ebert, Raleigh, & Lake, 1984). As with all studies of this kind, it is not known whether this difference involves an etiologic relationship between the neurotransmitter and the eating disorder, or whether it reflects a compensatory response due to the stress of weight loss. Stress is known to precipitate bulimic binges in individuals prone to them, and, based on animal studies (Leibowitz, 1984; Morley et al., 1983), a role for brain opiates and NE in this phenomenon may be proposed.

REFERENCES

Amir, S., & Amit, Z. (1979). The pituitary gland mediates acute and chronic pain responsiveness in stressed and non-stressed rats. *Life Science, 24,* 439–448.

Amir, S., Brown, Z. W., & Amit, Z. (1980). The role of endorphins in stress: Evidence and speculations. *Neuroscience & Biobehavioral Reviews, 4,* 77–86.

Antelman, S. M., Szechtman, H., Chin, P., & Fisher, A. E. (1975). Tail pinch-induced eating, gnawing and licking behavior in rats: Dependence on the nigrostriatal dopamine system. *Brain Research, 99,* 319–337.

Apfelbaum, M., & Mandenoff, A. (1981). Naltrexone suppresses hyperphagia induced in the rat by a highly palatable diet. *Pharmacology Biochemistry & Behavior, 15,* 89–91.

Armstrong, S. (1981). Periodicity of nocturnal feeding in the rat—what the gut tells the brain or what the brain tells the gut. *Behavioral & Brain Sciences, 4,* 575–576.

Atkinson, R. L. (1982). Naloxone decreases food intake in obese humans. *Journal of Clinical Endocrinology & Metabolism, 55,* 196–198.

Atrens, D. M., & von Vietinghoff-Riesch, F. (1972). The motivational properties of electrical stimulation of the medial and paraventricular hypothalamic nuclei. *Physiology & Behavior, 9,* 229–235.

Atweh, S. F., & Kuhar, M. J. (1977). Autoradiographic localization of opiate receptors in rat brain II: The brainstem. *Brain Research, 129,* 1–29.

Bellinger, L. L., Bernardis, L. L., & Williams, F. E. (1983). Naloxone suppression of food and water intake and cholecystokinin reduction of feeding is attenuated in weanling rats with dorsomedial hypothalamic lesions. *Physiology & Behavior, 31,* 839–846.

Bertierre, M. C., Mame Sy, T., Baigts, F., Mandenoff, A., & Apfelbaum, M. (1984). Stress and sucrose hyperphagia: Role of endogenous opiates. *Pharmacology Biochemistry & Behavior, 20,* 675–679.

Bhakthavatsalam, P., & Leibowitz, S. F. (1986a). α_2-Noradrenergic feeding rhythm in paraventricular nucleus: Relation to corticosterone. *American Journal of Physiology, 250,* R83–R88.

Bhakthavatsalam, P., & Leibowitz, S. F. (1986b). Morphine-elicited feeding: Diurnal rhythm, circulating corticosterone and macronutrient selection. *Pharmacology Biochemistry & Behavior, 24,* 911–917.

Bläsig, J., & Herz, A. (1980). Interactions of opiates and endorphins with cerebral catecholamines. In L. Szekeres (Ed.), *Adrenergic activators and inhibitors: Handbook of experimental pharmacology* (Vol. 54, pp. 463–497). New York: Springer-Verlag.

Bodnar, R. J., Kelly, D. D., Brutus, M., & Glusman, M. (1980). Stress-induced analgesia: Neural and hormonal determinants. *Neuroscience Biobehavioral Review, 4*, 87–100.

Booth, D. A., & Quartermain, D. (1965). Taste sensitivity of eating elicited by chemical stimulation of the rat hypothalamus. *Psychonomic Science, 3*, 525–526.

Bray, G. A. (1984). Hypothalamic and genetic obesity: An appraisal of the autonomic hypothesis and the endocrine hypothesis. *International Journal of Obesity, 8*, 119–137.

Carr, K. D., & Simon, E.J. (1983). Effects of naloxone and its quarternary analogues on stimulation-induced feeding. *Neuropharmacology, 22*, 127–130.

Cooper, S. J. (1983). Effects of opiate agonists and antagonists on fluid intake and saccharin choice. *Neuropharmacology, 22*, 323–328.

Cruce, J. A. F., Thoa, N. B., & Jacobowitz, D. M. (1976). Catecholamines in the brains of genetically obese rats. *Brain Research, 101*, 165–170.

Cytawa, J., Jurkowlaniec, E., & Bialowas, J. (1980). Positive reinforcement produced by noradrenergic stimulation of the hypothalamus of rats. *Physiology & Behavior, 25*, 615–619.

Dallman, M. F. (1984). Viewing the ventromedial hypothalamus from the adrenal gland. *American Journal of Physiology, 246*, R1–R12.

Daniel, D. R., Stanley, B. G., & Leibowitz, S. F. (1985). Paraventricular nucleus injection of the pancreatic polypeptide, NPY and PPY, selectively stimulate carbohydrate intake. *Proceedings of the Eastern Psychological Association, 56*, 30.

Duka, Th., Schubert, P., Schubert, M., Stroiber, R., & Herz, A. (1981). A selective distribution pattern of different opiate receptors in certain areas of rat brain as revealed by in vitro autoradiography. *Neuroscience Letters, 21*, 119–124.

Dum, J., Gramsch, C. H., & Herz, A. (1983). Activation of hypothalamic β-endorphin pools by reward induced by highly palatable food. *Pharmacology Biochemistry Behavior, 18*, 443–447.

Ferguson-Segall, M., Flynn, J. J., Walker, J., & Margules, D. L. (1982). Increased immunoreactive dynorphin and leu-enkephalin in posterior pituitary of obese mice (ob/ob) and super-sensitivity to drugs that act at kappa receptors. *Life Science, 31*, 2233–2236.

Frederickson, R. C. A., Wesche, D. L., Edwards, J. D., Harrell, C. E., & Burgis V. (1978). Mouse brain enkephalins: Studies of levels and synthesis correlated with nociceptive sensitivity. *Neuroscience Abstracts, 4*, 407.

Gambert, S. R., Garthwaite, T. L., Pontzer, C. H., & Hagen, T. C. (1980). Fasting associated with decrease in hypothalamic β-endorphin. *Science, 210*, 1271–1272.

Gibbs, J., & Smith, G. P. (1984). The neuroendocrinology of postprandial satiety. In L. Martin & W. F. Ganong (Eds.), *Frontiers in neuroendocrinology* (Vol. 8, pp. 223–246). New York: Raven Press.

Gibson, M. J., Liotta, A. S., & Krieger, D. T. (1981). The zucker fa/fa rat: Absent circadian corticosterone periodicity and elevated β-endorphin concentrations in brain and neurointermediate pituitary. *Neuropeptides, 1*, 349–362.

Goldman, C. K., Marino, L., & Leibowitz, S. F. (1985). Postsynaptic α_2-noradrenergic receptors in the paraventricular nucleus mediate feeding induced by norepinephrine and clonidine. *European Journal of Pharmacology, 115*, 11–19.

Goodman, R. R., Snyder, S. H., Kuhar, M. J., & Young, W. S. (1980). Differentiation of delta and mu opiate receptor localization by light microscopic autoradiography. *Proceedings of the National Academy of Science U.S.A., 77*, 6239–6243.

Gosnell, B. A., Morley, J. E., & Levine, A. S. (1986). Opiod-induced feedings: Localization of sensitive brain sites. *Brain Research, 369*, 177–184.

Grandison, L., & Guidotti, A. (1977). Stimulation of food intake by muscimol and beta endorphin. *Neuropharmacology, 16*, 533–536.

Grossman, S. P. (1962). Direct adrenergic and cholinergic stimulation of hypothalamic mechanisms. *American Journal of Physiology, 202*, 872–882.

Gunion, M. W., & Peters, R. H. (1981). Pituitary β-endorphin, naloxone, and feeding in several experimental obesities. *American Journal of Physiology, 241,* R173–R184.

Henry, J. L. (1982). Circulating opioids: Possible physiological roles in cerebral nervous function. *Neuroscience Biobehavioral Review, 6,* 229–245.

Hermann, G., & Novin, D. (1980). Morphine-inhibition of parabrachial taste units reversed by naloxone. *Brain Research Bulletin, 5*(S4), 169–173.

Holaday, J. W., Law, P. Y., Loh, H. H., & Li, C. H. (1979). Adrenal steroids indirectly modulate morphine and β-endorphin effects. *Journal of Pharmacology & Experimental Therapeutics, 208,* 176–183.

Holaday, J. W., Law, P. Y., Tseng, L. F., Loh, H. H., & Li, C. H. (1977). β-endorphin: Pituitary and adrenal glands modulates its action. *Proceedings of the National Academy of Science USA, 74,* 4628–4632.

Jhanwar-Uniyal, M., Factor, A. D., Bailo, M., Roland, C. R., & Leibowitz, S. F. (1985). Impact of adrenalectomy and food deprivation on α_1- and α_2-noradrenergic receptors in rat brain and on daily food intake. *Proceedings of the Eastern Psychological Association, 56,* 36.

Jhanwar-Uniyal, M., Fleischer, F., Levin, B. E., & Leibowitz, S. F. (1982). Impact of food deprivation on hypothalamic α-adrenergic receptor activity and norepinephrine (NE) turnover in rat brain. *Neuroscience Abstracts, 8,* 711.

Jhanwar-Uniyal, M., & Leibowitz, S. F. (1986a). Impact of on α_1 and α_2-noradrenergic receptors in the paraventricular nucleus and other hypothalamic areas. *Brain Research Bulletin, 17,* 889–896.

Jhanwar-Uniyal, M., & Leibowitz, S. F.(1986b). Impact of circulating corticosterone on α_1- and α_2-noradrenergic receptors in discrete brain areas. *Brain Research, 368,* 404–408.

Jhanwar-Uniyal, M., Roland, C. R., & Leibowitz, S. F. (1986). Diurnal rhythm of α_2-noradrenergic receptors in the paraventricular nucleus and other brain areas: Relation to circulating corticosterone and feeding behavior. *Life Science, 38,* 473–482.

Jhanwar-Uniyal, M., Woods, J. S., Levin, B. E., & Leibowitz, S. F. (1984). Cannula mapping and biochemical studies of the hypothalamic opiate and noradrenergic systems in relation to eating behavior. *Proceedings of the Eastern Psychological Association, 55,* 106.

Jones, J. G., & Richter, J. A. (1981). The site of action of naloxone in suppressing food and water intake in rats. *Life Science, 28,* 2055–2064.

Kavaliers, M., & Hirst, M. (1985). The influence of opiate agonists on day-night feeding rhythms in young and old mice. *Brain Research, 326,* 160–167.

Kaye, W. H., Ebert, M. H., Raleigh, M., & Lake, C. R. (1984). Abnormalities in CNS monoamine metabolism in anorexia nervosa. *Archives of General Psychiatry, 41,* 350–355.

Kaye, W. H., Pickar, D., Naber, D., & Ebert, M. H. (1982). Cerebrospinal fluid opioid activity in anorexia nervosa. *American Journal of Physiology, 139,* 643–649.

Kerdelhue, B., Karteszi, M., Pasqualini, C., Reinberg, A., Mezey, E., & Palkovits, M. (1983). Circadian variations in beta-endorphin concentrations in pituitary and in some brain nuclei of the adult male rat. *Brain Research, 261,* 243–248.

Khachaturian, H., Lewis, M. E., & Watson, S. J. (1983). Enkephalin systems in diencephalon and brainstem of the rat. *Journal of Comparative Neurology, 220,* 310–320.

Khachaturian, H., Watson, S. J., Lewis, M. E., Coy, D., Goldstein, A., & Akil, H. (1982). Dynorphin immunocytochemistry in the rat central nervous system. *Peptides, 3,* 941–954.

King, B. M., Castellanos, F. X., Kastin, A. J., Berzas, M. C., Mauk, M. D., Olson, G. A. & Olson, R. D. (1979). Naloxone-induced suppression of food intake in normal and hypothalamic obese rats. *Pharmacology Biochemistry & Behavior, 11,* 729–732.

Krieger, D. T., & Hauser, H. (1978). Comparison of synchronization of circadian corticosteroid rhythms by photoperiod and food. *Proceedeings of the National Academy of Science, USA, 75,* 1577–1581.

Kuhar, M. J., Pert, C. B., & Snyder, S. H. (1973). Regional distribution of opiate receptor binding in monkey and human brain. *Nature (London), 245*, 447–450.

Lanthier, D., Stanley, B. G., & Leibowitz, S. F. (1985). Feeding elicited by central morphine injection: Sites of action in the brain. *Proceedings of the Eastern Psychological Association, 56*, 30.

Leibowitz, S. F. (1975). Ingestion in the satiated rat: Role of alpha and beta receptors in mediating effects of hypothalamic adrenergic stimulation. *Physiology and Behavior, 14*, 743–754.

Leibowitz, S. F. (1978). Paraventricular nucleus: A primary site mediating adrenergic stimulation of feeding and drinking. *Pharmacology Biochemistry and Behavior, 8*, 163–175.

Leibowitz, S. F. (1980). Neurochemical systems of the hypothalamus. Control of feeding and drinking behavior and water-electrolyte excretion. In P. J. Morgane & J. Panksepp (Eds.), *Handbook of the hypothalamus* (Vol. 3A, pp. 297–437). New York: Dekker.

Leibowitz, S. F. (1984). Noradrenergic function in the medial hypothalamus: Potential relation to anorexia nervosa and bulimia. In K. M. Pirke & D. Ploog (Eds.), *The psychobiology of anorexia nervosa* (pp. 35–45). Berlin: Springer-Verlag.

Leibowitz, S. F. (1986). Brain monoamines and peptides: Role in the control of eating behavior. *Federal Proceedings, 45*, 1396–1403.

Leibowitz, S. F., Arcomano, A., & Hammer, N. J. (1978). Tranylcypromine: Stimulation of eating through α-adrenergic neuronal system in the paraventricular nucleus. *Life Science, 23*, 749–758.

Leibowitz, S. F., Brown, O., Tretter, J. R., & Kirschgessner, A. (1985a). Norepinephrine, clonidine, and tricyclic antidepressants selectively stimulate carbohydrate ingestion through noradrenergic system of the paraventricular nucleus. *Pharmacology Biochemistry Behavior, 23*, 541–550.

Leibowitz, S. F., Chang, K., & Oppenheimer, R. L. (1976). Feeding elicited by noradrenergic stimulation of the paraventricular nucleus: Effects of corticosterone and other hormone manipulations. *Neuroscience Abstracts, 2*, 292.

Leibowitz, S. F., Hammer, N. J., & Chang, K. (1983). Feeding induced by central norepinephrine injection is attenuated by discrete lesions in the hypothalamic paraventricular nucleus. *Pharmacology Biochemistry and Behavior, 19*, 945–950.

Leibowitz, S. F., & Hor, L. (1980). Behavioral effect of β-endorphine (β-EP) and norepinephrine (NE) in the hypothalamic paraventricular nucleus (PVN). *Neuroscience Abstracts, 6*, 318.

Leibowitz, S. F., & Hor, L. (1982). Endorphinergic and α-noradrenergic systems in the paraventricular nucleus: Effects on eating behavior. *Peptides, 3*, 421–428.

Leibowitz, S. F., Jhanwar-Uniyal, M., Dvorkin, B. & Makman, M. H. (1982). Distribution of α-adrenergic, β-adrenergic and dopaminergic receptors in discrete hypothalamic areas of rat. *Brain Research, 233*, 97–114.

Leibowitz, S. F., Jhanwar-Uniyal, M., & Roland, C. R. (1984a). Circadian rhythms of circulating corticosterone and α_2-noradrenergic receptors in discrete hypothalamic and extra-hypothalamic areas of the rat brain. *Neuroscience Abstracts, 10*, 294.

Leibowitz, S. F., Roland, C. R., Hor, L., & Squillari, V. (1984b). Noradrenergic feeding elicited via the paraventricular nucleus is dependent upon circulating corticosterone. *Physiology & Behavior, 32*, 857–864.

Leibowitz, S. F., Roossin, P., & Rosenn, M. (1984c). Chronic norepinephrine injection into the hypothalamic paraventricular nucleus produces hyperphagia and increased body weight in the rat. *Pharmacology Biochemistry and Behavior, 21*, 801–808.

Leibowitz, S. F., & Shor-Posner, G. (1986). Hypothalamic monoamine systems for control of food intake: Analysis of meal patterns and macronutrient selection. In *Psychopharmacology of eating disorders: Theoretical and clinical Developments*. (M. O. Carruba and J. E. Blundell, eds.) pp. 29–49. New York: Raven Press.

Leibowitz, S. F., & Stanley, B. G. (1986). Brain peptides and the control of eating behavior. In T. W. Moody (Ed.), *Neural and endocrine peptides and receptors*, (pp. 333–352). New York: Plenum Press.

Leibowitz, S. F., Weiss, G. F., Yee, F., & Tretter, J. R. (1985b). Noradrenergic innervation of the paraventricular nucleus: Specific role in control of carbohydrate ingestion. *Brain Research Bulletin, 14,* 561–567.

LeMagnen, J. (1981). The metabolic basis of dual periodicity of feeding in rats. *Behavioral & Brain Sciences, 4,* 561–607.

LeMagnen, J., Marfaing-Jallat, P., Miceli, D., & Devos, M. (1980). Pain modulating and reward systems: A single brain mechanism? *Pharmacology Biochemistry and Behavior, 12,* 729–733.

Levin, B. E., & Sullivan, A. C. (1979). Catecholamine levels in discrete brain nuclei of seven month old genetically obese rats. *Pharmacology Biochemistry and Behavior, 11,* 77–82.

Lichtenstein, S. S., Marinescu, C., & Leibowitz, S. F. (1984). Chronic infusion of norepinephrine and clonidine into the hypothalamic paraventricular nucleus. *Brain Research Bulletin, 13,* 591–595.

Lynch, W. C., & Libby, L. (1983). Naloxone suppresses intake of highly preferred saccharin solutions in food deprived and sated rats. *Life Science, 33,* 1909–1914.

MacLennan, A. J., Drugan, R. C., Hyson, R. L., Maier, S. F., Madden IV, J., & Barchas, J. D. (1982). Corticosterone: A critical factor in an opioid form of stress-induced analgesia. *Science, 215,* 1530–1532.

Mandenoff, A., Fumeron, F., Apfelbaum, M., & Margules, D. L. (1982). Endogenous opiates and energy balance. *Science, 215,* 1536–1537.

Manshardt, J., & Wurtman, R. J. (1968). Daily rhythm in the noradrenaline content of rat hypothalamus. *Nature (London), 217,* 574–575.

Margules, D. L. (1979a). The obesity of middle age: A common variety of Cushing's Syndrome due to a chronic increase in adrenocorticotrophin (ACTH) and beta-endorphin activity. *Neuroscience Biobehavioral Review, 3,* 107–111.

Margules, D. L. (1979b). Beta-endorphin and endoloxone: Hormones for the autonomic nervous system for the conservation or expenditure of bodily resources and energy in anticipation of famine or feast. *Neuroscience Biobehavioral Review, 3,* 155–162.

Margules, D. L., Moisset, B., Lewis, M., Shibuya, H., & Pert, C. B. (1978). β-endorphin is associated with overeating in genetically obese mice (ob/ob) and rats (fa/fa). *Science, 202,* 988–991.

Marks-Kaufman, R. (1982). Increased fat consumption induced by morphine administration in rats. *Pharmacology Biochemistry and Behavior, 16,* 949–955.

Marks-Kaufman, R., & Kanarek, R. (1981). Modifications nutrient selection induced by naloxone in rats. *Psychopharmacology, 74,* 321–324.

Martin, G. E., & Myers, R. D. (1975). Evoked release of [^{14}C] norepinephrine from the rat hypothalamus during feeding. *American Journal of Physiology, 229,* 1547–1555.

Mash, D. C., Soliman, K. F. A., & Walker, C. A. (1980). Circadian variations of beta endorphin in specific areas of the rat brain. *Federal Proceedings, 39,* 605.

McCabe, J. T., DeBellis, M., & Leibowitz, S. F. (1984). Clonidine-induced feeding: Analysis of central sites of action and fiber projections mediating this response. *Brain Research, 309,* 85–104.

McGivern, R., Berka, C., Berntson, G. B., Walker, J. M., & Sandman, C. A. (1979). Effect of naloxone on analgesia induced by food deprivation. *Life Science, 25,* 885–888.

McGivern, R. F., & Berntson, G. G. (1980). Mediation of diurnal fluctuations in pain sensitivity in the rat by food intake patterns: Reversal by naloxone. *Science, 210,* 210–211.

McKay, L. D., Kenney, N. J., Eden, N. K., Williams, R. H., & Woods, S. C. (1981). Intracerebroventricular beta-endorphin increases food intake of rats. *Life Science, 29,* 1429–1434.

McLean, S., & Hoebel, B. G. (1982). Opiate and norepinephrine-induced feeding from the paraventricular nucleus of the hypothalamus are dissociable. *Life Science, 31,* 2379–2382.

McLean, S., & Hoebel, B. G. (1983). Feeding induced by opiates into the paraventricular hypothalamus. *Peptides, 4,* 287–292.

Morley, J. E., & Levine, A. S. (1980). Stress induced eating is mediated through endogenous opiates. *Science, 209,* 1259–1261.

Morley, J. E., & Levine, A. S. (1981). Dynorphin-(1–13) induces spontaneous feeding in rats. *Life Science, 29,* 1901–1903.

Morley, J. E., Levine, A. S., Yim, G. K., & Lowy, M. T. (1983). Opioid modulation of appetite. *Neuroscience Biobehavioral Review, 7,* 281–305.

Moss, R. L., Urban, I., & Cross, B. A. (1972). Microelectrophoresis of cholinergic and aminergic drugs on paraventricular neurons. *American Journal of Physiology, 223,* 310–318.

Mucha R. F., & Iversen, S. D. (1986). Increased food intake after opioid microinjections into nucleus accumbens and ventral tegmental area of rat. *Brain Research, 397,* 214–224.

Muehlethaler, M., Gaehwiler, B. H., & Dreifuss, J. J. (1980). Enkephalin-induced inhibition of hypothalamic paraventricular neurons. *Brain Research, 197,* 264–268.

Myers, R. D., & McCaleb, M. L. (1980). Feeding: Satiety signal from intestine triggers brain's noradrenergic mechanism. *Science, 209,* 1035–1037.

O'Brien, C. P., Stunkard, A. J., & Ternes, J. W. (1982). Absence of naloxone sensitivity in obese humans. *Psychonomic Medicine, 44,* 215–218.

Olson, G. A., Olson, R. D., & Kastin, A. J. (1984). Endogenous opiates: 1983. *Peptides, 5,* 975–992.

Oltmans, G. A. (1983). Norepinephrine and dopamine levels in hypothalamic nuclei of the genetically obese mouse (ob/ob). *Brain Research, 273,* 369–373.

Palmer, M. R., Seiger, A., Hoffer, B. J., & Olson, L. (1983). Modulatory interactions between enkephalin and catecholamines: Anatomical and physiological substrates. *Federal Proceedings, 42,* 2934–2945.

Pearson, J., Brandeis, L., Simon, E., & Hiller, J. (1980). Radioautography of binding of tritiated diprenorphine to opiate receptors in the rat. *Life Science, 26,* 1047–1052.

Pert, C. B., Kuhar, M. J., & Snyder, S. H. (1975). Autoradiographic localization of the opiate receptor in the rat brain. *Life Science, 16,* 1849–1854.

Pittman, Q. J., Hatton, J. D., & Bloom, F. E. (1980). Morphine and opioid peptides reduce paraventricular neuronal activity: Studies on the rat hypothalamic slice preparation. *Proceedings of the National Academy of Science, USA, 77,* 5527–5531.

Recant, L., Voyles, N. R., Luciano, M., & Pert, C. B. (1980). Naltrexone reduces weight gain, alters "β-endorphin," and reduces insulin output from pancreatic islets of genetically obese mice. *Peptides, 1,* 309–313.

Roland, C. R., Bhakthavatsalam, P., & Leibowitz, S. F. (1986). Interaction between corticosterone and α2-noradrenergic system of the paraventricular nucleus in relation to feeding behavior. *Neuroendocrinology, 42,* 296–305.

Roland, C. R., Oppenheimer, R. L., Chang, K., & Leibowitz, S. F. (1985). Hypophysectomy disturbs the noradrenergic feeding system of the paraventricular nucleus. *Psychoneuroendocrinology, 10,* 109–120.

Rosenfeld, J. P., & Rice, P. E. (1979). Diurnal rhythms in nociceptive thresholds of rats. *Physiology & Behavior, 23,* 419–420.

Rossier, J., French, E. D., Rivier, C., Ling, N., Guillemin, R., & Bloom, F. E. (1977). Foot shocked induced stress increases β-endorphin levels in blood but not brain. *Nature (London), 270,* 618–620.

Rossier, J., Rogers, J., Shibasaki, T., Guillemin, R., & Bloom, F. E. (1979). Opioid peptides and α-melanocyte-stimulating hormone in genetically obese (ob/ob) mice during development. *Proceedings of the National Academy of Science, USA, 76,* 2077–2080.

Sanger, D. J. (1981). Endorphinergic mechanisms in the control of food and water intake. *Appetite, 2,* 193–208.

Sawchenko, P. E., Gold, R. M., & Leibowitz, S. F. (1981). Evidence for vagal involvement in the eating elicited by adrenergic stimulation of the paraventricular nucleus. *Brain Research, 225,* 249–269.

Schlemmer, R. F., Casper, R. C., Narasimhachari, N., & Davis, J. M. (1979). Clonidine-induced hyperphagia and weight gain in monkeys. *Psychopharmacology, 61*, 233–234.

Sclafani, A., & Toris, J. (1981). Influence of diet palatability on the noradrenergic feeding response in the rat. *Pharmacology Biochemistry and Behavior, 15*, 15–19.

Scott, P., Jawaharlal, K., & Hoebel, B. G. (1984). Feeding induced with kappa and mu agonists injected in the region of the paraventricular nucleus (PVN) in rats. *Proceedings of the Eastern Psychological Association, 55*, 106.

Shor-Posner, G., Azar, A. P., Filart, R., Tempel, D. & Leibowitz. (1986a) Morphine-stimulated feeding: Analysis of macronutrient selection and paraventricular nucleus lesions. *Pharmacology Biochemistry and Behavior, 24*, 931–939.

Shor-Posner, G., Azar, A. P., Jhanwar-Uniyal, M., Filart, R., & Leibowitz, S. F. (1986b). Destruction of noradrenergic innervation to the paraventricular nucleus: Deficits of food intake, macronutrient selection, and compensatory eating after food deprivation. *Pharmacology Biochemistry and Behavior, 25*, 381–392.

Shor-Posner, G., Grinker, J. A., Marinescu, C., & Leibowitz, S. F., (1985). Role of hypothalamic norepinephrine in control of meal patterns. *Physiology and Behavior, 35*, 209–214.

Simon, E. (1975). Opiate receptor binding with 3H-etorphine. *Neuroscience Research Program Bulletin, 13*, 43–50.

Siviy, S. M., & Reid, L. D. (1983). Endorphinergic modulation of acceptability of putative reinforcers. *Appetite, 4*, 249–257.

Slangen, J. L., & Miller, N. E. (1969). Pharmacological tests for the function of hypothalamic norepinephrine in eating behavior. *Physiology Behavior, 4*, 543–552.

Smythe, G. A., Bradshaw, J. E., & Vining, R. F. (1983). Hypothalamic monoamine control of stress-induced adrenocorticotropin release in the rat. *Endocrinology, 113*, 1062–1071.

Stachowiak, M., Bialowas, J., & Jurkowski, M. (1978). Catecholamines in some hypothalamic and telencephalic nuclei of food-deprived rats. *Acta Neurobiologiae Experimentalis, 38*, 157–165.

Stanley, B. G., Hoebel, B. G., & Leibowitz, S. F. (1983). Neurotensin: Effects of hypothalamic and intravenous injections on feeding and drinking in rats. *Peptides, 4*, 493–500.

Stanley, B. G., Lanthier, D., & Leibowitz, S. F. (1984). Feeding elicited by the opiate peptide D-Ala-2-Met-enkephalinamide: Sites of action in the brain. *Neuroscience Abstracts, 10*, 1103.

Stein, L., & Belluzzi, J. D. (1979). Brain endorphins: Possible role in reward and memory formation. *Federal Proceedings, 38*, 2468–2472.

Sternbach, H. A., Annitto, W., Pottash, A. L. C., & Gold, M. S. (1982). Anorexic effects of naltrexone in man. *The Lancet, 1*, 388–389.

Swanson, L. W., & Sawchenko, P. E. (1983). Hypothalamic integration: Organization of the paraventricular and supraoptic nuclei. *Annual Review of Neuroscience, 6*, 269–324.

Swanson, L. W., Sawchenko, P. E., Rivier, J., & Vale, W. W. (1983). Organization of ovine corticotropin-releasing factor immunoreactive cells and fibers in the rat brain: An immunohistochemical study. *Neuroendocrinology, 36*, 165–186.

Tanaka, M., Kohno, Y., Nakagawa, R., Ida, Y., Iimori, K., Hoaki, Y., Tsuda, A., & Nagasaki, N. (1982). Naloxone enhances stress-induced increases in noradrenaline turnover in specific brain regions in rats. *Life Science, 30*, 1663–1669.

Tanaka, M., Kohno, Y., Tsuda, A., Nakagawa, R., Ida, Y., Iimori, K., Hoaki, Y., & Nagasaki, N. (1983). Differential effects of morphine or noradrenaline release in brain regions of stressed and non-stressed rats. *Brain Research, 275*, 105–115.

Tepperman, F. S., & Hirst, M. (1983). Effect of intrahypothalamic injection of [D-Ala2, D-Leu5] enkephalin on feeding and temperature in the rat. *European Journal of Pharmacology, 96*, 243–249.

Tepperman, F. S., Hirst, M., & Gowdey, W. (1981). A probable role for norepinephrine in feeding after hypothalamic injection of morphine. *Pharmacology Biochemistry Behavior, 15*, 555–558.

Terenius, L. (1980). Opiate receptors: Problems of definition and characterization. In G. Pepeu, M. J. Kuhar, & S. J. Enna (Eds.), *Receptors for neurotransmitters and peptide hormones* (pp. 321–328). New York: Raven Press.

Thornhill, J. A., & Saunders, W. (1984). Ventromedial and lateral hypothalamic injections of naloxone or naltrexone suppress the acute food intake of food-deprived rats. *Appetite, 5,* 25–30.

Unnerstall, J. R., Kopajtic, T. A., & Kuhar, M. J. (1984). Distribution of α_2-agonist binding sites in the rat and human central nervous system: Analysis of some functional, anatomic correlates of the pharmacologic effects of clonidine and related adrenergic agents. *Brain Research Reviews, 7,* 69–101.

Van der Gugten, J. & Slangen, J. L. (1977). Release of endogenous catecholamines from rat hypothalamus in vivo related to feeding and other behaviors. *Pharmacology Biochemistry & Behavior, 7,* 211–219.

Van Vugt, D. A., & Meites, J. (1980). Influence of endogenous opiates on anterior pituitary function. *Federal Proceedings, 39,* 2533–2538.

Wilkinson, C. W., Shinsako, J., & Dallman, M. F. (1979). Daily rhythms in adrenal responsiveness to adrenocorticotropin are determined primarily by the time of feeding in the rat. *Endocrinology, 104,* 350–359.

Wise, C. D., & Stein, L. (1969). Facilitation of brain self-stimulation by central administration of norepinephrine. *Science, 163,* 299–301.

Wise, R. A. (1978). Catecholamine theories of reward: A critical review. *Brain Research, 152,* 215–247.

Woods, J. S., & Leibowitz, S. F. (1985). Hypothalamic sites sensitive to morphine and naloxone: Effects on feeding behavior. *Pharmacology Biochemistry & Behavior. 23,* 431–438.

8

THE FUNCTIONAL
BOWEL DISORDERS

Herbert Weiner
Brain Research Institute
and School of Medicine
University of California
Los Angeles

INTRODUCTION

It is an ironic and historical accident that medicine has consistently sought a local anatomical explanation for disease—a tradition begun by Hippocrates, carried forward by Mundinus (in his search for the bodily location of the soul), Vesalius, Morgagni, Bichat, and Virchow. A radical criticism of this traditional point of view can be found in Sir Francis Bacon's (1561–1626) writings. He wrote in 1605:

> In the inquirie which is made by anatomie, I finde much deficience: for they enquire of the parts, and their substances, figures, and collocations. But they enquire not of the diversities of the parts; the secrecies of the passages; and the seats and nestlings of the humours; nor much of the footsteps and impressions of diseases. . .
>
> Another article of this knowledge is the inquirie touching the affections: for as in medicining of the body it is in order first to know the diverse complexions and constitutions, secondlye the diseases, and lastly the cures.
>
> —The Two Bookes of the Proficience and Advancement of Learning

Until about 100 years ago and to the present with very few exceptions, physicians sought to explain all symptoms and disturbances in function in terms of changes in structure. One of the first to throw serious doubt on this sequence was Gustav von Bergmann (1878–1955) who stated categorically that structural change could result from changes in function. As a corollary of this, changes in physiological function can only be studied in living organisms, not in dead tissue.

To illustrate this thesis: Until the latter part of the 19th century, innumerable papers were written about dyspepsia. The ubiquitous nature and unpleasantness of this symptom is attested to by Bayard Taylor's (1825–1878) poignant statement, "It is better to live unknown than to die of dyspepsia." Dyspepsia (emanating from the stomach) was viewed as the cause of neurasthenia and hysteria until this hypothesis was reversed by Jean Martin Charcot (1825–1915), Carl Anton Ewald (1845–1915), and Adolf von Strümpell (1853–1926), all of whom maintained that neurasthenia, hysteria, and anxiety were the antecedents of dyspepsia—a thesis which continues to the present. But the old argument persists: The search for the elusive anatomical lesion for "functional" bowel disorders never ends. When disturbances of physiological function are found, they are treated as "things unto themselves"—local phenomena. Social and psychological factors are dismissed as irrelevant, and the single cause for this disorder is sought. Because the pain is abdominal, and diarrhea and constipation are important complaints, the many associated symptoms pointing to an illness of a person not his gut are dismissed as "nonspecific" or irrelevant.

It is a remarkable fact that the two most common groups of gastrointestinal complaints—irritable bowel syndrome (IBS) and dyspepsia—were virtually neglected by gastroenterologists until 35 years ago because anatomical lesions—peptic ulcer, cholecystitis, infection, and inflammation—were consistently being sought in the upper and lower gastrointestinal tract to account for their symptoms. The desultory concern with these very common disorders (see, however, Alexander, 1950; White, Cobb, & Jones, 1939) was also manifested by the early prophets of psychosomatic medicine, who did not seem to consider their symptoms as proper subject matter of their interests.

The investigations of Almy begun in 1947 and the key paper in 1962 by Chaudhary and Truelove brought IBS to the attention of physicians, to its psychological components, and to those interested in behavioral approaches to the relief of its symptoms.

IRRITABLE BOWEL SYNDROME

There is no subject in medicine that is in a more confused state than IBS. In fact, there is no agreed upon definition or subclassification of this syndrome, which goes by a variety of descriptive names.

In the English and Irish literature, the functional gastrointestinal disorders (Lennard-Jones, 1983) and IBS (Fielding, 1977, 1978, 1984) are names for symptoms and disturbances which emanate from every part of the alimentary tract, from the mouth to the anus. Other British authors (Chaudhary & Truelove, 1962) and most American gastroenterologists prefer to confine the syndrome to the colon; they focus their attention on symptoms of pain, diarrhea, constipation, etc. (e.g., Drossman, Powell, & Sessions, 1977; Latimer, 1983; Schuster, 1983).

There is increasing evidence, however, for the belief that when the predominant symptoms emanate from the colon, more general disturbances of function occur throughout the alimentary tract. This statement is based on several lines of evidence: (a) Lower esophageal sphincter pressure (13.8 vs. 23.8 cm H_2O) is lower in patients with IBS than in control subjects (Whorwell, Clouter, & Smith, 1981). (b) Jejunal motility is decreased (Thompson, Laidlaw, & Wingate, 1979). Migratory motor complexes are normally as frequent during the day as at night. But in one patient with an irritable colon, jejunal motor complexes were reduced. Abdominal pain was then associated with an irregular nocturnal pattern of contraction, which did not terminate in a motor complex. (No sleep stage recordings were done.) (c) Transit time from mouth to cecum and through the entire gut of a solid meal in patients with IBS whose symptoms were mainly diarrhea was twice as fast as in normal subjects. The transit time for constipated patients was, however, considerably longer (Read, 1980). Note, however, that using another technique (radio-opaque pellets rather than food) and in a mixed group of patients (with IBS and other gastrointestinal diseases), no difference in transit time was found by Taylor and his colleagues (Taylor, Darby, Hammond, & Basu, 1978a; Taylor, Darby, & Hammond, 1978b).

As one reviews the literature, one finds that in IBS the entire alimentary tract is symptomatic at one time or another, but additionally patients with IBS have many other symptoms of distress. They are ill in general, not only in particular regions of the gut.

INCIDENCE AND PREVALENCE OF IBS

The ubiquity of IBS (or the so-called functional disturbances of the gut) is attested to by the fact that in a non-random, English sample, 20.6% had the experience of abdominal pain six times in 1 year. In 13% of the sample, the pain was believed to emanate from the region of the colon. Six percent had painless constipation, whereas 3.7% had diarrhea (Thompson & Heaton, 1979). In a U.S. sample of a "healthy" population, the figures for the prevalence of abdominal pain in 1 year were similar to the English sample, and the prevalence of symptoms of IBS was 17% (Drossman, Sandler, McKee, & Lovitz, 1982). The lifetime prevalence rate has been calculated to be 50%–75% (Texter & Butler, 1975), of whom only 10% are ever seen by a physician (Wadsworth, Butterfield, & Blaney, 1971). Nonetheless, more than half (or more) of the clientele of gastroenterologists in the U.S. suffer from one or other form of IBS (Drossman et al., 1977).

In 1976, the U.S. Digestive Disease Commission reported that 115,000 patients were discharged with the diagnoses of psychogenic gastrointestinal disorders or

IBS as the primary reason for hospitalization. In another 103,000 patients, these categories were applied as a secondary diagnosis. Together, the syndrome accounted for 450,000 hospital days (Mendeloff, 1983). Yet the fact remains that most surveys such as those carried out by DHEW do not include the two diagnostic categories among surveys of the incidence of prevalence of diseases of the digestive tract.

FUNCTIONAL DISTURBANCES OF THE ESOPHAGUS

Patients with disturbances in esophageal motility may also complain of dyspepsia ("heartburn"). While 87% of patients with predominantly colonic symptoms of IBS may also have dyspeptic symptoms due to acid regurgitation, heartburn, and epigastric pain (Dotevall, Svedlund, & Sjodin, 1982).

The symptoms of esophageal motility disturbances are, in a diminishing order of frequency, difficulty in swallowing with or without chest pain, nausea or "heartburn," chest pain or heartburn alone, or a "lump" in the throat (Clouse & Lustman, 1983).

"Globus"

Globus is a very common symptom, present in about 50% of a population (Thompson & Heaton, 1982). The lump may be associated with difficulty in and pain on swallowing, emanating from the upper esophagus, an excessive perception of the glossal papillae, and a complaint of "bad breath" (Fielding, 1984). On the other hand, the "lump" may be present between meals and not be associated with any swallowing difficulty.

No consensus exists as to the psychological correlates of globus. Originally considered to be the prototypical hysterical symptom, it is now believed to occur more frequently in depressed and obsessional patients (Lehtinen & Puhakka, 1976). Grieving persons commonly experience a sensation of tightness in the throat and swallowing difficulty. [Other authors (Cohen, 1973; Stacher, 1983) deny any relationship of globus to the emotions.]

Globus is not a homogeneous symptom because it may also occur with gastroesophageal reflux (Hunt, Connell, & Smiley, 1970); in this instance it is probably associated with a reflex endeavor to clear the esophagus of gastric acid.

Gastroenterologists have sought a single cause for globus: Its very heterogeneity has led to disagreements—it has no *one* "cause." Schuster (1983) considered globus to be due to a heightened awareness of cricopharyngeal contraction. Jacobs and Kirkpatrick (1964) believed that it is merely due to an increase in the "webs and folds" of the hypopharynx in 86% of patients complaining of globus; but they do not tell us what the origin of this increase is.

Aerophagia

Little is known about a tendency to swallow saliva and air during, or not during, the drinking of liquids or the eating of food. Almy (1983) defined aerophagia as a "habit pattern" associated with anxiety and other emotions which may produce pain in the neck or behind the lower end of the sternum. The swallowing of air is often followed not only by pain but by nausea and eructations.

However, there are many other reasons why gaseousness and eructation may occur: diseases of the upper gastrointestinal and biliary tract, sinusitis, the gulping of liquids and bolting of food, the drinking of carbonated liquids and alcohol, the use of bicarbonate, bacterial fermentation, and abnormal intestinal bacterial flora or unusual substrates for normal flora (Roth, 1973).

In most instances, air is swallowed through a relaxed upper esophageal sphincter, either at will or unknown to the patient. It then accumulates in the stomach. At times, the lower esophageal sphincter is tonically contracted (Almy, 1983), allowing less air to be expelled by mouth than was originally swallowed; leading to postprandial fullness and dilatation, bloating, substernal or precordial pressure, shortness of breath, hiccupping or flatulence, and even to a hiatus hernia (Roth, 1973).

Gastroesophageal Reflux and Reflux Esophagitis

Gastroesophageal reflux (GER) occurs in virtually everyone but may only become symptomatic in some persons, in which case it is manifested as "heartburn," substernal pain, waking at night with acid in the mouth, or coughing. It may lead to esophagitis and even to esophageal strictures (Dent et al., 1980). Characteristically, the pain is relieved by sitting up or by taking neutralizing antacids. But reflux can also occur in the upright as well as the recumbent position.

Usually, the esophagus is cleared of acids by a reflex, peristaltic wave; in those subject to esophagitis, it is less efficient than in normal persons, especially while asleep (Johnson & DeMeester, 1974; Orr, Robinson, & Johnson, 1981). In addition, such persons have a lower resting tone of the lower esophageal sphincter (Orr, 1983). But the matter may be even more complex, as the work of Dent and his co-workers (Dent et al., 1980) highlights; they showed that in sleep there is little relationship between refluxing and the resting pressure of the lower sphincter. Rather, patients with GER at night awaken too transiently and do not clear their esophagus as readily of acid, nor do they constrict the sphincter protectively.

The question of the correlation of symptoms of GER and anatomical evidence of esophagitis is not settled either. Some claim that the extent of thickening of the basal layer of the epithelium of the esophagus and the appearance of subepithelial papillae near its surface correlates well with symptoms (Ismail-Beigi, Horton, & Pope, 1970), but others do not think so (Goldman, Rasch, Wilts, &

Finkel, 1967; Sladen, Riddell, & Willoughby, 1975). Polymorphonuclear leukocytes may be present near the surface of the esophagus in esophagitis, but are also seen in 57 percent of normal persons (Weinstein, Bogoch, & Bowes, 1975). Yet esophagitis may go on to ulceration in some, usually with severe symptoms of pain and burning.

Diffuse Esophageal Spasm

Intermittent substernal pain and dysphagia are daily symptoms of this form of spasm. In one half of all patients, spasm is brought on by meals (Benjamin, Gerhardt & Castell, 1977; Castell, 1976; Cohen, 1979; Vantrappen & Hellemans, 1983). In other patients, it is not necessarily associated with swallowing.

In this form of spasm, nonperistaltic, repetitive waves occur especially in the lower portions of the esophagus. These waves may be long in duration and high in amplitude. In about one third of all patients, the lower esophageal sphincter does not relax during these waves (DiMarino & Cohen, 1974); in the remainder it does.

Different abnormalities of esophageal motility have also been observed:"tetanic" responses to a single swallow (Gillies, Nicks, & Skyring, 1967; Roth & Fleshler, 1964), spontaneous contractions independent of the act of swallowing, and interrupted peristalsis. The lower sphincter may be under higher pressures or be hyperreactive at normal pressures (Gillies et al., 1967; Graham, 1978).

Thus, a variety of motility disturbances may be associated with esophageal spasm. Spasms can also be produced by gastric acid. It may be "stress related" or occur for unknown reasons in elderly patients (Ingelfinger, 1958; Schuster, 1983) and during pregnancy (Nagler & Spiro, 1961).

Symptomatic Peristalsis

A variant of an esophageal motility disorder is associated with a normal, progressive, peristaltic wave of increased amplitude and/or duration that produces substernal ("angina-like") pain and dysphagia. Pain is associated with the pressure wave and can be precipitated by ergonovine (London et al., 1981).

Motility Disturbances and Chest Pain

The importance of esophageal motility disturbances, particularly of esophagitis, diffuse spasm, and symptomatic peristalsis cannot be overemphasized because they may mimic ischemic heart disease (Bennett & Atkinson, 1966; Brand, Martin, & Pope, 1977; Davies, Jones, & Rhodes, 1982).

In 100 consecutive, emergency-room patients with anterior chest pain, 77 had symptoms of angina pectoris. In 61 of these, the pain was due to ischemic heart disease, and in 16 it was due to an esophageal motility disturbance. In 4 of the

16, the disturbance consisted of diffuse esophageal spasm, and 8 had esophagitis on endoscopy. Acid perfusion of the esophagus reproduced the pain in 5 patients (Davies et al., 1982).

But the matter becomes even more complex because chest pain can occur with normal esophageal manometrics, and no chest pain may occur despite diffuse spasm, high-amplitude, or long-lasting esophageal peristaltic waves. Dysphagia may also occur with normal manometric tracings. When abnormal tracings are seen, diffuse spasm occurs in one quarter of patients and high-amplitude, long-lasting waves in the remainder (Brand et al., 1977).

Physiology, Pharmacology, and Psychophysiology of Esophageal Function

The usual stepwise primary and secondary peristaltic movements of the esophagus and its sphincters are regulated and coordinated by brain-stem and reticular mechanisms which are, in turn, under volitional control. Little is as yet known about what other and humoral factors might affect esophageal motility. However, the lower esophageal resting pressure is raised by metoclopromide and cholinergic agonists (Mellow, 1977). Esophageal spasm may be induced by alpha-adrenergic agonists in some predisposed persons. This sphincter's resting pressure is lowered by secretin (perhaps by inhibiting gastrin), nicotine, alcohol, anticholinergics, and the female sex steroids.

It has been known for years that nonpropulsive esophageal waves may occur with stress (Jacobson, 1927; Rubin, Nagler, Spiro, & Pilot, 1962) and are reduced by relaxation and during sleep. On the other hand, heightened emotional tension enhances dysphagia when esophageal motility is disturbed (Rubin et al., 1962). Sounds above 1000 Hz produce nonpropulsive contractions of the esophagus which habituate and are part of the "defense" reaction (Stacher, 1983).

Additionally, it has been shown that aerophagia can be eliminated (Johnson, DeMeester, & Haggitt, 1978), and a reduced resting pressure of the lower esophageal sphincter can be increased by biofeedback (Schuster, Nikoomanesh, & Wells, 1973).

Esophageal Contraction Abnormalities and Psychopathology

In a recent paper by Clouse and Lustman (1983), esophageal manometry was carried out on 50 patients, of whom 25 were found to have contraction abnormalities. (The reason for referral was that 13 had chest pain only, 31 complained of dysphagia with chest pain or heartburn, and 2 complained of heartburn alone.) Four kinds of manometric abnormalities were discovered in the 25 patients: (a) 5 had diffuse spasm; (b) 18 had an increase in mean wave duration and amplitude, abnormal motor responses, and triple-peaked waves; (c) 1 had esophageal refluxing; and (d) 1 had a distal esophageal ring. Twenty-one of these 25 patients had diagnosable depression (13), anxiety disorder (9), phobias (7), somatization disorder (5), or alcoholism or drug dependency (4), singly or in combination, compared with only 8 of 25 patients with normal manometric patterns, a "nonspecific" motility disturbance, reflux esophagitis, or achalasia.

The percentage of patients with discernible psychopathology, interestingly enough, is the same as those with irritable colon syndrome (Alpers, 1981, 1983).

FUNTIONAL DISTURBANCES OF THE STOMACH

Non-ulcer Dyspepsia

The symptoms of dyspepsia are nausea and/or vomiting, eructation, heartburn, retrosternal pain, epigastric bloating and/or pain, early satiety, and occasionally weight loss. They are often aggravated by eating food. But the subject of nonulcer dyspepsia is truly confusing. No agreed-upon classification exists. The diagnosis rests on the absence of one of the many forms of gastritis; liver, heart, kidney, and gall bladder disease; and alcoholism, peptic ulceration, or failure to respond to a drug such as cimetidine. An increasingly frequent cause is the use of nonsteroidal anti-inflammatory drugs.

According to some authors, the only true discriminant between non-ulcer dyspepsia and peptic ulcer is that patients with the former are younger, tend to complain of nausea and vomiting, and do not have epigastric pain at night nor a family history of peptic ulcer disease (Crean et al., 1982; Horrocks & deDombal, 1978). The usual symptoms of non-ulcer dyspepsia enumerated above are frequently accompanied by loose or frequent stools, lower abdominal pain relieved by defecation, and abdominal distention (Hill & Blendis, 1967; Möllman, Bonnevie, Gudmand-Hoyer, & Wulff, 1976; Manning, Thompson, Heaton, & Morris, 1978). These additional symptoms are only reported in some series; when they are, they clearly suggest that some forms of non-ulcer dyspepsia are part of a more general (IBS) syndrome.

Sixty percent of 775 patients with dyspepsia do not have a peptic ulcer or other structural diseases. Forty-five percent of 200 patients with nonulcer dyspepsia have normal gastric mucosa, 36% have slight mucosal surface erosions, 14.5% have chronic atrophic gastritis, and 4.5% show chronic superficial gastritis (Williams, Edwards, Lewis, & Coghill, 1957). Dyspeptic patients who do and those who do not have gastritis cannot be differentiated by virtue of their symptoms alone. Furthermore, gastritis may be present, but only 65% to 70% of patients complain of symptoms (Edwards and Coghill, 1968; Kreuning, Bosman, Kuiper, van der Wal, & Lindman, 1978; Volpicelli, Yardley, & Hendrix, 1977).

Until recently, these data were subject in all likelihood to a sampling error: A single mucosal biopsy may miss patches of gastritis. Multiple biopsy samples need to be taken. In those patients with non-ulcer dyspepsia, the gastritis, when present consisted of polymorphonuclear infiltration of the gastric epithelium and lamina propria. But antibodies against parietal cells or impairment of Vitamin B_{12} absorption are both absent in this form of gastritis.

This gastritis is often associated with a duodenitis for which there are no agreed-upon anatomical criteria. It may antecede or occur with or without peptic duodenal ulceration; it may be localized or diffuse to include the esophagus (Gregg & Garabedian, 1974). In Piris and Whitehead's (1975) study, 12 of 18 patients with non-ulcer dyspepsia when compared with controls had a greater number of gastrin (G-) containing cells in the gastric antrum. Only 4 of these 12 had a superficial gastritis, and 9 had a duodenitis with normal serum gastrin levels. The remaining 6 patients had atrophic gastritis of various degrees, 4 had duodenitis; the number of antral gastrin cells was the same as in the control subjects, but elevated serum gastrin levels were present.

Thus, in this small group of patients with non-ulcer dyspepsia, heterogeneity exists, both anatomically and physiologically. But the authors of this study say nothing about the history of the patients' symptoms, lives, diet or drug intake, or whether the symptoms were produced by liquids, solids, or a particular component of food.

The question of whether liquids or solids produce symptoms is no trivial matter; recent studies suggest that the tonic activity of the gastric fundus is mainly responsible for the emptying of liquids, whereas the grinding and emptying of solids is carried out by the antrum (Kelly, 1983). It is then of some interest that in a report of a single patient (with treated pernicious anemia) with long-standing dyspepsia, normal fundic activity and tone were described. But this patient's response to a solid-liquid meal consisted of low amplitude distal antral contraction with little duodenal activity. Gastric emptying of the meal was much delayed (Rees, Miller & Malagelada, 1980). Clearly a single case study does not prove anything; nor is this patient a representative one. However, as techniques are developed for measuring gastric motility, emptying and transit time, and electrical activity, such studies should help to classify and clarify the nature of non-ulcer dyspepsia in its various forms.

A different kind of abnormality was found in one half of 70 non-ulcer dyspeptics, who were especially prone to nausea on awakening, often associated with retching, dry heaves, and vomiting of bile (Chey, You, Lee, & Menguy, 1983). They tolerated liquids better than solids. Eleven of the 31 patients also had lower abdominal cramps or pain, diarrhea and/or constipation—symptoms of IBS. Instead of showing the usual rhythmic 3–4 cycle per minute (c.p.m.) pacesetter potential recorded from the antrum of the stomach, two different kinds of changes were seen in patients: (a) an irregular 5 c.p.m. rhythm (tacchyar-rhythmia); and (b) a regular 7 c.p.m. rhythm followed by silent periods (tachygastria). Retropropagation of slow waves also occurred. A third anomaly was seen in 2 patients: an intermittent 1–2 c.p.m. pacesetter potential (You, Chey, Lee, Menguy, & Bortoff, 1981; You, Lee, Chey, & Menguy, 1980).

Thus, in patients with this form of dyspepsia, several kinds of gastric motility disturbances are seen. Furthermore, they do not as a group respond uniformly to drugs, such as domperidone.

Nervous Dyspepsia

What, then, is meant by the designation "nervous dyspepsia" (Truelove & Reynell, 1972)? It is supposed to be "stress related," and its symptoms are said to be "more or less like those of peptic ulcer." Its diagnosis is made by exclusion; gastroenterologists caution that repeated examinations are needed, a doubt lingers on in their minds that an anatomical gastroduodenal lesion will eventually be revealed. In view of the fact that there is no cogent way of differentiating nonulcer dyspepsia and nervous dyspepsia from each other and that the former may also be "stress related," why should two designations be preserved?

FUNCTIONAL DISTURBANCES OF THE COLON

Irritable Colon Syndrome

It is well recognized that patients with IBS of the colonic variety or its various synonyms (mucous and spastic colitis, nervous diarrhea, colon neurosis, membranous enteritis, dyssynergia, functional or irritated bowel syndrome, etc.) mainly suffer from clusters of symptoms: colicky abdominal pain (in 85%–90%) which is often much enhanced by eating (in 75%) and relieved by a bowel movement; constipation and/or diarrhea (in 80%); gas, mucus in the stool (in 25%); and weight loss (20%) (Drossman et al., 1977; Fielding, 1984).

Characteristically, the physician focuses on these symptoms while failing to take note of the fact that a considerable proportion of patients also complain of globus, nausea and vomiting, bloating sensations after meals, headache, backache, flushing, fatigue, anxiety and depression, sighing respiration, and hyperventilation (Drossman et al., 1977). They frequently have cool and sweaty palms and brisk reflexes. They smile (often in embarrassment), describe their symptoms vaguely, and have a fear of cancer (50%). They have had abdominal operations to excess (Chaudhary & Truelove, 1962; Fielding, 1984). These facts should alert physicians to the fact that IBS is an illness of persons not only of the gut.

Nonetheless, the physician should be aware of the fact that diarrhea may be the result of lactase deficiency (McMichael, Webb, & Dawson, 1965; Weser, Rubin, Ross, & Sleisinger, 1965) or malabsorption of bile salts (Thayson & Pedersen, 1976) as a cause of diarrhea. Yet, lactase deficiency may occur without symptoms (Peña & Truelove, 1972).

In addition, chronically constipated persons may medicate themselves with laxatives, producing anatomical changes (loss of haustration and damage to the myenteric plexus) in the colon (Smith, 1968; Thompson, 1980). In fact, about 30% of all IBS patients have a history of regular or occasional laxative use (Chaudhary & Truelove, 1962). And 26% may date the onset of their symptoms from the time of having an infectious form of "dysentery" (Chaudhary & Truelove, 1962).

It is often forgotten that DaCosta (1871) reported what is now called IBS. He also described "soldier's heart" (the "hyperventilation syndrome"). Both syndromes were found in soldiers exposed to the danger of battle. But no conclusions were drawn by later physicians from the self-evident connection of fear and bowel disturbances.

It remained for Chaudhary and Truelove (1962) in their series of 130 patients to identify a series of psychological factors which were associated with the onset or exacerbations of this chronic, yet intermittent disorder. They could be identified in 77% of patients with a spastic colon and in 87.5% of patients with painless diarrhea. They were more apparent in women patients, who were more likely to be concerned about their children or their marriages. They were chronic worriers or fearful people. The men were more likely to be concerned about their work. Of interest also is that an interaction was found between IBS patients with a history of dysentery and psychological factors; when both were present, the prognosis was considerably worse.

Another approach consists of identifying psychiatric illness in patients with IBS, rather than describing events in the patient's life at onset. The identification of such illness does not tell us, however, what role it plays: Is it an antecedent or consequent condition to bowel symptoms which may be painful, embarrassing, or inconvenient? If associations are found, what do they really mean or explain? Nonetheless, such studies tell of a frequent association of psychiatric illness and IBS. Increased levels of anxiety (Esler & Goulston, 1973) and depression (Hislop, 1971) are found in IBS patients. In Hislop's series (1971), 80% were depressed. Young, Alpers, Norland, and Woodruff (1976) found evidence of psychoneurotic symptoms in 72 percent of patients with IBS, in contrast to an incidence of 18% in a comparison group of patients with other forms of bowel disease.

Diarrhea alone, independent of the IBS, occurs in 14 percent of patients with anxiety neurosis and neurocirculatory asthenia (Wheeler, White, Reed, & Cohen, 1950). In view of the much greater aggregation of anxiety disorders and IBS, some additional factor must exist. This is suggested by a series of recent studies carried out in St. Louis: Seventy-two percent of such patients had a clinically diagnosable psychiatric disorder. Patients whose IBS was characterized mainly by diarrhea could be classified independently as suffering from an anxiety neurosis or somatization disorder. When constipation and pain predominated, they were either depressed or suffering from a somatization disorder. In two thirds of the patients, psychiatric symptoms anteceded the bowel symptoms. Patients with other chronic bowel diseases had an 18% incidence of psychiatric disorders (Alpers, 1981, 1983).

Psychogenic Abdominal Pain

Another group of patients suffers mainly from abdominal pain, called psychogenic (Drossman, 1982). However, they have other pains, too—headache, joint, and back pain—and they complain of fatigue. In addition, 25% at least have symptoms of the colonic form of IBS. (The accounts of these patients incline the reader to believe that this is a variant of IBS).

In Drossman's series of 24 patients, 20 were young women with recurrent abdominal pain of 6 months duration or more. They fell into four main psychiatric categories: They were either histrionic, pain-prone, hypochondriacal, or depressed. Of particular interest was that in two out of three patients the abdominal pain had begun in a setting of bereavement or separation, a finding that confirms Gomez and Dally's (1977) observations.

Nothing in these studies was said about a history of bereavement or illness in childhood, which we have known since Mendeloff and his colleagues' studies (Mendeloff, Monk, Siegel, & Lilienfeld, 1970) to be more frequent in IBS patients than an inflammatory bowel disease or in a healthy control population.

The Physiology and Psychophysiology of the Irritable Colon Syndrome

The topic of the physiology of the colonic variety of the IBS falls into a number of different categories: attempts to understand the basis of its symptoms; attempts to identify some especial physiological feature of the IBS which might help as a diagnostic criterion; or attempts to explain its pathophysiology, etiology, or pathogenesis. Unfortunately, none of these aims has been accomplished.

Pain. The cramping abdominal pain which is a feature of IBS is believed to be a correlate of small bowel or colonic hypermotility (Connell, Jones, & Rowlands, 1965; Holdstock, Misiewicz, & Waller, 1959; Horowitz & Farrer, 1962; Mendeloff, Monk, Siegel, & Lilienfeld, 1970). But the matter may be more complex than merely a matter of motility. Patients with IBS may have a lower pain tolerance or, alternatively, a heightened perception of pain. Although they frequently complain of gaseous bloating accompanied by pain, the quantity and quality of intestinal gas is the same as in normal subjects (Lasser, Bond, & Levitt, 1975; Levitt & Bond, 1983). However, experimentally distending the colon with 60 to 160 cc of air is likely to produce pain in many more IBS patients (55 percent) than in normal (6%) subjects (Ritchie, 1973; Whitehead,

Engel, & Schuster, 1980)—a finding that was not confirmed by Latimer et al. (1979, 1981). The perception of pain appears to be the same in IBS patients than in normal persons, but the tolerance to it differs (Whitehead et al., 1980). This conclusion is supported by the fact that some patients with functional abdominal pain may be pain-prone; in future studies of this kind, patients might well be classified according to their various psychological profiles.

Motility disturbances. Another line of work begun by Almy and his colleagues (Almy & Tulin, 1947; Almy, Kern, & Tulin, 1949a; Almy, Hinkle, Berle, & Kern, 1949b; Almy, Abbot, & Hinkle, 1950) indicated that constipated patients with IBS were prone to increased colonic (sigmoid) motility (frequency, amplitude, and duration), whereas in those with diarrhea, motility was decreased— observations that have repeatedly been confirmed by other investigators (Bloom et al., 1968; Chaudhary & Truelove, 1961; Misiewicz, Connell, & Pontes, 1966; Waller, Misiewicz, & Kiley, 1972; Wangel & Deller, 1965). These patterns can be induced by meals which in some IBS patients are particularly likely to lead to diarrhea. However, many different drugs and toxins which produce diarrhea in animals and man are associated with hypomotility, whereas obstipating agents and patients with simple constipation have hypermotile colonic patterns (Powell, 1977; Truelove, 1966).

The matter may again be more complex. The response of the colon to fecal matter or air may be different in IBS than in the normal person. The response of distending the rectosigmoid colon with 20 cc of air in a stepwise manner produces in normal persons an immediate single contraction. In IBS patients (not further specified) the response is delayed and multiple without regard to the activity or inactivity of the illness. In other words, dilation of the colon in IBS patients produces tetanic contractions for reasons poorly understood (Whitehead et al., 1980).

However, these findings have not been replicated consistently. Connell et al. (1965) could find no differences in colonic motility between patients with the "spastic" form of IBS and patients with duodenal ulcer. But they did find that patients who suffered abdominal pain after meals showed a doubling of colonic motility after eating but did not differ significantly from the "spastic" colon or ulcer groups. And Murrell and Deller (1967) could find no differences in resting colonic motility or the responses of the colon to bradykinin in normal subjects when compared with various forms of IBS.

Latimer (1983) has pointed out, on the basis of his review of nine separate studies in this area, that consistent differences have not been found between normal persons and those with IBS when patients with painless diarrhea or diarrhea-prone patients are excluded. Based on his own recent work and that with his colleagues (Latimer et al., 1979), comparing "psychoneurotic," normal subjects, and IBS patients during baseline monitoring, a neutral stimulus, and stressful interview, meal, and intramuscular neostigmine (0.5 mg), he has concluded that no contractile differences exist, partly because of the marked individual variation in motor activity in each group (Latimer et al., 1981).

Myoelectrical activity of the colon.   The colon has functions different from those of the rest of gut. Whereas only two types of basic electrical activity are known in the upper gut, the colon has four kinds (Sarna, 1983). But only two of these four activities have been studied in IBS: a slow (2.5–4 c.p.m.) and a faster (6–9 c.p.m.) basic electrical rhythm (Christensen, 1971; Daniel, 1975; Misiewicz, 1975). Normally 10% to 15% of a unit of time is occupied by the slower variety and the remainder by the faster one. In patients with IBS, the proportion of slow electrical activity is increased to 40% to 50%, leading to increased segmental motor activity at this lower frequency (Snape, Carlson, & Cohen, 1976; Snape, Carlson, Matarazzo, & Cohen, 1977; Snape & Cohen, 1979; Taylor, Duthie, Smallwood, Brown, & Linkens, 1974). Pentagastrin and cholecystokinin enhance and glucagon diminishes the incidence of these low-frequency waves in normal persons and in IBS patients (Snape et al., 1977; Taylor et al., 1974; Taylor, Duthie, Smallwood, & Linkens, 1975). However, the increased incidence of the slow waves is unrelated to the symptoms of IBS because it occurs in patients who suffer either from diarrhea, constipation, or are asymptomatic (Taylor et al., 1978a, 1978b).

As Latimer (1983) has pointed out, Snape and his colleagues (1976) claimed that the peak distributions of the two frequencies were discontinuous. Taylor et al. (1978a) found a continuous spectrum of frequencies, and the peak frequencies were simultaneously present.

These findings are of great interest but have not always been confirmed. No differences were detected in IBS patients and controls with respect to the incidence of low-frequency myoelectric activity (Latimer et al., 1979; Sarna, Bardakjian, Waterfall, Lind, & Daniel, 1980). Or, there may be heterogeneity among patients with regard to various parameters of the *duration* of spike-bursting electrical activity rather than in their frequency in IBS (Bueno, Fioramonti, Rukebusch, Frexinos, & Coulomb, 1980).

Therefore, the matter of a *specific* myoelectric abnormality in IBS is by no means settled.

Effects of meals in IBS.   A subgroup of patients exists in whom meals bring on abdominal pain and/or diarrhea. Despite claims to the contrary, the role of meals in producing such symptoms remains unsettled. Wangel and Deller (1965) found that food enhanced colonic motility in normal persons and patients, although in those who suffered from diarrhea, the effect was less than in those who had pain—a result that is diametrically opposite to that found by Waller et al. (1972). On the other hand, and to compound the confusion, Sullivan, Cohen, and Snapes (1978) and Snape and Cohen (1979) maintained that patients show a delay in the onset of colonic motility with a 1000-calorie meal which lasts much longer (80 vs. 50 minutes) than in normal persons and is associated with myoelectric activity at a predominant frequency of 6–7 c.p.m. (rather than at 10–11 c.p.m.) which is also of greater duration.

Effects of monoamines.   Although Latimer (1983) could find no special effect of neostigmine on colonic motility in patients with IBS, others have found that parasympathomimetic agents do increase sigmoid activity in patients with "spastic" colons and painless diarrhea (Chaudhary & Truelove, 1961) and in normal control patients (Wangel & Deller, 1965). In fact, the effect of neostigmine is by no means settled (Champion, 1973; Connell, Gaafer, Hassanein, & Jones, 1964; Misiewicz et al., 1966); and, when it occurs, it may also be seen in patients with diverticulosis (Chowdhury, Dinoso, & Lorber, 1976; Painter & Truelove, 1964).

Sometimes, only segmental rectosigmoid motility is observed (in 67% of 24 patients) with constipation, regardless of whether it was associated with diverticulosis or IBS; it was abolished by atropine (and glucagon; Chowdhury et al., 1976). On the other hand, serotonin may produce diarrhea and colonic hypomotility in subjects with constipation and diarrhea (Murrell & Deller, 1967).

Effects of prostaglandins.   The prostaglandins (both of the E and F series) may also decrease motility and cause diarrhea (Hung, Delawari, & Misiewicz, 1975; Konturek, 1978). Prostaglandin E_2 (PGE_2) levels in jejunal fluid in patients with IBS of various kinds have been measured: 2 of 15 with alternating diarrhea and constipation, and 10 of 17 patients with chronic "nervous" diarrhea had significantly elevated levels. In 6 of the latter group of patients, indomethacin decreased stool volume and frequency; and in 2 it lowered PGE_2 levels (Bukhave & Rask-Madsen, 1980). Elevated levels of PGs have also been found in the blood of children with diarrhea (Dodge, Handi, Burns, & Yamashiro, 1981) and in the stools of food-intolerant patients with IBS (Jones, McLaughlan, Shorthouse, Workman, & Hunter, 1982).

Gut peptides.   A potential role for gut peptides is suspected in IBS; some alter gut motility and are also released by food. For example, gastric inhibitory polypeptide (GIP) is released by protein and carbohydrate, and cholecystokinin (CCK) by fat and protein. Both of these and calcitonin, glucagon, secretin, neurotensin, substance P, and vasoactive intestinal peptide (VIP) induce intestinal fluid and electrolyte secretion. They could produce diarrhea. At the same time, these peptides have opposite effects on motility: gastrin, CCK, and motilin increase it, and secretin, glucagon, GIP, VIP, and pancreatic polypeptide (PP) diminish it (Harvey, 1979).

Nonetheless, no confirmed evidence exists as yet that levels of any of these gut hormones are altered in IBS. Neither in the fasting nor in the postprandial state were blood levels of gastrin, insulin, GIP, PP, motilin, enteroglucagon, or neurotensin significantly different than in control subjects (Besterman et al., 1981). Yet in another study, motilin and PP were raised in response to a waterload in patients with the constipation and diarrhea of IBS (Preston, Adrian, Chris-tofides, Lennard-Jones, & Bloom, 1983). It is, of course, possible that blood levels are normal but that the local effects of the peptides are not; that the intestinal muscle or mucosal cells have a heightened sensitivity to one or other of these peptides or that their interactive or regulatory effects on motility and secretion are altered.

Cholecystokinin is known to increase small intestinal and colonic motor activity in animals and man (Dinoso, Meshkinpour, Lorber, Gutierrez, & Chey, 1973; Glossi, Messini, Del Duca, Ricci, & Messini, 1966; Gutierrez, Chey, & Dinoso, 1974). In patients wtih IBS, marked increases in duration and amplitude of colonic contractions occurred almost exclusively in 8 patients who complained of abdominal pain on eating. The peptide reproduced the pain in 4 of the 8 patients. Only one of the remaining patients (whose principal complaint was pain unrelated to eating) had such an increase in motility (Harvey & Read, 1973).

However, Chowdhury et al. (1976) found that a hyperactive colonic segment in constipated IBS and other patients was unaffected by CCK and secretin. Thus CCK may only play a role in abdominal pain induced by eating and have no part in any other symptom of IBS. It would, therefore, be of great interest, should this first study be confirmed to determine whether some IBS patients only have pain or other symptoms with fatty, carbohydrate, or protein meals. Such an analysis, if carried out, might provide some further leads to our understanding of the syndrome.

Although morphine is the most powerful constipating agent known and produces hypermotility (Painter & Truelove, 1964), no studies in IBS have been carried out on endorphins or their antagonists.

Psychophysiology.   That emotions may change gastrointestinal motility, mucosal blood flow, or mucous secretion has been known at least since the time of Pavlov (1910) and Cannon (1929). These observations were significantly extended in normal human beings by Almy et al. (1947, 1949a, 1950) and many others. Specific correlations between increases in colonic contraction and mucosal engorgement and pain, fear, anger, excitement, tenseness, withholding, and coping were found. Giving up and hopelessness produced a diminution of contractions (Chaudhary & Truelove, 1961; Connell, 1962; Wangel & Deller, 1965). Indeed, morbidly depressed patients are constipated, but if giving up, depression, and hopelessness produce diminished colonic contractions, such patients should have diarrhea! In all likelihood, the changes associated with the emotions have no specificity, occurring in all persons: normal persons, those with IBS, and those with ulcerative colitis (Almy et al., 1949a,b; Chaudhary & Truelove, 1961).

Furthermore, marked individual differences are seen in response to the eliciting of strong, short-term emotions (Almy et al., 1950; Latimer et al., 1981) in IBS patients and normal subjects. In fact, the laboratory may not be the place in which these relationships can or should be sought. On the other hand, emotion and food may produce the same responses in patients with IBS of various categories (Wangel & Deller, 1965).

Studies on the psychophysiology of the colon have not identified any specific characteristic of IBS patients. But no other kinds of studies to date have done so either. Thus, one must conclude that pain or emotion may change colonic motility over the short term. The common occurrence of anxiety and depression in patients as traits does not, however, explain the etiology or pathogenesis of IBS.

CONCLUSION

In the introduction to this chapter, it was pointed out that there is a long tradition in medicine to seek out the singular anatomical basis for symptoms and disease. When no anatomical basis can be found, the traditional model of disease is not applicable, and conceptual disarray and confusion ensue. When minor anatomical deviations in organs are found, hope is reestablished, and these deviations become the sole explanation for disturbances in function; in actual fact, they may be the result of a disturbance in function, not the antecedent of it. The IBS is an example of the conceptual confusion that traditional medical thought brings about.

In reviewing this area of medicine, several conclusions force themselves upon the reader:

1. The symptoms of IBS do not point to a local but to a general disturbance of the entire alimentary canal.
2. The symptoms of IBS are additionally embedded in a matrix of symptoms of pain and distress which are characteristic of an illness of a person, not a diseased portion of the gut.
3. The search for a single cause for any one symptom of IBS is fruitless because each of the main categories of symptoms—globus, esophageal motility disturbances, diffuse esophageal spasm, esophageal reflux, dyspepsia, and the colonic syndrome—is characterized by several different physiological disturbances.

   Even in the case of esophageal refluxing of acid, the local disturbance is not singular. Both a disturbance in acid clearing and a lowered esophageal pressure need to be present, but neither is sufficient to produce symptoms unless a more general disturbance in the arousal mechanism (from sleep), centrally regulated, also exists.

4. There are no unique or consistent disturbances in the function of the colon in IBS. Also, several different patterns of functional disturbance have been described in the irritable colon syndrome. These, in turn, suggest that the disturbances are neither unitary, nor local—at the effector terminal. Rather, they suggest disturbances of the regulation and modulation of motility occurring in interneurons at several levels—the enteric, spinal, brain stem, etc.

5. The emotional disturbances described in IBS do not alone or uniquely produce the disturbances in function. They must interact with some predisposition which, in turn, could, as Chaudhary and Truelove (1962) first described, be of an infectious nature (including a viral one). On the other hand, early social experiences could alter gut function. The predisposition could take the form of altered receptor sensitivity or number, or changes in membrane potential to a host of neural and humoral influences regulating motility in various parts of the gut. (It is not likely, however, that the answer will be found by measuring blood levels of various peptides, etc.)

What needs to be done to further our knowledge in this important area?:

1. A detailed behavioral analysis of each IBS patient, as Engel (1983) has advocated, which seeks to determine the characteristics of symptoms, their antecedents, and their contingencies. Such an analysis would pay particular attention to the specific (and recurrent) social context in which symptoms occur, including the manner with which it was coped and the availability of supports. The analysis should include details about the composition of the diet.

2. A detailed longitudinal history of each patient, including a family history.

3. Studies of children with abdominal pain, diarrhea, or constipation (Stone & Barbero, 1970) with particular emphasis on the context in which symptoms occur. Long-term follow-up studies should provide information as to whether and when such symptoms recur in adolescence and early adulthood.

4. Studies of the differences between those patients with IBS who seek medical help (10 percent) and those who do not. How do they differ socially, psychologically, physiologically? Are those who seek help devoid of supports?

5. Development of techniques for studying dyspeptic patients in order to characterize subgroups by measuring serum gastrin, proteases, gastric electrical activity, motility patterns, and transit time to fluids and liquids.

In the case of the irritable colon syndrome, studies of various responses of subgroups to the local application of peptides. Techniques should be developed for studying all four kinds of colonic myoelectric activity and the five kinds of motor activity (nonpropulsive, haustral, multi-haustral, mass propulsive, and peristaltic).

6. Psychophysiological studies within and between individuals to determine whether the responses to psychological stimuli, drugs, or peptides are state-dependent. If so, they might account for the marked individual differences noted by Latimer (1983).

7. Once various subgroups of IBS are characterized, psychophysiological, behavioral interventions should be attempted to determine which are most effective in what subform.

REFERENCES

Alexander, F. G. (1950). *Psychosomatic medicine*. New York: W. W. Norton.

Almy, T. P. (1983). Clinical features and diagnosis of functional GI disorders. In W. Y. Chey (Ed.), *Functional disorders of the digestive tract* (pp. 7–11). New York: Raven Press.

Almy, T. P., Abbot, F. K., & Hinkle, L. E. (1950). Alterations in colonic function in man under stress. IV. Hypomotility of the sigmoid colon and its relationship to the mechanism of functional diarrhea. *Gastroenterology, 15*, 95–103.

Almy, T. P., Hinkle, L. E., Berle, B., & Kern, F. (1949b). Alterations in colonic function in man under stress: Experimental production of sigmoid spasm in patients with spastic constipation. *Gastroenterology, 12*, 437–449.

Almy, T. P., Kern, F., & Tulin, M. (1949a). Alterations in colonic function in man under stress: Experimental production of sigmoid spasm in healthy persons. *Gastroenterology, 12*, 425–436.

Almy, T. P., & Tulin, M. (1947). Alterations in colonic function in man under stress: Experimental production of changes simulating the "irritable colon." *Gastroenterology, 8*, 616–626.

Alpers, D. H. (1981). Irritable bowel syndrome—still more questions than answers. *Gastroenterology, 80*, 1068.

Alpers, D. H. (1983). Functional gastrointestinal disorders. *Hospital Practice, 18*, 139–153.

Bacon, F. (1605). *The two books of proficience and advancement of learning*. London: Tomes.

Benjamin, S. B., Gerhardt, D. C., & Castell, D. O. (1977). High amplitude peristaltic esophageal contractions associated with chest pain and/or dysphagia. *Gastroenterology, 77*, 478–483.

Bennett, J. R., & Atkinson, M. (1966). The differentiation between oesophageal and cardiac pain. *Lancet, 2*, 1123–1127.

Besterman, H. S., Sarson, D. L., Rambaud, J. C., Stewart, J. S., Guerkin, S., & Bloom, S. R. (1981). Gut hormone responses in the irritable bowel syndrome. *Digestion, 21*, 219–224.

Bloom, A. A., LoPresti, P., & Farrar, J. T. (1968). Motility of the intact human colon. *Gastroenterology, 54*, 232–240.

Brand, D. L., Martin, D., & Pope, II, C. E. (1977). Esophageal manometrics in patients with angina-like chest pain. *Digestive Diseases and Science, 22*, 300–304.

Bueno, L., Fioramonti, J., Rukebusch, Y., Frexinos, J., & Coulomb, P. (1980). Evaluation of colonic myoelectrical activity in health and functional disorders. *Gut, 21*, 480–485.

Bukhave, K., & Rask-Madsen, J. (1980). An approach to evaluation of local intestinal PG production and clinical assessment of its inhibition by indomethacin in chronic diarrhea. *Advances in Prostaglandin and Thromboxane Research, 8*, 1627–1631.

Cannon, W. B. (1929). *Bodily changes in pain, hunger, fear and rage*. New York: Appleton–Century–Crofts.

Castell, D. O. (1976). Achalasia and diffuse esophageal spasm. *Archives of Internal Medicine, 136,* 571–579.

Champion, P. (1973). Some cases of the irritable bowel syndrome studied by intraluminal pressure recordings. *Digestion, 9,* 21–29.

Chaudhary, N. A., & Truelove, S. C. (1961). Human colonic motility: A comparative study of normal subjects, patients with ulcerative colitis and patients with irritable colon syndrome. *Gastroenterology, 40,* 1–17.

Chaudhary, N. A., & Truelove, S. C. (1962). The irritable colon syndrome: A study of the clinical features, predisposing causes and prognosis in 130 cases. *Quarterly Journal of Medicine, 31,* 307–323.

Chey, W. H., You, C. H., Lee, K. Y., & Menguy, R. (1983). Gastric dysrhythmia: Clinical aspects. In W. Y. Chey (Ed.), *Functional disorders of the digestive tract* (pp. 175–181). New York: Raven Press.

Chowdhury, A. R., Dinoso, V. P., & Lorber, D. H. (1976). Characterization of a hyperactive segment at the rectosigmoid function. *Gastroenterology, 71,* 584–588.

Christensen, J. (1971). The control of gastrointestinal movements: Some old and new views. *New England Journal of Medicine, 285,* 85–98.

Clouse, R. E., Lustman, P. J. (1983). Psychiatric illness and contraction abnormalities of the esophagus. *New England Journal of Medicine, 309,* 1337–1342.

Cohen, B. R. (1973). Emotional considerations in esophageal disease. In A. E. Lindner (Ed.), *Emotional factors in gastrointestinal disease* pp. 37–44. Amsterdam: Excerpta Medica.

Cohen, S. (1979). Motor disorders of the esophagus. *New England Journal of Medicine, 301,* 184–192.

Connell, A. M. (1962). The motility of the pelvic colon. II: Paradoxical motility in diarrhea and constipation. *Gut, 3,* 342–348.

Connell, A. M., Gaafer, M., Hassanein, M. A., & Jones, F. A. (1964). Motility of the pelvic colon. III: Motility response in patients with symptoms following amoebic dysentery. *Gut, 5,* 443–447.

Connell, A. M., Jones, F. A., & Rowlands, E. N. (1965). Motility of the pelvic colon. IV: Abdominal pain associated with colonic hypermotility after meals. *Gut, 6,* 105–112.

Crean, G. P., Card, W. I., Beattie, A. D., Holden, R. J., James, W. B., Knill-Jones, R. P. Lucas, R. W., & Spiegelhalter, D. (1982). Ulcer-like dyspepsia. *Scandinavian Journal of Gastroenterology (Suppl.), 79,* 9–15.

DaCosta, J. M. (1871). Membranous enteritis. *American Journal of Medical Science, 124,* 321–338.

Daniel, E. E. (1975). Electrophysiology of the colon. *Gut, 16,* 298–329.

Davies, H. A., Jones, D. B., & Rhodes, J. (1982). "Esophageal angina" as the cause of chest pain. *Journal of the American Medical Association, 249,* 2274–2278.

Dent, J., Dodds, W. J., Friedman, R. H., Sekiguchi, T., Hogan, W. J., Arndorfer, R. C., & Petrie, D. J. (1980). Mechanism of gastroesophageal reflux in recumbent asymptomatic human subjects. *Journal of Clinical Investigation, 65,* 226–267.

DiMarino, A. J., Jr., & Cohen, S. (1974). Characteristics of lower esophageal sphincter function in symptomatic diffuse esophageal spasm. *Gastroenterology, 66,* 1–6.

Dinoso, V. P., Meshkinpour, H., Lorber, S. H., Gutierrez, J. G., & Chey, W. Y. (1973). Motor responses of the sigmoid colon and rectum to exogenous cholecystokinin and secretion. *Gastroenterology, 65,* 438–444.

Dodge, J. A., Handi, I. A., Burns, G. M., & Yamashiro, Y. (1981). Toddler diarrhea and prostaglandins. *Archives of Diseases of Children, 56,* 705–707.

Dotevall, G. J., Svedlund, J., & Sjodin, I. (1982). Symptoms in irritable bowel disease. *Scandinavian Journal of Gastroenterology, (Suppl.), 79,* 16–19.

Drossman, D. A. (1982). Patients with psychogenic abdominal pain: Six years' observation in the medical setting. *American Journal of Psychiatry, 139,* 1549–1557.

Drossman, D. A., Powell, D. W., & Sessions, J. T., Jr. (1977). The irritable bowel syndrome. *Gastroenterology, 73*, 811–822.

Drossman, D. A., Sandler, R. S., McKee, D. C., & Lovitz, A. J. (1982). Bowel patterns among subjects not seeking health care: use of a questionnaire to identify a population with bowel dysfunction. *Gastroenterology, 83*, 529–534.

Edwards, F. C., & Coghill, N. F. (1968). Clinical manifestations of patients with chronic atrophic gastritis, gastric ulcer and duodenal ulcer. *Quarterly Journal of Medicine, 37*, 337–360.

Engel, B. T. (1983). Fecal incontinence and encopresis: A psychophysiological analysis. In R. Hölzl & W. E. Whitehead (Eds.), *Psychophysiology of the gastrointestinal tract* (pp. 301–310). New York: Plenum Press.

Esler, M. D., & Goulston, K. J. (1973). Levels of anxiety in colonic disorders. *New England Journal of Medicine, 288*, 16–20.

Fielding, J. (1977). A year in outpatients with the irritable bowel syndrome. *Irish Journal of Medical Science, 146*, 162–166.

Fielding, J. (1978). Clinical and radiological manifestation of the irritable bowel syndrome. *Journal of the Irish College of Physicians and Surgeons, 8*, 11–15.

Fielding, J. F. (1984). Clinical recognition of stress-related gastrointestinal disorders in adults. In R. E. Ballieux, J. F. Fielding, & A. L'Abbate (Eds.), *Breakdown in human adaptation to stress* Vol. II, pp. 799–806. Boston: Martinus Nijhoff.

Gillies, M., Nicks, R., & Skyring, A. (1967). Clinical manometric and pathological studies in diffuse esophageal spasm. *British Medical Journal, 2*, 527–530.

Glossi, F. B., Messini, B., Del Duca, T., Ricci, M., & Messini, M. (1966). Peristaltic activity of the colonic mass in sequence after the administration of "Cecekin." *Clinica Therapeutica, 37*, 117–121.

Goldman, M. S., Rasch, M. S., Jr., Wilts, D. S., & Finkel, M. (1967). The incidence of esophagitis in peptic ulcer disease. *American Journal of Digestive Diseases, 12*, 994–999.

Gomez, J., & Dally, P. (1977). Psychologically mediated abdominal pain in surgical and medical outpatient clinics. *British Medical Journal, 1*, 1451–1453.

Graham, D. Y. (1978). Hypertensive lower esophageal sphincter: A reappraisal. *Southern Medical Journal, 71*, 31–37.

Gregg, J. A., & Garabedian, M. (1974). Duodenitis. *American Journal of Gastroenterology, 61*, 177–184.

Gutierrez, J. G., Chey, W. Y., & Dinoso, V. P. (1974). Actions of cholecystokinin and secretin on the motor activity of the small intestine in man. *Gastroenterology, 67*, 35–41.

Harvey, R. F., & Read, A. E. (1973). Effect of cholecystokinin on colonic motility and symptoms in patients with the irritable-bowel syndrome. *Lancet, 1*, 1–3.

Harvey, R. H. (1979). Effects of hormones in normal subjects and patients with the irritable bowel syndrome. *Practical Gastroenterology, 3*, 10–15.

Hill, O. W., & Blendis, L. (1967). Physical and psychological evaluation of "nonorganic" abdominal pain. *Gut, 8*, 221–229.

Hislop, I. G. (1971). Psychological significance of the irritable colon syndrome. *Gut, 12*, 452–457.

Holdstock, D. J., Misiewicz, J. J., & Waller, S. L. (1969). Observations on the mechanism of abdominal pain. *Gut, 10*, 19–31.

Horowitz, L., & Farrar, J. T. (1962). Intraluminal small intestinal pressure in normal patients and in patients with functional gastrointestinal disorders. *Gastroenterology, 42*, 455–464.

Horrocks, J. C., & deDombal, F. T. (1978). Clinical presentation of patients with dyspepsia: Detailed symptomatic study of 360 patients. *Gut, 19*, 19–26.

Hunt, P. S., Connell, A. M., & Smiley, T. B. (1970). The cricopharyngeal sphincter in gastric reflux. *Gut, 11*, 303–306.

Hunt, R. H., Delawari, J. B., & Misiewicz, J. J. (1975). The effect of intravenous prostaglandin F_2a and E_2 on the motility of the sigmoid colon. *Gut, 16*, 47–49.

Ingelfinger, F. J. (1958). Esophageal motility. *Physiological Reviews, 38*, 533–583.

Ismail-Beigi, F., Horton, P. F., & Pope, C. E. II. (1970). Histological consequences of gastroesophageal reflux in man. *Gastroenterology, 58*, 163–174.

Jacobs, A., & Kirkpatrick, G. S. (1964). The Paterson-Kelly syndrome. *British Medical Journal, 2*, 79–82.

Jacobson, E. (1927). Spastic esophagus and mucous colitis. *Archives of Internal Medicine, 30*, 433–445.

Johnson, L. F., & DeMeester, T. R. (1974). Twenty-four hour pH monitoring of the distal esophagus, a quantitative measure of gastroesophageal reflux. *American Journal of Gastroenterology, 62*, 325–332.

Johnson, L. F., DeMeester, T. R., & Haggitt, E. C. (1978). Esophageal epithelial response to gastroesophageal reflux: a quantitative study. *American Journal of Digestive Diseases, 23*, 498–509.

Jones, V. A., McLaughlan, P., Shorthouse, M., Workman, E., & Hunter, J. O. (1982). Food intolerance: A major factor in the pathogenesis of irritable bowel syndrome. *Lancet, 2*, 1115–1117.

Kelly, K. A. (1983). Physiology of gastric motility and emptying. In W. Y. Chey (Ed.), *Functional disorders of the digestive tract* (pp. 143–149). New York: Raven Press.

Konturek, S. H. (1978). Prostaglandins and gastrointestinal secretion in motility. *Advances in Experimental Medicine and Biology, 106*, 297–307.

Kreuning, J., Bosman, F. T., Kuiper, G., vander Wal, A. M., & Lindman, J. (1978). Gastric and duodenal mucosa in healthy subjects. *Journal of Clinical Pathology, 31*, 69–77.

Lasser, R. B., Bond, J. H., & Levitt, M. D. (1975). The role of intestinal gas in functional abdominal pain. *New England Journal of Medicine, 293*, 524–526.

Latimer, P. R. (1983). Colonic psychophysiology: Implications for functional bowel disorders. In R. Hölzl & W. E. Whitehead (Eds.), *Psychophysiology of the gastrointestinal tract* (pp. 263–288). New York: Plenum Press.

Latimer, P. R., Campbell, D., Latimer, M., Sarna, S. K., Daniel, E. E., & Waterfall, W. E. (1979). Irritable bowel syndrome: A test of the colonic hyperalgesia hypothesis. *Journal of Behavioral Medicine, 2*, 285–295.

Latimer, P. R., Sarna, S. K., Campbell, D., Latimer, M. R., Waterfall, W. E., & Daniel, E. E. (1981). Colonic motor and myoelectrical activity: a comparative study of normal subjects, psychoneurotic patients and patients with irritable bowel syndrome (IBS). *Gastroenterology, 80*, 893–901.

Lehtinen, V., & Puhakka, H. (1976). A psychosomatic approach to the globus hystericus syndrome. *Acta Psychiatrica Scandinavica, 53*, 21.

Lennard-Jones, J. E. (1983). Current concepts: Functional gastrointestinal disorders. *New England Journal of Medicine, 308*, 431–435.

Levitt, M. D., & Bond, J. H. (1983). The role of intestinal gas in functional abdominal pain. In W. Y. Chey (Ed.), *Functional disorders of the digestive tract* (pp. 245–249). New York: Raven Press.

London, R. L., Ouyang, A., Snape, W. J., Jr., Goldberg, S., Hirschfeld, J. W., & Cohen, S. (1981). Provocation of esophageal pain by ergonovine or edrophonium. *Gastroenterology, 81*, 10–14.

Manning, A. P., Thompson, W. G., Heaton, K. W., & Morris, A. F. (1978). Towards positive diagnosis of the irritable bowel. *British Medical Journal, 2*, 653–654.

McMichael, H. B., Webb, J., & Dawson, A. M. (1965). Lactase deficiency in adults: Cause of functional diarrhea. *Lancet, 1*, 717–720.

Mellow, M. (1977). Diffuse esophageal spasm. Manometric follow-up and response to cholinergic stimulation and cholinesterase inhibition. *Gastroenterology, 77*, 472–477.

Mendeloff, A. I. (1983). Epidemiology of functional gastrointestinal disorders. In W. Y. Chey (Ed.), *Functional disorders of the digestive tract* (pp. 13–19). New York: Raven Press.

Mendeloff, A. I., Monk, M., Siegel, C. I., & Lilienfeld, A. (1970). Illness experience and life stresses in patients with irritable colon and with ulcerative colitis. *New England Journal of Medicine, 282*, 14–17.

Misiewicz, J. J. (1975). Colonic motility. *Gut, 16*, 311–315.

Misiewicz, J. J., Connell, A. M., & Pontes, F. A. (1966). Comparison of the effect of meals and prostigmine on the proximal and distal colon in patients with and without diarrhea. *Gut, 7*, 468–473.

Möllman, K-M., Bonnevie, O., Gudmand-Hoyer, E., & Wulff, H. R. (1976). Nosography of x-ray negative dyspepsia. *Scandinavian Journal of Gastroenterology, 11*, 193–197.

Murrell, T. G. C., & Deller, D. J. (1967). Intestinal motility in man: The effects of bradykinin on the motility of the distal colon. *American Journal of Digestive Diseases, 12*, 568–576.

Nagler, R., & Spiro, H. M. (1961). Heartburn in late pregnancy. Manometric studies of esophageal motor function. *Journal of Clinical Investigation, 40*, 954–970.

Orr, W. C. (1983). Studies of esophageal function during waking and sleep. In R. Hölzl, & W. E. Whitehead (Eds.), *Psychophysiology of the gastrointestinal tract* (pp. 5–20). New York: Plenum Press.

Orr, W. C., Robinson, M. G., & Johnson, L. F. (1981). Acid clearance during sleep in the pathogenesis of reflux esophagitis. *Digestive Diseases and Science, 26*, 423–427.

Painter, N. S., & Truelove, S. C. (1964). The intraluminal pressure patterns in diverticulosis. III: The effect of prostigmine. *Gut, 5*, 365–369.

Pavlov, I. P. (1919). *The work of the digestive glands.* Translated by W. H. Thompson. London: Griffin.

Peña, A. S., & Truelove, S. C. (1972). Hypolactasia and the irritable colon syndrome. *Scandinavian Journal of Gastroenterology, 7*, 433–438.

Piris, J., & Whitehead, R. (1975). Quantitation of G-cells in fibreoptic biopsy specimens and serum gastrin levels in healthy normal subjects. *Journal of Clinical Pathology, 28*, 636–638.

Powell, D. W. (1977). Intestinal motility: The irritable bowel syndrome. *Gastroenterology, 73*, 812–814.

Preston, D. M., Adrian, T. E., Christofides, N. D., Lennard-Jones, J. E., & Bloom, S. R. (1983). Gut hormone response in functional bowel disease. *Scandinavian Journal of Gastroenterology 18 (Suppl. 82)*, 199–200.

Read, N. W. (1980). Disordered transit of a meal through the small and large bowel in the irritable bowel syndrome. *Gut, 21*, A906.

Rees, W. D. W., Miller, L. J., & Malagelada, J-R. (1980). Dyspepsia, antral motor dysfunction, and gastric stasis of solids. *Gastroenterology, 73*, 360–365.

Ritchie, J. (1973). Pain from distension of the pelvic colon by inflating a balloon in the irritable colon syndrome. *Gut, 14*, 125–132.

Roth, H. P., & Fleshler, B. (1964). Diffuse esophageal spasm. *Annals of Internal Medicine, 61*, 914–923.

Roth, J. L. A. (1973). Aerophagia. In A. E. Lindner (Ed.), *Emotional factors in gastrointestinal illness* (pp. 16–36). Amsterdam: Excerpta Medica.

Rubin, J., Nagler, R., Spiro, H. M., & Pilot, M. L. (1962). Measuring the effect of emotions on esophageal motility. *Psychosomatic Medicine, 24*, 170–176.

Sarna, S. (1983). The control of colonic moltility. In W. Y. Chey (Ed.), *Functional disorders of the gastrointestinal tract* (pp. 277–285). New York: Raven Press.

Sarna, S. K., Bardakjian, B. L., Waterfall, W. E., Lind, J. F., & Daniel, E. E. (1980). The organization of human colonic electrical control activity. In J. Christensen (Ed.), *Gastrointestinal motility* (pp. 302–310). New York: Raven Press.

Schuster, M. M. (1983). Disorders of the esophagus: Application of psychophysiological methods to treatment. In R. Hölzl & W. E. Whitehead (Eds.), *Psychophysiology of the gastrointestinal tract* (pp. 33–42). New York: Plenum Press.

Schuster, M. M., Nikoomanesh, P., & Wells, D. (1973). Biofeedback control of lower esophageal sphincter contraction. *Rendiconti Gastroenterologia, 5*, 14–18.

Sladen, G. E., Riddell, R. H., & Willoughby, J. M. T. (1975). Oesophagoscopy, biopsy, and acid perfusion test in diagnosis of "reflux oesophagitis." *British Medical Journal, 1*, 71–76.

Smith, B. (1968). Effect of irritant purgatives on the myenteric plexus in man and mouse. *Gut, 9*, 139–143.

Snape, W. J., Carlson, G. M., & Cohen, S. C. (1976). Colonic myoelectric activity in the irritable bowel syndrome. *Gastroenterology, 70*, 326–330.

Snape, W. J., Carlson, G. M., Matarazzo, S. A., & Cohen, S. (1977). Evidence that abnormal myoelectrical activity produces colonic motor dysfunction in the irritable bowel syndrome. *Gastroenterology, 72*, 383–387.

Snape, W. J., & Cohen, S. (1979). How colonic motility differs in normal subjects and patients with IBS. *Practical Gastroenterology, 3*, 21–25.

Stacher, G. (1983). The responsiveness of the esophagus to environmental stimuli. In R. Hölzl, & W. E. Whitehead (Eds.), *Psychophysiology of the gastrointestinal tract* (pp. 21–31). New York: Plenum Press.

Stone, R. T., & Barbero, G. J. (1970). Recurrent abdominal pain in childhood. *Pediatrices, 45*, 732–741.

Sullivan, M. A., Cohen, S., & Snape, W. J. (1978). Colonic myoelectrical activity in irritable-bowel syndrome: Effect of eating and anticholinergics. *New England Journal of Medicine, 298*, 878–883.

Taylor, I., Darby, C., Hammond, P., & Basu, P. (1978a). Is there a myoelectrical abnormality in the irritable colon syndrome? *Gut, 19*, 391–395.

Taylor, I., Darby, C., & Hammond, P. (1978b). Comparison of rectosigmoid myoelectrical activity in the irritable colon syndrome during relapses and remissions. *Gut, 19*, 923–929.

Taylor, I., Duthie, H. L., Smallwood, R., Brown, B. H., & Linkens, D. A. (1974). The effect of stimulation on the myoelectrical activity of the rectosigmoid in man. *Gut, 15*, 599–607.

Taylor, I., Duthie, H. L., Smallwood, R., & Linkens, D. (1975). Large bowel myoelectrical activity in man. *Gut, 16*, 808–814.

Texter, E. C., Jr., & Butler, R. C. (1975). The irritable bowel syndrome. *American Family Physician, 11*, 169–173.

Thayson, E. H., & Pedersen, L. (1976). Idiopathic bile salt catharsis. *Gut, 17*, 965–970.

Thompson, D. G., Laidlaw, J. M., & Wingate, D. L. (1979). Abnormal small bowel motility demonstrated by radiotelemetry in a patient with irritable colon. *Lancet, 1*, 1321–1323.

Thompson, W. G. (1980). Laxatives: Clinical pharmacology and rational use. *Drugs, 19*, 49–58.

Thompson, W. G., & Heaton, K. W. (1979). Functional bowel disorders in apparently healthy people. *Gastroenterology, 79*, 283–288.

Thompson, W. G., & Heaton, K. W. (1982). Heartburn and globus in apparently healthy people. *Canadian Medical Association Journal, 126*, 46–48.

Truelove, S. C. Movement of the large intestine. *Physiological Reviews, 46*, 457–512.

Truelove, S. C., & Reynell, P. C. (1972). *Diseases of the digestive system* (2nd Ed). Oxford: Blackwell Scientific Publications.

Vantrappen, G., & Hellemans, J. (1983). Esophageal motility disorders. In W. Y. Chey (Ed.), *Functional disorders of the digestive tract* (pp. 117–124). New York: Raven Press.

Volpicelli, N. A., Yardley, J. H., & Hendrix, T. R. (1977). The association of heartburn with gastritis. *American Journal of Digestive Diseases, 22*, 333–339.

Wadsworth, M. E. J., Butterfield, W. J. H., & Blaney, R. (1971). *Health and sickness: The choice of treatment*. London: Tavis Publications.

Waller, S. L., Misiewicz, J. J., & Kiley, N. (1972). Effect of eating on motility of the pelvic colon in constipation and diarrhea. *Gut, 13*, 805–811.

Wangel, A. G., & Deller, D. J. (1965). Intestinal motility in man. III: Mechanisms of constipation and diarrhea with particular reference to th irritable bowel syndrome. *Gastroenterology, 48*, 69–84.

Weinstein, W. M., Bogoch, E. R., & Bowes, K. L. (1975). The normal human esophageal mucosa: A histological reappraisal. *Gastroenterology, 68*, 40–44.

Weser, E., Rubin, W., Ross, L., & Sleisinger, M. H. (1965). Lactase deficiency in patients with "irritable colon syndrome." *New England Journal of Medicine, 273*, 1070–1075.

Wheeler, E. O., White, P. D., Reed, E. W., & Cohen, M. E. (1950). Neurocirculatory asthenia (anxiety neurosis, effort syndrome, neurasthenia): A twenty year follow-up study of one hundred and seventy-three patients. *Journal of the American Medical Association, 142*, 878–889.

White, B. V., Cobb, S., & Jones, C. M. (1939). *Psychosomatic Medicine Monographs: I. Mucous colitis.* Washington, DC: National Research Council.

Whitehead, W. E., Engel, B. T., & Schuster, M. M. (1980). Irritable bowel syndrome: Physiological and psychological differences between diarrhea-predominant and constipation-predominant patients. *Digestive Diseases and Science, 25*, 404–413.

Whorwell, P. J., Clouter, C., & Smith, C. L. (1981). Oesophageal motility in the irritable bowel syndrome. *British Medical Journal, 282*, 1101–1102.

Williams, A. W., Edwards, F., Lewis, T. H. C., & Coghill, N. F. (1957). Investigation of non-ulcer dyspepsia by gastric biopsy. *British Medical Journal, 1*, 372–377.

You, C. H., Chey, W. H., Lee, K. T., Menguy, R., & Bortoff, A. (1981). Gastric and small intestinal myoelectric dysrhythmia associated with chronic intractable nausea and vomiting. *Annals of Internal Medicine, 95*, 449–451.

You, C. H., Lee, K. Y., Chey, W. Y., & Menguy, R. (1980). Electrogastrographic study of patients with unexplained nausea, bloating and vomiting. *Gastroenterology, 79*, 311–314.

Young, S. J., Alpers, D. H., Norland, C. C., & Woodruff, R. A. (1976). Psychiatric illness and the irritable bowel syndrome: Practical implications for the primary physician. *Gastroenterology, 70*, 162–166.

9

PEPTIC ULCER DISEASE
Are Some Regulatory Disturbances Acquired During Postnatal Development?

Sigurd H. Ackerman
New York Hospital-Cornell Medical Center

The links among behavior, brain, and organ pathology have been intensively studied in the case of peptic ulcer disease. Systematic observations establishing these links began to be made very early in the history of modern medicine. In 1841, Rokitansky presented clear evidence, based on anatomical data, that some forms of ulcer disease may have a neurogenic origin, especially involving the vagus nerve (Cushing, 1932). In 1845, Maurice Schiff showed that experimental ulcers could be produced in animals by unilateral lesions of the optic thalamus (Cushing, 1932). Prior to that, Beaumont (1833) had already published his observations on a patient with a gastric fistula, in which he described changes in the stomach associated with changes in emotional state.

Work over the next century and a half made these initial observations incontrovertible. There is little doubt that external stimuli and central nervous system (CNS) processes contribute to the normal regulation of gastric function and to the occurrence of some forms of peptic ulcer disease.

More recently, the question of vulnerability to ulcer disease also began to be addressed systematically. Could one identify specific states or traits that affect the likelihood that ulcer disease would occur in this person but not that one, or at this time but not some other time? There are many ways to formulate this question. From the point of view of the behavioral sciences, one important part of the question is whether differences in life history—other things being equal—could affect vulnerability to ulcer disease.

The study of acute gastric erosions in the rat—so-called experimental stress ulcers—have provided some insight into the issue of vulnerability. These lesions are fairly easy to produce. They occur readily, for example, if rats are physically restrained, especially in the cold; or if they are subjected to electrical shocks, especially in an approach-avoidance conflict paradigm.

About 25 years ago, a number of investigators began to study the effects of early experience on vulnerability to experimental ulcer disease (Ader, 1971). They found that vulnerability to gastric stress ulcer in the adult rat could be modified by many interventions or circumstances during development. These include daily handling, premature separation from the mother, restricted food intake, and differences in housing density. Although it was clear that circumstances early in life could have long-term effects on gastric stress ulcer susceptibility, it was not at all clear how this could happen (i.e., by what intervening mechanisms or processes).

As we began to study these intervening processes, much of our attention became focused on the developmental physiology of the stomach, and especially on the complexities of the regulation of acid secretion during postnatal development. The ontogeny of acid secretion in the rat is neither linear nor regular. Parts of the system come in piecemeal, or experimental interventions which delay the maturation of one part do not affect the maturation of another. The regulation of acid secretion, as it appears in the adult rat, is, therefore, the end result of a complex set of physiological adjustments which take place during postnatal development. Elements must come in or out at the right time during development, and up-regulation or down-regulation of systems must occur at the right time and to the right degree.

There is increasing evidence that similar regulatory adjustments also take place during postnatal development in humans. The fact that the regulation of acid secretion in most adults falls within a "normal" range suggests that these developmental processes occur successfully in most children. On the other hand, some adults, especially persons with duodenal ulcer (DU), have specific disturbances in the regulation of acid secretion. Many persons with DU (30–40%) have a higher than normal maximal acid output, and some have a high basal output. Various persons with DU have an increase in food-stimulated release of gastrin and acid, a decrease in inhibition by acid of the food-stimulated release of gastrin and acid, an increase in the sensitivity of parietal cells to secretagogues, and an increased parietal cell mass (Soll & Isenberg, 1983). Some persons have antral G-cell hyperplasia (Calam et al., 1979); others have an increased acid secretory response to ingested Ca^{++} (Barclay, Maxwell, Grossman, & Solomon, 1983).

Some occurrences of these regulatory disturbances in adults appear to be powerfully influenced by genetic factors, although the evidence is still inferential. Elevated serum pepsinogen I (PG-I) is inherited as an autosomal dominant trait. Elevated PG-I is associated with a high peak acid output. Overall, there is a strong correlation between serum PG-I levels and betazol-stimulated peak acid output ($r = 0.74$; Samloff, Secrist, & Passaro, 1975). Parenthetically, elevated PG-I also markedly increases the risk for DU.

Other occurrences of regulatory disturbances in adults could be state dependent. We know, for example, that low-level electrical stimulation of the anterior hypothalamus in rhesus monkeys produces an increase in the sensitivity of the acid secretory response to histamine without changing basal output or the maximal response. This increased sensitivity to histamine terminates when the electrical stimulation is terminated (Hall & Smith, 1969).

Yet another possibility—the one that I will address here—is that some of the acid secretory disturbances found in persons with DU might be acquired during postnatal development. If the normal maturation of acid secretion is a complex affair in which new regulatory interactions are introduced and older ones wane, then, in the course of these complex adjustments, errors can occur; "mistakes" can be made. Some errors might be introduced because of unfavorable environmental circumstances, and their effects might persist as disturbances in the regulation of acid secretion, such as the ones seen in adult patients with DU.

There is a straightforward way to address this possibility experimentally. If we characterize in detail the normal developmental transitions in the regulation of acid secretion, we will also know where this development could go wrong. We might then be able to identify the specific kinds of developmental errors which could lead to disturbances analogous to those seen in adult DU patients. Finally, we might be able to induce such developmental disturbances experimentally. I will present some preliminary work which takes advantage of this strategy.

THE ONTOGENY OF RESPONSIVENESS
TO PARIETAL CELL AGONISTS

Gastric acid comes from the parietal cell. The current thinking is that there are three types or classes of parietal cell surface receptors, each responsive to a different agonist; namely, histamine, gastrin, and acetylcholine. Thus, total acid output from a parietal cell is partly regulated by the availability of one, two, or all three of the specific ligands (Soll, 1978).

There is also evidence that stimulation of these separate receptors does not increase acid output additively, but rather synergistically. There are apparently potentiating interactions among these sites so that the maximum response to the three agonists together is greater than the sum of their separate effects (Soll, 1982). These parietal cell receptors can also be antagonized separately (e.g., somatostatin inhibits only the gastrin receptor).

In the rat, these receptor systems are not all functional at birth. Rather, each receptor system appears to achieve physiologic competence at a characteristic time during postnatal development.

We studied the ontogeny of acid secretion in the pentobarbitol-anesthetized rat by continuously perfusing the innervated gastric lumen with saline and titrating the amount of H^+ in each 10-minute sample to pH 7.0 with .01N NaOH. In the 15-day-old rat, histamine diphosphate (2–12 mg/kg/hr, i.v.) did not stimulate acid secretion, whereas both pentagastrin (120 μg/kg/hr) and the cholinergic stimulant, bethanechol (1 mg/kg/hr), produced three- to fivefold increases (Table 9.1). By day 21, histamine also produced a four- to fivefold increase in H^+ secretion (Ackerman, 1982).

Histamine affects both H-1 and H-2 receptors, although only H-2 receptors are found in parietal cells. We therefore attempted to replicate our observations on histamine using the selective H-2 receptor agonist, impromidine. Using 13- to 14-day-old pups (24–29 g), we found that the response to impromidine (0.9 μmol/kg/hr) was no different from the response to saline. However, in the same rats, the infusion of pentagastrin (120 μg/kg/hr) produced a fourfold increase in H^+ secretion (Figure 9.1). We also found that, at this age, impromidine did not potentiate the effects of pentagastrin and that cimetidine, an H-2 receptor antagonist, did not attenuate the effects of pentagastrin.

These findings show that in the rat, pentagastrin and a cholinergic agonist can stimulate acid secretion at a time during development when histamine (or impromidine) does not. Also at this phase of postnatal development, the histamine and gastrin "systems" do not interact.

If one studies rats younger than 12 days, neither pentagastrin nor bethanechol are stimulants to acid secretion. By the fourth postnatal week, the parietal cell is responsive to pentagastrin, bethanechol, and histamine and to the potentiating effects of their interactions. Thus, in the rat, there appears to be an orderly developmental progression in the responsiveness of the parietal cell to gastrinergic, cholinergic, and histaminergic agonists (Ackerman, 1982).

In humans, too, there appears to be a postnatal ontogeny in the regulation of acid secretion, although the data here are more preliminary than the animal data. During the neonatal period and early infancy, acid secretion probably occurs first in response to vagal stimulation, then to gastrin, and lastly to histamine. Neonates can increase acid secretion significantly over basal level in response to food, a response which is probably vagally mediated (Hyman, Harada, Everett,

TABLE 9.1
Effects of Three Secretagogues on Acid Output in 2-Week-Old Rat Pups

| Substance | Dose | N | Acid Output | |
			Basal	Stimulated
Histamine	8 mg/kg/h	10	7.62 ± 1.94	10.06 ± 0.61^a
Pentagastrin	120 μg/kg/h	14	6.78 ± 0.81	23.0 ± 0.3^b
Bethanechol	1 mg/kg/h	8	5.14 ± 0.7	27.1 ± 4.58^b

Note: Values (microequivalent per hour) are means $\pm$ standard errors.
$^a p > 0.10$, analysis of variance.
$^b p < 0.01$.

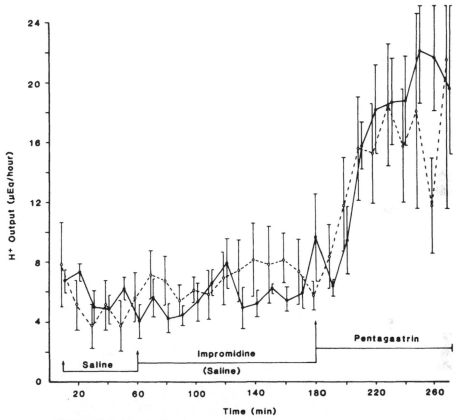

FIGURE 9.1 Effects of impromidine (0.9 μmol/kg/hr) and pentagastrin (120 μg/kg/hr) on H⁺ secretion in 13- to 14-day-old rat pups. Rats received saline (solid line; $n = 8$) or impromidine (dashed line; $n = 8$) during the second and third hours of gastric perfusion. Thereafter, all rats received pentagastrin. The effect of pentagastrin is significantly different from that of saline ($p < 0.0001$, analysis of variance), but the effect of impromidine is not.

& Ament, 1983). However, for the first 48 hours of life, there is a low basal rate of acid secretion, despite a high level of serum gastrin (Euler et al., 1977), and the low basal rate does not increase in response to exogenous pentagastrin (Euler, Byrne, Meis, Leake, & Ament, 1979). A secretory response to betazole does not occur until after the fourth week of life (Agunod, Yamaguchi, Lopez, Luhby, & Glass, 1969).

We do not know whether environmental or behavioral factors can intrude on this developmental progression to produce enduring disturbances in the regulation of acid secretion, but it is not hard to imagine that they might. For example, in the rat, antral gastrin (Lichtenberger & Johnson, 1975) and gastrin receptor binding (Takeuchi, Peitsch, & Johnson, 1981) both rise rapidly to adult levels at the time of weaning. This rapid rise can be delayed or attenuated if the onset of weaning is delayed. The long-term consequences are not known, but could such a delay or attenuation in the rise of gastrin lead to a long-lasting compensatory increase in the production of other agonists or to an up-regulation of parietal cell sensitivity to gastrin? If so, then the altered relationships could look, in the adult, like some of the regulatory disturbances found in patients with DU.

THE ONTOGENY OF BASAL AND MAXIMAL ACID OUTPUT

Another characteristic of the ontogeny of acid secretion in the rat is relevant to this line of reasoning. The rate of acid secretion does not increase linearly from infancy to adulthood. Instead, the greatest rate of basal and stimulated acid output occurs in the immediate post-weaning period and thereafter decreases to adult levels (Ackerman & Shindledecker, 1984).

We measured basal acid output (BAO) and maximally stimulated acid output (MAO) at three different ages: day 15 (1 week pre-weaning), day 30 (1 week post-weaning), and day 100 (adulthood). We determined the MAO in response to six different acid secretory stimulants. These included pentagastrin (120 μg/kg/hr), bethanechol (1 mg/kg/hr), histamine (8 mg/kg/hr), impromidine (0.9 μmole/kg/hr), pyloric ligation (4 hr), and low ambient temperature (core temperature reduced to 29°C). All of the data were collected from anesthetized, lumen-perfused rats as described in the previous section (except that, following pyloric ligation, the rats were conscious and gastric secretion was collected after 4 hours).

The results are shown in Figure 9.2. We found that both BAO and MAO increase through the first four weeks of life. Then, between postnatal day 30 and postnatal day 100, there is a 50% decrease in BAO and a two- to eightfold decrease in MAO, the size of the effect depending on the secretory stimulant used. These values are adjusted for age-related increases in the mass of the gastric fundus.

When changes in fundic mass are considered separately from changes in acid output, the data show that a 30-day-old rat, with only one fourth of the fundic mass of a 100-day-old rat, can secrete 2–3 times more H^+ ions/hr than a 100-day-old rat (Ackerman & Shindledecker, 1984).

We have tried to determine the mechanisms which account for this age-related decline in the rate of acid secretion after day 30. I have already indicated that the decline in acid secretion is not due to senescence of the mass of the gastric fundus as a whole. Another possibility is that it may be attributable to age-related changes in parietal cell mass. However, in morphometric studies (carried out with D. M. Jacobs) we found this not to be the case. Using an image analyzer, we obtained measures of parietal cell number, size, and volume density at 15,

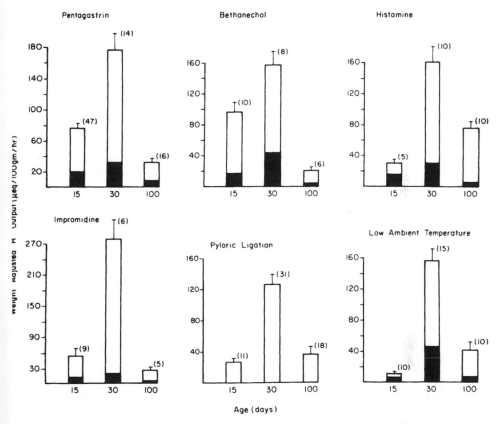

FIGURE 9.2   Acid output (mean ± SE) corrected for body weight (μeq./100 g body wt/h), at three different ages. Data from six different acid secretory stimuli are shown separately. *Black bar*, basal output; *white bar*, maximal output for that stimulus. Pentagastrin dose, 120 μg/kg/h; bethanechol, 1 mg/kg/h; histamine diphosphate, 8 mg/kg/h; impromidine, 0.9 μmol/kg/h; pyloric ligation, 4h; low ambient temperature, until core temperature = 29°C. Number of animals is shown in parentheses.

30, and 100 days of age. None of these measures correspond to the ontogeny of basal or maximal H^+ secretion (Jacobs & Ackerman, 1984).

The decline in acid output does not appear to be regulated by corresponding changes in available endogenous secretagogues or antagonists. There is no decrease, after day 30, in gastric mucosal histamine (Issac & Sapperstein, 1977), histidine decarboxylase (Aures & Hakanson, 1968), antral gastrin (Lichtenberger & Johnson, 1975), or antral gastrin binding (Takeuchi et al., 1981). The ontogeny of secretory antagonists such as somatostatin and secretin is not known.

Another possibility is that the developmental changes in acid output might correspond to changes in parietal cell sensitivity to secretory stimulants. This proved to be the case. We established a dose-response curve for pentagastrin at each of the three ages, through a dose range of 2–120 μg/kg/hr. The slope of the log-dose regression lines was virtually identical from 15- and 100-day-old rats, whereas the slope of the regression line for 30-day-old rats was significantly higher (Table 9.2).

We also obtained inferential evidence that vagal tone may be greater in 30-day-old rats than in either 15- or 100-day-old rats. We injected graded doses of atropine (0.1–4 mg/kg) intravenously during the continuous intravenous infusion of pentagastrin (75 μg/kg/hr) in anesthetized rats. Atropine failed to suppress pentagastrin-stimulated acid secretion in 15-day-old rats, produced only a 10% suppression in 100-day-old rats, and produced a 35% suppression in 30-day-old rats. The slopes of the regression lines for dose responses were significantly different for the three ages. These differences in the effect of atropine suggest that a substantial portion of the pentagastrin-stimulated acid output in 30-day-old, anesthetized rats is attributable to background vagal drive, whereas background vagal activation makes little or no contribution to the acid output at the other ages.

These preliminary data suggest the tentative conclusion that for conscious rats also, tonic vagal activity may be greatest in the post-weaning period. Increased vagal tone may account for the higher BAO around postnatal day 30. Moreover, both the increased sensitivity to pentagastrin and the greater MAO at this age may be attributable to tonic cholinergic potentiation of other acid secretory stimuli.

Vagal activity is readily modified by external stimuli. Thus, it is possible, in principle, that environmental factors in the postnatal period could prevent the normal developmental decline in tonic vagal activity. In that case, the adult animal would have an increased BAO and MAO and an increased sensitivity to gastrin, analogous to the disturbance in acid secretion seen in some persons with DU. Indeed, increased vagal tone probably does occur in a subset of persons with DU (Grand, Watkins, & Forti, 1976), although its genesis is not known.

TABLE 9.2
Sensitivity of Acid Secretory Response to Pentagastrin in Rats of Three
Different Ages

Age (days)	N	H^+ Increase/Log Dose	t	F
15	15	16.7	4.44*	
30	27	41.4	8.55*	91.22*
100	18	17.1	8.79*	

Note: Data summarized from linear regression analysis.
*p < .0001.

There are indications that increases and decreases in the rate of acid secretion also occur during postnatal development in humans (Agunod et al., 1969; Euler et al., 1977; Feldman, Richardson, & Fordtran, 1980; Miller, 1941; Miyoshi, Ohe, Inagama, Inoue, & Shirakawa, 1980), although the data from several studies are not sufficiently systematic or consistent with each other to allow one to characterize these changes with any confidence. In general, the data suggest that there are developmental changes in the rate of acid secretion in humans. It remains to be seen whether these changes can be permanently disturbed by interventions during postnatal development.

PREMATURE WEANING AND EXPERIMENTAL STRESS ULCER

The discussion so far is predicated on the assumption that the regulation of acid secretion could be modified during development so as to produce long-lasting changes of biological significance. An example which supports such an assumption comes from the study of experimental gastric erosions. Premature separation of a rat pup from its mother (around postnatal day 15) is a developmental circumstance that has long-lasting effects on both body temperature regulation and susceptibility to restraint-induced gastric erosions (RGEs). By the fifth postnatal week (the pre-pubertal period), rats ordinarily have achieved stable body temperature regulation and are relatively resistant to the occurrence of RGEs. In our laboratory, 24 hours of food deprivation followed by 24 hours of restraint produces no effect on the body temperature of 30-day-old, normally reared rats and only a 10–20% incidence of RGEs.

In contrast, prematurely separated rats subjected to food deprivation and restraint at this age have a marked fall in core body temperature (usually 4–6°C) (Ackerman, Hofer, & Weiner, 1978) and a high rate of RGE occurrence (about 90%; Ackerman, Hofer, & Weiner, 1975). Prematurely separated rats continue to have a greater RGE susceptibility than normals until after 100 days of age (Ackerman et al., 1975).

Body temperature regulation is closely linked to RGE susceptibility in that early-separated rats do not develop an excess of RGEs if hypothermia during restraint is prevented, whereas normally reared rats have a high incidence of RGEs if hypothermia is experimentally induced during restraint (Ackerman et al., 1978).

Body temperature regulation is also closely linked to the regulation of acid secretion. In anesthetized, normally reared rats, a fall in body temperature of 6°C produces an increase in acid output that is comparable to the peak response to pentagastrin (Ackerman, 1981; Figure 9.3). This response, which is abolished by vagotomy, is seen in both 30-day-old and 100-day-old rats. The relevant physiological mechanisms may be more related to body temperature regulation

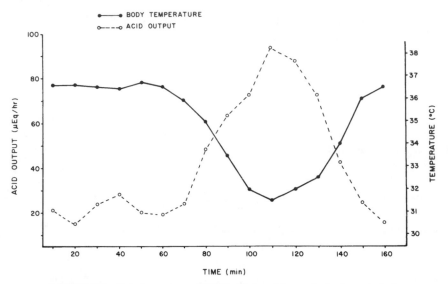

FIGURE 9.3   Data from a normal (21-S), 30-day-old, anesthetized rat. As body temperature is systematically lowered from 36.5°C to 31.5°C by external cooling and then elevated to normal by external warming, acid output correlates inversely ($r = 0.96$, $p < 0.001$).

than to body temperature per se. Thus, in conscious rats, a fall in ambient temperature from 22°C to 10°C produces a two- to threefold increase in acid output, even if gastric temperature is held constant experimentally and core temperature remains normal. In any case, a fall in core temperature is a sufficient condition for an increase in acid output.

The point here is that premature maternal separation in the rat, through its long-lasting effects on body temperature regulation, has enduring effects on the regulation of acid secretion. Because prematurely separated rats are more likely to become hypothermic under a variety of experimental conditions, they are more likely to have increases in acid secretion. Whether these effects on acid secretion contribute to the increased RGE susceptibility of prematurely separated rats is not yet clear.

CONCLUSION

The regulation of acid secretion during the postnatal period in the rat is different from that of the adult. Early in development, responses to gastrin and acetycholine appear to predominate over responses to histamine. Basal and maximal acid output increase through the postweaning period and then decline as the rat reaches adulthood. These acid secretory changes may correspond to an increase and then decline of tonic vagal activity. In humans, also, it is likely that developmental changes in the regulation of acid secretion take place during the postnatal period.

The identification of a normal ontogeny of acid secretion raises the possibility that abnormalities may occur as development unfolds. In particular, abnormalities might be induced during the postnatal period by circumstances in the external environment. In the rat, premature separation from the mother is one such circumstance which, under special conditions, can have persistent effects on the regulation of acid secretion.

These experimental data lead to the hypothesis that some of the disturbances in acid secretion seen in adult patients with duodenal ulcer may have been acquired during postnatal development. If this hypothesis is correct, these same disturbances may also be preventable.

REFERENCES

Ackerman, S. H. (1981). Premature weaning, thermoregulation, and the occurrence of gastric pathology. In H. Weiner, M. Hofer, & A. J. Stunkard (Eds.), *Brain, behavior and bodily disease* (67–85). (ARNMD Research Publication). New York: Raven Press.

Ackerman, S. H. (1982). The ontogeny of gastric H^+ secretion in the rat: Evidence for multiple response systems. *Science, 217*, 75–77.

Ackerman, S. H., Hofer, M. A., & Weiner, H. (1975). Age at maternal separation and gastric erosion susceptibility in the rat. *Psychosomatic Medicine, 37*, 180–184.

Ackerman, S. H., Hofer, M. A., & Weiner, H. (1978). Early maternal separation increases gastric ulcer risk by producing a latent thermoregulatory disturbance. *Science, 201*, 373–376.

Ackerman, S. H., & Shindledecker, R. D. (1984). Maturational increases and decreases in acid secretion in the rat. *American Journal of Physiology, 247*, G638–G644.

Ader, R. (1971). Experimentally induced gastric lesions. In H. Weiner (Ed.), *Advances in psychosomatic medicine. Vol. 6: Duodenal ulcer* (pp. 1–39). New York: Karger.

Agunod, M., Yamaguchi, N., Lopez, R., Luhby, A. L., & Glass, G. B. J. (1969). Correlative study of hydrochloric acid, pepsin, and intrinsic factor secretion in newborns and infants. *American Journal of Digestive Diseases, 14*, 400–414.

Aures, D., & Hakanson, R. (1968). Histidine decarboxylase and DOPA decarboxylase in the stomach of the developing rat. *Experientia, 15*, 666–668.

Barclay, G., Maxwell, V., Grossman, M., & Solomon, T. E. (1983). Effects of graded amounts of intragastric calcium on acid secretion, gastrin release, and gastric emptying in normal and duodenal ulcer subjects. *Digestive Diseases and Sciences, 28*, 385–391.

Beaumont, W. (1833). In *Experiments and observations on the gastric juice and the physiology of digestion*. Plattsburg, NY: F. P. Allen.

Calam, J., Taylor, I. L., Dockray, G. J., Semkin, E., Cooke, A., Rotter, J., & Samloff, I. M. (1979). A subgroup of duodenal ulcer (DU) patients with familial G-cell hyperfunction and hyperpepsinogenemia. *Gut, 20*, A934.

Cushing, H. (1932). Peptic ulcers and the interbrain. *Surgery Gynecology Obstetrics, 55*, 1–34.

Euler, A. R., Byrne, W. J., Cousins, L. M., Ament, M. E., Leake, R. D., & Walsh, J. H. (1977). Increased serum gastrin concentrations and gastric acid hyposecretion in the immediate newborn period. *Gastroenterology, 72*, 1271–1273.

Euler, A. R., Byrne, W. J., Meis, P. J., Leake, R. D., & Ament, M. E. (1979). Basal and pentagastrin-stimulated acid secretion in newborn human infants. *Pediatric Research, 13*, 36–37.

Feldman, M., Richardson, C. T., & Fordtran, J. S. (1980). Effect of sham feeding on gastric acid secretion in healthy subjects and duodenal ulcer patients: Evidence for increased vagal tone in some ulcer patients. *Gastroenterology, 79*, 796.

Grand, R. J., Watkins, J. B., & Forti, D. M. (1976). Development of the human gastrointestinal tract. A review. *Gastroenterology, 70*, 790–810.

Hall, W. H., & Smith, G. P. (1969). Gastric secretory response to chronic hypothalamic stimulation in monkeys. *Gastroenterology, 57*, 491–499.

Hyman, P. E., Harada, T., Everett, S., & Ament, M. E. (1983). Food-stimulated gastric acid secretion in the neonate. *Gastroenterology, 84*(5), 1193.

Issac, L., & Sapperstein, R. L. (1977). Gastric histamine metabolism in the aging rat. *Biochemical Pharmacology, 26*, 585–588.

Jacobs, D. M., & Ackerman, S. H. (1984). Differential growth rate of rat gastrin mucosal cells during postnatal ontogeny. *American Journal of Physiology, 247*, G645–650.

Lichtenberger, I., & Johnson, J. R. (1975). Gastrin in the ontogenetic development of the small intestine. *American Journal of Physiology, 227*, 390–395.

Miller, R. A. (1941). Observations on the gastric acidity during the first month of life. *Archives of Disease in Children, 16*, 22–30.

Miyoshi, A., Ohe, K., Inagama, T., Inoue, M., & Shirakawa, T. (1980). A statistical study of the age distribution of gastric secretion in patients with peptic ulcer. *Hiroshima Journal of Medical Sciences, 29*, 21–28.

Samloff, I. M., Secrist, D. M., & Passaro, E., Jr. (1975). A study of the relationship between serum group I pepsinogen levels and gastric acid secretion. *Gastroenterology, 69*, 1196–1200.

Soll, A. H. (1978). The interaction of histamine with gastrin and carbamylcholine on oxygen uptake by isolated mammalian parietal cells. *Journal of Clinical Investigation, 61*, 381–389.

Soll, A. H. (1982). Potentiating interactions of gastric stimulants on [^{14}C]aminopyrine accumulation by isolated canine parietal cells. *Gastroenterology, 83*, 216–223.

Soll, A. H., & Isenberg, J. I. (1983). Duodenal ulcer disease. In M. H. Sleisinger & J. S. Fordtran (Eds.), *Gastrointestinal disease*. Philadelphia: Saunders.

Takeuchi, K., Peitsch, W., & Johnson, L. R. (1981). Mucosal gastrin receptor. V. Development in newborn rats. *American Journal of Physiology, 240*, G163–G169.

10

DISCONTROL OF APPETITE AND SATIETY— SOCIAL AND PSYCHOLOGICAL FACTORS IN OBESITY
What We Don't Know

C. Peter Herman
University of Toronto

Any survey of social and psychological factors in obesity must immediately come to terms with the question, *Are* there any social or psychological factors in obesity? After all, obesity is essentially an anatomical or physiological condition; what reason do we have to suppose that social or psychological factors play any role at all in its development and maintenance? Perhaps obesity is determined genetically, as is often alleged; humans and other species tend to resemble their parents, anatomically and physiologically, even when reared apart (see Foch & McClearn, 1980, for a review). If you want to be thin, arrange to have thin relatives.

Even if obesity is not entirely a matter of genetic endowment, we do not necessarily have to invoke social or psychological mechanisms in order to account for its development and maintenance. For instance, we have been told (Knittle & Hirsch, 1968) that early nutritional experience may affect anatomical development so as to increase or decrease the likelihood that an obese body state will ensue. Thus, even if you are not destined from birth to be fat, you may become fat even in the absence of social or psychological influences.

As regards more short-term influences, we know that manipulations of the palatability of the organism's regular diet may affect the body weight (and perhaps the degree of adiposity) that is maintained (Peck, 1978). Could such changes in weight or adiposity occur strictly because the palatability of the diet per se affects set point and its metabolic defenses directly, with no behavioral mediation? Peck's (1978) proposal has been taken up again recently by Bennett and Gurin (1982) in their attempt to explain *everything* in terms of set point, and while their argument is not absolutely compelling, it does have some charm.

All things considered, then, it is possible to argue that social and psychological factors are overrated as determinants of obesity. One can easily imagine making a case for obesity as a strictly biological phenomenon, with the various social and psychological factors alleged to be responsible for it playing the role of an explanatory smoke screen. This line of argument has some appeal to me because I am often called upon to explain the importance of social and psychological variables to people for whom the terms "social" and "psychological" represent an admission of ignorance. The prospect of going over to the strictly biological camp, and denying a role to social or psychological factors, is particularly appealing because the defense of social and psychological variables in obesity is not all that easy, as we shall see.

In this chapter I argue that social and psychological factors have not been convincingly demonstrated to play a role in the etiology of obesity. To forestall any misinterpretation of this conclusion, though, I should add that it would be an extremely difficult task, methodologically, to conduct such a convincing demonstration; thus, the absence of a convincing demonstration should probably not lead us to infer that social and psychological factors are *not* involved in the development of obesity. The jury is still out.

By the same token, we must be cautious about ascribing too much explanatory power to biological predispositions. The current Zeitgeist regards such physiological constraints as what might be termed "causes by default." That is, researchers—and increasingly, the lay public—tend to assume that obesity stems from biological origins, unless some other cause is demonstrably present. Therefore, because social and psychological factors have not been established as contributors to obesity, we fall back on biological explanations. And even when social or psychological factors seem to play a role, it can always be argued that they exert an influence only insofar as that influence operates in the direction to which biology is already predisposed. This seems somewhat unfair since the biological camp has not provided a comprehensive account of the etiology of obesity either. Physiological correlates do not constitute explanations, nor do heritabilities. And the likelihood that different people get fat for different reasons renders monolithic explanations highly suspect. This paper's focus on the short-comings of social and psychological causes of obesity, then, should not be read as an endorsement of biological models; rather, my goal is to emphasize the difficulties involved in drawing any conclusions about the etiology of obesity.

So let us consider the case for social and psychological factors. At least in some trivial senses, social and psychological factors are obviously involved in obesity. For instance, it is obvious that there are significant social and psychological consequences of obesity. In our society, at least, one cannot help but notice the powerful reactions that obesity elicits in other people, reactions which, for the most part, are expressions of a negative stereotype. I will not belabor this point other than to suggest that most of the efforts currently under way to convince fat people and everyone else that "big is beautiful" are as yet pathetically unsuccessful. Obese people are seen—and see themselves—as ugly and ineffectual. If they *were* effectual, they wouldn't be so fat and ugly.

But, of course, identifying social and psychological consequences of obesity is not really what we had in mind. The question is, really, Do social and psychological factors contribute to obesity? One approach to answering this question that appeals to me, if only by virtue of its perversity, is to assert the importance of psychological factors in obesity by definition. There is some distinguished precedent for this tactic. Bruch (1973) identified "thin-fat" patients, who to all appearances were thin but who on the "inside" (i.e., psychologically) were really fat. Nisbett (1972) identified a group of "superfats," who were fatter than fat, but who did not behave in the typical obese fashion; psychologically, they were normal.

While it is intriguing to think about biological fatness as distinct from psychological fatness, such thinking ultimately founders on the fact that when we say that someone "acts fat," we really mean that he acts as we would expect him to act if he were fat. But that so-called "fat behavior" is not really one of the defining characteristics of obesity; it remains simply a correlate. (It is interesting to contrast obesity with a condition occasionally regarded as its opposite—anorexia nervosa—where behavioral and psychological factors are very much a part of the definition of the condition. And bulimia, of course, is defined exclusively in terms of behavioral and psychological factors.)

Are there any nontrivial senses in which psychological or social factors might contribute to obesity? The answer is a qualified "yes"; and I believe that there are two channels through which such factors might operate.

The first channel is what I would reluctantly call the "psychosomatic channel." My reluctance to use this term is due to the term's having acquired a long history of misapplication to obesity. Historically (e.g., Kaplan & Kaplan, 1957), the so-called "psychosomatic" hypothesis has proposed that obesity results from overeating, which, in turn, is attributable to eating's effect on anxiety (and vice versa). I consider this a misapplication of the term "psychosomatic" because the effect of the psyche is not directly on the body, as in the case of asthma, hives, or ulcers. Stress does not produce obesity directly in this model; instead, it produces overeating, which in turn leads to obesity. The mediation of the psychosomatic effect by behavior disqualifies it, in my view, from the true psychosomatic domain. (There are also any number of empirical problems with the psychosomatic hypothesis, but these need not concern us yet.)

A true psychosomatic channel would operate such that one's psychological state had a direct effect on some bodily process that, say, altered one's metabolic rate and thereby produced obesity. Whether stress affects metabolic as well as behavioral end points is, at present, an open question, but it obviously should not be dismissed as a possibility. It seems unlikely to me that social influences operate through a psychosomatic channel, although one could imagine that the presence of other people might be stressful or relaxing, which might in turn affect metabolic rate. The interesting question thus remains: Can psychological or social factors contribute to obesity without the mediation of overeating?

Another mechanism that might produce obesity, and which seems to fall into the psychosomatic category, is the so-called cephalic-phase response. In this model, the anticipation of palatable food releases anticipatory digestive hormones; if the anticipatory response is unduly powerful, this may shift the metabolic balance in favor of obesity. The classic instance is the individual who gets fat merely by seeing—or even just thinking about—tasty food. This has been a chronic complaint of dieters from time immemorial, or at least since dieting became a voluntary activity.

The cephalic-phase hypothesis of obesity (Powley, 1977) suggests that, for a variety of reasons, including VMH lesions, organisms may show exaggerated cephalic-phase responses, which in turn are conducive to obesity. Note that in the purest version of this theory, the organism may get fat without eating any more than usual, because of its anabolic condition. Another version has the organism eating more as well, in response to hunger promptings which in turn result from the unnatural hormonal state. Unfortunately, the evidence that exaggerated cephalic-phase responses account for human obesity is scanty at best.

Some evidence has been presented (e.g., Rodin, 1978) that some people do indeed exhibit exaggerated hormonal reactions to the sight, smell, and cognitive anticipation of attractive food. But such people are not necessarily obese, and we cannot blithely assume that they will become so. And, in any case, the presence of exaggerated cephalic-phase responses in obese people is hardly proof that their obesity resulted from those hormonal reactions; causality remains terribly difficult to establish without manipulative control over the putative causal factor.

In our own lab (Klajner, Herman, Polivy, & Chhabra, 1981), we have demonstrated that dieters show exaggerated salivary responses to palatable food. This could mean that if they were to let themselves go, they might overeat to the point of gaining significant amounts of weight; but we have no way of determining this. Another implication, based on the "pure" interpretation of the cephalic-phase model, is that dieters may be anabolic; they may even weigh more than they otherwise would. We happen to believe—without a great deal of evidence—that dieting may well produce anabolism and make dieters weigh more on metabolic grounds. Whether this anabolism exactly opposes the weight that dieters lose by restricting their intake—that is, whether physiology "corrects" behavior—is at this point an unresolved question. It may turn out to be the case that dieters become anabolic through the rigors of dieting without losing significant weight at all; the net result may be that they end up weighing more than if they had not begun to diet in the first place (Polivy & Herman, 1983).

Anyone expecting a straightforward discussion of the social and psychological factors in obesity must be growing irritated by this point. Is there no simple mechanism whereby psychological and social factors can contribute to obesity?

Indeed, why spend so much time considering so-called pure "psychosomatic" effects when we know that social and psychological factors can produce overeating, which is the second and more obvious channel leading to obesity? The reason for this roundabout approach is somewhat embarrassing, but it ultimately cannot be avoided. The truth of the matter is that we have virtually no evidence regarding the two premises that underlie our belief that social and psychological factors contribute to obesity by making people overeat.

The first premise is that such social or psychological factors operate in the real world with enough consistency to produce significant long-term increments in eating. And the second premise is that significant, long-term overeating affects weight or obesity. Regrettably, it remains the case that most of our data are collected in short-term observations of eating from which we simply cannot extrapolate with any confidence. The fact that a social or psychological factor can be demonstrated to be effective in increasing eating in a particular context proves neither that it operates consistently as a general influence on eating nor that such overeating, even if it were to be observed, would produce significant weight gain.

Perhaps the preceding analysis is too abstract; let us flesh out the argument with some examples. For illustrative purposes, we shall consider three classes of social and psychological factors alleged to contribute to obesity: social imitation or modeling, externality, and stress. These examples are not meant to exhaust the range of psychosocial explanations for obesity that have been offered, but they are in many ways representative and depart from some of the more traditional clinical interpretations in that there has actually been some experimental research conducted on their behalf.

SOCIAL INFLUENCE

Probably the simplest example of a social influence on eating is the tendency for people to adjust their eating to correspond to that exhibited by others. When experimental confederates eat a lot, experimental subjects tend to eat a lot; when the confederates do not eat much, neither do the subjects (e.g., Nisbett & Storms, 1974). This imitative effect is not precise: Depending on exactly how much the confederates eat, the subjects will match them closely or not so closely. But the major effect—confederates who eat more generally induce subjects to eat more— is incontestable across a broad range of experimental conditions.

It is not difficult to imagine how such social influence might contribute to obesity. An individual who regularly happens to eat in the company of a lumberjack might be expected to end up weighing a great deal more than one who regularly eats in the company of a ballerina. Certainly it is a truism of dieting that having to eat in the company of nondieters puts a strain on a dieter (see Polivy, Herman, Younger, & Erskine, 1979, for an experimental analogue); the dieter's loved ones are encouraged to help set a good example.

But while people's susceptibility to social influence is indisputable, the implications of the phenomenon are very hotly disputed. From the standpoint of the hypothetical pure social psychologist, the implication might be that obesity is a socially induced condition. People get fat because they eat too much, and they eat too much because they track the eating of others who eat too much. Even if we leave aside the obvious problem of why the others eat too much in the first place, we are left with a number of perplexities.

First, how are we to reconcile this social influence model of overeating with what we know about the physiological control of eating? Even a social psychologist is vaguely aware that hunger and satiety—or whatever physiological needs underlie these phenomenal experiences—are influential in the control of eating. Thus, the individual who is famished or the individual who is absolutely stuffed cannot be expected to track the eating of other people who are not teetering on the edge of a physiological crisis. By the same token, though, the notion that physiologically determined hunger and satiety promptings account for all the variance in eating is demonstrably false, as the social influence studies show. In short, eating is vulnerable to social influence, but probably the extent to which social influence affects eating is constrained by physiology. We have been attempting to develop a model of eating (see Herman & Polivy, 1984) that is designed precisely to take into account the role of psychosocial factors within the range of influence permitted by physiological boundaries. Without going into detail, I can nevertheless reassure you that the quantitative aspects of such a model are quite far from specification. Although we know that social factors are effective up to a point, we can't really say how effective or up to what point.

Let us grant, though, what is undoubtedly true: Social influences can make people eat more, at least under certain conditions. Two major problems remain, though, before this fact can be extrapolated into an explanation of the etiology of obesity. First, is there any evidence that some individuals encounter consistent social pressure in the direction of overeating and obesity? The simple answer to this question is "no." This is not to assert that it is implausible that consistent social pressure might operate on a particular individual in the direction of overeating and weight gain; rather, I simply want to emphasize that the sorts of ecological studies of human eating behavior that would provide direct evidence are lacking. At present, we have a small but persuasive literature concerning the power of experimentally manipulated social influence on single occasions. We lack evidence that naturally occurring social influence situations are as powerful as what we have produced in the laboratory—although I do not doubt that natural situations are in fact occasionally quite potent—and we lack evidence that such influences tend to occur with the degree of consistency and repetition that would be necessary to produce obesity.

The second problem is that we have no assurance that consistent overeating causes obesity. The notion that overeating causes obesity, and that obesity is caused by overeating, remains the single most common etiological maxim in our culture, if not in our laboratories. But the fact remains that the data are extremely ambiguous. Over the past 15 years or so, we have been provided with a number of alternative views of obesity, in which overeating, as traditionally defined, is not the culprit. One view asserts that obesity is biologically determined and maintained; fat organisms need not overeat in order to get fat or stay fat, since their bodies are designed to achieve and maintain elevated weight or adiposity levels almost regardless of what goes on at the behavioral level. A second, more complex, view suggests that organisms may overeat in order to get fat. Note that in this view, overeating is not the primary problem, with obesity the unfortunate result; rather, the organism is somehow intended biologically to be fat, and overeating is simply a behavioral mechanism in the service of the biological demand.

Whether obesity is characterized by overeating or not, then, we cannot safely conclude that overeating is an independent cause of obesity. At most, it may be a mechanism by which an organism that is programmed to be obese achieves its natural stature. And, in many cases, overeating and obesity may be entirely independent. Again, we lack the sort of large-scale, natural environment studies which might establish the sorts of empirical relations under debate. More troublesome, in my view, is the persistent absence of a convincing method for determining one's biological set point. Ironically, the elusiveness of a good measure of set point has worked to its advantage, since an individual's set point can now be located wherever the researcher considers convenient until evidence proves otherwise. Thus, until such time as an indisputable measure of set point is provided, even the observation of persistent overeating leading to obesity remains subject to the interpretation that set point demands caused the overeating, which in turn facilitated the achievement of the obese state. Essentially, then, an elevated set point may be asserted as the ultimate cause of obesity, even if we obtain direct evidence of overeating as a proximal cause.

To return to our example of social influence, we are in somewhat of a quandary. We do not know whether social influence is capable of producing the sort of chronic overeating necessary to account for obesity. In fact, we do not even know if overeating *is* necessary to acount for obesity; and to the extent that it is, it may be that overeating (socially induced or otherwise) may be promoted in some way by the biological need for a higher weight or level of adipose stores.

To further complicate the issue, we must consider some preliminary evidence that some individuals are more susceptible to social influence than are others. Although the data are not entirely consistent, there is some indication that fat people may be more susceptible to social influence than are people of normal weight (e.g., Herman, Olmsted, & Polivy, 1983). As usual, such cross-sectional studies are difficult to interpret, since it is the person who is not yet fat who ought to be the real focus of our theoretical concern. Is the obese, socially influenceable eater obese *because* he is socially influenceable (and often under the influence of overeaters)? Or is he socially influenceable in the overeating direction because his body wants him to gain even more weight and uses every trick available, including heightened responsiveness to others' eating? Sometimes it seems that not even the accumulation of relevant data will suffice to disentangle these alternatives.

EXTERNALITY

Let us turn our attention briefly to a consideration of another reputed psychological influence—externality. There is still considerable debate about precisely what is meant by this term (Herman et al., 1983; Rodin, 1978), but there is general agreement that it refers to an exaggerated tendency to eat in response to environmental triggers. The mere sight of attractive food cues would be a good example of such a trigger.

Whether externality is considered to be a psychological factor will depend, of course, on what your definition of "psychological" is. In Schachter's original formulation (see, e.g., Schachter & Rodin, 1974), externality described a virtual reflex arc, passing from the stimulus through the perceptual organs and eventuating in a consummatory response. In fact, it seemed to apply fairly nicely to the way I think about the eating behavior of an amoeba; so I am not sure whether it really ought to be considered a traditional psychological factor, along the lines of, for instance, an oral dependency. Nevertheless, whatever externality may be, obese people are alleged to be characterized by it. And in one view, it is their externality that accounts for their obesity, inasmuch as anyone who is external is bound to become obese in our culture, where attractive food cues abound.

The alleged causal role of externality in obesity has undergone many challenges in the past decade. While externality still has some appeal as a phenomenon, as a causal agent its role has been severely circumscribed. Schachter himself traced the origins of externality back to what he suspected might be a "functional lesion of the VMH" (Schachter, 1971), but he went no further. Nisbett (1972) suggested that the functional VMH lesion was itself attributable to the organism's attempt to maintain a weight below set point. In his view, externality was not a primary etiologic factor, but rather a mechanism in the service of establishing a higher weight, as dictated by a biological set point. Externality was to be seen more as an agent than as an independent cause of obesity. That externality was more prevalent in obese people was not due so much to externality's causing obesity as to obese people's being more likely to enagage in deliberate weight loss attempts in defiance of set-point considerations. Externality represents nature's way of getting back at fat people who try, by dieting, to avoid their biological destiny.

We (Herman et al., 1983) have added what I hope will be a final twist to this convolution by arguing that externality and susceptibility to social influence are really two ways of looking at the same phenomenon. Externality and social compliance both characterize fat people, but neither is a true cause of obesity. In our view, the obese person, especially the obese person who attempts to diet— which is to say, most obese people—is characterized by uncertainty as to how to behave, especially when it comes to eating. Once the dieting mentality is adopted and normal physiological regulatory signals are dismissed as irrelevant to the weight-loss task at hand, the obese dieter no longer really knows when to eat or when not to eat. As a result, he or she becomes vulnerable to all sorts of suggestions provided by the environment. Signals from the social environment are typically classified as social influence variables; cues from the nonsocial, but edible, environment are regarded as externality variables. In both cases they provide behavioral guidance to the fat dieter who has lost touch with the normal, virtually automatic regulatory guidelines which are built into us physiologically and modulated by lifelong conditioning processes. Such automatic regulatory guidelines are severely disrupted by adherence to conflicting guidelines gleaned from diet books (Polivy & Herman, 1985).

Our contention, then, amounts to the proposal that dieting makes people compliant or external. These psychological properties of obese people are attributable to obese people being, for the most part, dieters. On the other hand, it may be that being compliant or external is what leads a fat person to undertake dieting in the first place so that only fat dieters ought to exhibit these traits. Or perhaps being deviant leads to a measure of compliance or externality in all fat people who live in a culture that derogates fat. (See Herman et al., 1983, for a discussion of these alternatives.) Unfortunately, it is easy for speculation to become idle in the absence of data bearing on causality.

STRESS

We seem to be no closer than before to identifying definite social or psychological causes of obesity. Before we abandon the attempt, though, let us consider one more candidate—stress. Stress as a proposed etiologic factor has a relatively ancient history in obesity theory and has appeared in many guises. The psychoanalytic view had stress interacting with an oral fixation to produce overeating and obesity (e.g., Cameron, 1963). Also, the symbolic consolations of a fat physique played a prominent role in the psychoanalytic account of obesity. For instance, obesity's resemblance to pregnancy, its connotations of physical power, or its value as a shield from social or other forms of intercourse were all interpreted as psychic dividends of obesity and thus contributory to the obese state (Bruch, 1973; see also Orbach, 1978, for a feminist perspective sharing some basic psychoanalytic assumptions). The psychoanalytic view, interestingly, often failed to distinguish between overeating and obesity, assuming that one entailed the other. ("Chronic overweight is nearly always a result of overeating. Endocrine and metabolic disorders are seldom involved.", Cameron, 1963, p. 689).

As we have seen, the "psychosomatic" view, which is really a variant on the basic psychoanalytic theme, postulates that stress produces overeating, owing to the anxiety-reducing effects of eating. Put differently, people in whom eating has an anxiety-reducing effect may be expected to become obese. Or perhaps eating has such an effect on everyone, but some people are more anxious and thus more likely to overeat. These alternatives are never quite as clear as they should be. Nor are the data. There is some indication, empirically, that fat people and/or dieters tend to eat more when stressed, whereas so-called normal people are likely to eat less (presumably because of the sympathomimetic, appetite-dampening physiological effects of stress). This general finding has been severely qualified, however, with some researchers (e.g., McKenna, 1972) obtaining the effect only when certain types of foods are available, and others (e.g., Slochower, 1976) noting that the effect appears only when certain types of stress are involved. The most important qualification, however, is that these studies are almost invariably one-shot laboratory investigations, from which extrapolations to substantial weight gain are extremely hazardous.

As with social influence or externality, we do not know whether stress-induced eating ever achieves the regularity required to produce a massive increase in caloric intake. And again, we do not know whether even a massive increase in intake will eventuate in significant weight gain, given the possible countervailing pressures that physiology may bring to bear. As before, we must be aware of the possibility that the vulnerability of some people to stress-induced eating may be yet another mechanism in the armamentarium of set-point defense. In our laboratory, it is dieters who show greater emotional response to stressors and who are more likely to eat in response to stress (Herman & Polivy, 1975; Polivy, Herman, & Warsh, 1978). Might these aberrations be defenses intent on restoring weight to its set-point level?

We (Polivy & Herman, 1976) conducted one study in which we demonstrated that clinical depression was associated with significant weight gain in dieters. However, our interpretation was that dieters, when they become depressed, may stop dieting as assiduously as before. The net result may be that they will regain previously lost weight. This is a long way from an explanation of obesity.

CONCLUSIONS

I have emphasized the gaps in our knowledge about the role of social and psychological factors in obesity. Indeed, I have argued that we are not in a position to grant such factors any definite causal role in the development of obesity. Most of my arguments have been premised on the assumption that physiological theories of obesity are adequate to account for it. Social and psychological factors may act as agents of physiology, serving to help achieve or restore the elevated weight that is dictated by set-point considerations.

This assumption is unabashedly reductionistic. It is easy to grant, for it puts me in the company of "real" scientists who are sure of the value of their approach. Unfortunately, though, this assumption, like the old psychoanalytic assumptions and the newer social psychological assumptions, is not as easy to defend as one would hope. The fact of the matter is that we do not really know why people get fat. It is certainly arguable that some of them are destined, biologically, to be fat. Among lower species, it would not surprise me if virtually all instances of obesity were expressions of genetic purpose. [There are a few interesting sorts of overeating that seem superficially to depart from the strict genetic view, such as cafeteria-feeding-induced obesity (see Sclafani, 1980); but even such examples can probably be reinterpreted, with a little ingenuity, within a framework of biological weight regulation.]

In humans, there remains some considerable doubt about the two assumptions that I have identified in this paper as underlying a social or psychological etiology of obesity. We do not know whether the acute effects of social or psychological pressures ever become so chronic as to produce the sort of extended overeating that obesity presumably demands. Above, I cast doubt on whether such chronicity obtained. Now, it seems only fair to cast doubt on the assumption that it doesn't obtain. We simply do not know. This is also true for the physiological regulation of weight.

We can well imagine that all excursions of weight are either demanded physiologically or counteracted physiologically, through a myriad of mechanisms involving hormones, energy expenditure, and even behavior. But by the same token, we cannot assert with assurance that dedicated overeating will not produce obesity, at least in some people.

How well defended is set point? My surveys of my colleagues leave me confused about what the consensus is on this issue. Is one to be impressed with the stability of weight or with its variability? Exactly how stable *is* human weight? Schachter (1982) reported that many of his friends and colleagues had lost tremendous amounts of weight and kept it off with little or no trouble. This report flew in the face of conventional wisdom and aroused the customary critiques of Schachter's data, methods, and purposes. Without wishing to share the castigation that Schachter suffers, I must nevertheless point out that the matter is still open to debate. Maybe weight is more malleable than a rigid set-point interpretation would have it. And maybe social and psychological factors play a prominent role in changing weight.

In our laboratory, we have focused on a phenomenon that we have termed "counter-regulation," in which dieters eat more after a calorically rich preload than after no preload at all (see Herman & Polivy, 1980, for a review). We have attributed this disinhibition to the collapse of the normal dietary restraint that characterizes dieters. Rich caloric preloads will certainly undermine one's capacity and thus one's motivation to stay on a rigid diet. But when we say that the observed "overeating" is caused by the preload-induced motivational collapse, we intend this only in a permissive sense. If one is no longer dieting, then one *may* eat.

But what is it that drives the overeating we observe in our disinhibited dieters? At one time, when we accepted the set-point analysis without much skepticism, we assumed that our dieters were below set point. Thus, if their eating was disinhibited, it would then be driven by the hunger that being below set point necessarily entails. At the very least, we viewed such disinhibited eating as somehow ponderostatic, a corrective to the physiological insult of dieting. Nowadays, we are not so sure. We have no real evidence that our dieters are below set point. If significant weight loss is really as hard to achieve as Schachter's critics contend, then it seems unlikely that our standard dieters could be all that deprived, especially inasmuch as most of them experience repeated episodes of disinhibited eating. And if dieters are not particularly deprived, then the assumption that their disinhibited eating is driven by long-standing hunger seems unwarranted. So why do they overindulge, if they are not genuinely hungry? At present, we are not certain; but it seems likely to us that factors other than the defense of body weight play an important role.

Elsewhere (Polivy & Herman, 1985), we have suggested that disinhibited eating is under the control of psychological and environmental factors that have little to do with physiological regulatory needs. Indeed, we have argued that the dieter, in attempting to overcome the normal physiological constraints against weight loss, may develop an eating pattern that is largely unresponsive to physiological pressures. Part of the price involved in the dieter's Faustian bargain (no allusion to Irving Faust is intended) is that physiological constraints on weight gain (as well as weight loss) may be abrogated, and psychological and social factors may gain the upper hand in the control of eating and weight. Admittedly, this proposal is speculative; but such speculation is not contradicted by facts, since the facts are themselves so suspect.

It is important to remember that granting a role to social or psychological factors in the development of obesity does not require that one abandon the notion that weight is regulated or that set-point defenses operate. What is required is an appreciation of the possibility that such physiological regulatory mechanisms may not be omnipotent. The dedicated overeater may be able to gain weight beyond the demands of set point or even beyond its preferred limits. Until we know more about the mechanisms and parameters of set-point defense in humans, it would be unwise to rule out a significant role for social and psychological factors in obesity.

REFERENCES

Bennett, W., & Gurin, J. (1982). *The dieter's dilemma*. New York: Basic Books.
Bruch, H. (1973). *Eating disorders*. New York: Basic Books.
Cameron, N. (1963). *Personality development and psychopathology*. Boston: Houghton-Mifflin.

Foch, T. T., & McClearn, G. E. (1980). Genetics, body weight, and obesity. In A. J. Stunkard (Ed.), *Obesity* (pp. 48–71). Philadelphia: Saunders.

Herman, C. P., Olmsted, M. P., & Polivy, J. (1983). Obesity, externality, and susceptibility to social influence: An integrated analysis. *Journal of Personality and Social Psychology, 45,* 926–934.

Herman, C. P., & Polivy, J. (1975). Anxiety, restraint, and eating behavior. *Journal of Abnormal Psychology, 84,* 666–672.

Herman, C. P., & Polivy, J. (1980). Restrained eating. In A. J. Stunkard (Ed.), *Obesity* (pp. 208–225). Philadelphia: Saunders.

Herman, C. P., & Polivy, J. (1984). A boundary model for the regulation of eating. In A. J. Stunkard & E. Stellar (Eds.), *Eating and its disorders* (pp. 141–156). New York: Raven.

Kaplan, H., & Kaplan, H. S. (1957). The psychosomatic concept of obesity. *Journal of Nervous and Mental Disease, 125,* 181–201.

Klajner, F., Herman, C. P., Polivy, J., & Chhabra, R. (1981). Human obesity, dieting, and anticipatory salivation to food. *Physiology and Behavior, 27,* 195–198.

Knittle, J. L., & Hirsch, J. (1968). Effect of early nutrition on the development of rat epididymal fat pads: Cellularity and metabolism. *Journal of Clinical Investigation, 47,* 2091–2098.

McKenna, R. J. (1972). Some effects of anxiety level and food cues on the eating behavior of obese and normal subjects. *Journal of Personality and Social Psychology, 22,* 311–319.

Nisbett, R. E. (1972). Hunger, obesity, and the ventromedial hypothalamus. *Psychological Review, 79,* 433–453.

Nisbett, R. E., & Storms, M. D. (1974) Cognitive and social determinants of food intake. In H. London & R. E. Nisbett (Eds.), *Thought and feeling* (pp. 190–208). Chicago: Aldine.

Orbach, S. (1978). *Fat is a feminist issue.* London: Paddington.

Peck, J. W. (1978). Rats defend different body weights depending on palatability and accessibility of their food. *Journal of Comparative and Physiological Psychology, 92,* 555–570.

Polivy, J., & Herman, C. P. (1976). Clinical depression and weight change: A complex relation. *Journal of Abnormal Psychology, 85,* 338–340.

Polivy, J., & Herman, C. P. (1983). *Breaking the Diet Habit.* New York: Basic.

Polivy, J., & Herman, C. P. (1985). Dieting and bingeing: A causal analysis. *American Psychologist, 40,* 193–201.

Polivy, J., Herman, C. P., & Warsh, S. (1978). Internal and external components of emotionality in restrained and unrestrained eaters. *Journal of Abnormal Psychology, 87,* 497–504.

Polivy, J., Herman, C. P., Younger, J. C., & Erskine, B. (1979). Effects of a model on eating behavior: The induction of a restrained eating style. *Journal of Personality, 47,* 100–117.

Powley, T. L. (1977). The ventromedial hypothalamic syndrome, satiety, and a cephalic phase hypothesis. *Psychological Review, 84,* 89–126.

Rodin, J. (1978). Has the distinction between internal versus external control of feeding outlived its usefulness? In G. A. Bray (Ed.), *Recent advances in obesity research* (Vol. II, pp. 75–85). London: Newman.

Schachter, S. (1971). Some extraordinary facts about obese humans and rats. *American Psychologist, 26,* 129–144.

Schachter, S. (1982). Recidivism and self-cure of smoking and obesity. *American Psychologist, 37,* 436–444.

Schachter, S., & Rodin, J. (1974). *Obese humans and rats.* New York: Halsted.

Sclafani, A. (1980). Dietary obesity. In A. J. Stunkard (Ed.), *Obesity* (pp. 166–181). Philadelphia: Saunders.

Slochower, J. (1976). Emotional labeling and overeating in obese and normal weight individuals. *Psychosomatic Medicine, 38,* 131–139.

11

THE REGULATION OF BODY WEIGHT
AND THE TREATMENT
OF OBESITY

Albert J. Stunkard
University of Pennsylvania

Obesity is hard to treat; there is no question about it. A decade ago, it could be said that "Most people will not enter treatment for obesity; of those who do enter such treatment most will drop out of it; of those who remain in treatment most will not lose very much weight and of those who lose weight, most will regain it. Furthermore, most will pay a high price for trying" (Stunkard, 1975, p. 196).

The treatment of obesity has improved since that gloomy pronouncement. Nevertheless, it is still true that drop-out rates remain high, weight losses are modest, and the maintenance of these losses infrequent. One thing, however, has changed during the past years. The explanation for this sorry state of affairs has undergone a 180-degree change of direction, and today we understand far better than we did before why it is so hard to treat obesity. The change in our understanding is one from a primarily psychogenic explanation of obesity to a primarily somatogenic one.

THE PSYCHOGENIC EXPLANATION

Although it was never stated as a testable hypothesis, the psychogenic theory of obesity informed the treatment for obesity for many years. This theory held that obesity resulted from an emotional disorder in which food intake, and particularly excessive food intake, relieved the anxiety and depression to which obese persons were unusually susceptible (Fenichel, 1945; Kaplan & Kaplan, 1957). Psychoanalytic theorists traced the origins of this disorder to the oral stage of libidinal development, ascribing it to either a deprivation or an excess of oral supplies. The resulting fixation of libido at the oral stage rendered obese persons unusually susceptible to the conflicts and frustrations of adult life. In the face of these conflicts, obese persons were seen as unusually prone to regression to the oral stage, and thus to excessive eating. Psychogenic explanations of obesity traditionally have been couched in terms of libido theory; for some reason, ego psychology was never seriously applied to the problem of obesity.

This theory neatly accommodated the five clinical problems of obesity noted above. Not entering treatment, dropping out of it, and failing to lose weight were seen as resulting from a disinclination on the part of obese persons to risk the loss of the oral supplies on which they were so dependent. The "dieting depressions" (Stunkard, 1957) to which obese persons are prone were seen as a consequence of losing these supplies, and the regaining of weight as a result of the overeating undertaken to restore the supplies. For many years the psychogenic hypothesis seemed to be a perfectly adequate explanation of these problems, leaving no need to look elsewhere. When new explanations came, it was from physiology and a study of the regulation of body weight. These explanations have turned the earlier psychogenic hypothesis on its head: The emotional disorders so closely linked to obesity are now seen as the result, rather than the cause, of obesity, particularly the result of attempts to control obesity by dieting.

THE SOMATOGENIC HYPOTHESIS:
THE REGULATION OF BODY WEIGHT

Normal-weight Animals and Humans

The idea that the regulation of body weight might be a determinant of obesity was a long time in coming. For many years discussions of the origins of obesity started with what seemed to be a truism: Obesity results from a disorder in the regulation of body weight. Nothing seemed to be more obvious. The wild fluctuations in the body weights of obese persons posed a sharp contrast to the stability of the weights of experimental animals and of many humans of normal weight. This contrast was even more striking when the remarkable regulatory ability of experimental animals was examined.

Perturbations of the body weight of experimental animals produced by a variety of experimental manipulations are predictably followed by a return to the previous weight when the source of the perturbation is removed. For example, rats made obese by force feeding (Cohn & Cohn, 1962), or by insulin injections (Hoebel & Teitelbaum, 1966) will subsequently lower their body weight to control levels when the manipulations are stopped. Similarly, rats made underweight by food restriction will increase their body weight to control levels when permitted to return to ad libitum feeding (Hamilton, 1969). Furthermore, they respond to changes in the caloric density of their diet by increasing or decreasing food intake so as to maintain a stable body weight (Adolph, 1947). The evidence for regulation of body weight in these animals is thus based not only on their ability to maintain a constant body weight under usual conditions, but to defend that body weight against attempts to raise or lower it.

Demonstrations of the remarkable ability of some animals to regulate their body weight are provided by the examples of migration and hibernation. These animals can not only maintain a constant body weight under usual circumstances, but they can also perform extraordinary feats of anticipatory regulation. Prior to its 600-mile flight across the Caribbean Sea, the ruby-throated hummingbird undergoes a period of premigratory hyperphagia which produces fat stores sufficient to provide energy for this long flight, plus a reserve sufficient for excess flying time in the event of adverse wind conditions (Odum, 1960). Similarly, golden-mantled ground squirrels undergo a period of prehibernatory hyperphagia that produces fat stores sufficient to provide energy for several winter months, plus a reserve sufficient for their survival during an unexpectedly prolonged winter (Pengelley & Fisher, 1963).

The evidence for the regulation of body weight in organisms of normal weight is not confined to animals. Two experiments with humans indicate that people of normal weight can also regulate body weight with considerable accuracy. A classic experiment (Keys, Brozek, Henschel, Mickelson, & Taylor, 1950) during World War II investigated the effects of severe caloric deprivation on young, adult male volunteers. Restricting their caloric intake to 50% of its normal value for 24 weeks reduced the body weight of these volunteers to 75% of its usual value. When they were subsequently allowed to eat as much as they wished, their body weight increased to its preexperimental level and stopped there.

Sims and Horton (1968) carried out a complementary experiment of the effects of excessive food intake on a similar group of young, adult male volunteers of normal weight. These men consumed diets containing two to three times their usual caloric intake until their body weights reached 125% of their initial values. Thereafter, when they were permitted to eat as much as they wished, they restricted their food intake, and their body weights fell to their preexperimental levels. Evidently, the precise regulation of body weight of so many animals also characterizes humans of normal weight.

Fat Rats

As evidence for the regulation of body weight mounted, the regulatory capacities of obese animals came under scrutiny. The first study dealt a severe blow to the regulatory disorder theory of obesity. When rats which had been made obese by hypothalamic lesions were tested for their ability to regulate body weight, it was found that they, too, contrary to long-standing beliefs, regulated body weight! Figure 11.1 depicts one of the first studies of the regulation of body weight by a hypothalamic obese rat (Hoebel & Teitelbaum, 1966). After body weight had reached an asymptote at its high postoperative level, force feeding produced

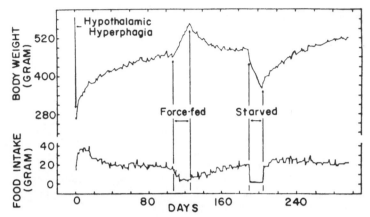

FIGURE 11.1   Effects of force feeding and starvation on food intake and body weight of a rat with ventromedial hypothalamic lesions (Hoebel & Teitelbaum, 1966).

further increases in weight. When force feeding was discontinued, body weight returned to its previous level. Similarly, Figure 11.1 shows that weight lost by starvation was promptly regained when the animal was given free access to food.

The hypothalamic rat (and genetic strains of obese rats) (Cruce et al., 1974) thus regulates body weight. But, if regulation is not impaired, why is it obese? One suggestion is that its obesity results from an elevation in the set point about which its body weight is regulated (Mrosovsky & Powley, 1977). Hypothalamic obese rats, according to this view, are not fat simply because they overeat; they overeat in order to become fat.

This theory was tested by an ingenious experiment (Hoebel & Teitelbaum, 1966). Figure 11.2 shows the production of obesity by insulin injections in Rat #3. When its weight had reached 475 grams, the ventromedial hypothalamus was destroyed. Two alternative outcomes were:

1. Food intake and body weight might increase if neural damage to a satiety area released its inhibitory effect.
2. Food intake and body weight might *not* increase if body weight was already regulated at a new, elevated set point.

Figure 11.2 shows that the experiment supported the second alternative: Following hypothalamic damage, there was no increase in body weight. The existence of a set point at about 475 grams was further substantiated by the consequences of a period of starvation and weight loss. When the rat was allowed free access to food, its body weight returned promptly to its previous level. Indeed, the rate of weight gain from its starvation-induced nadir was approximately the same as

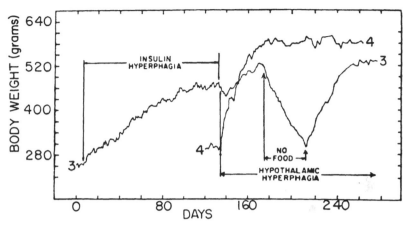

FIGURE 11.2   Failure of a rat to increase body weight following ventromedial hypothalamic lesions when obesity had already been produced by chronic insulin injection. The usual course of increase in body weight following such lesions is seen in the second rat. Food intake not shown (Hoebel & Teitlelbaum, 1966).

that of Rat #4, which shows the more usual course of hypothalamic obesity in which weight gain promptly follows hypothalamic damage.

Thin Rats

Rats can also be rendered *underweight* by hypothalamic lesions, this time in the lateral hypothalamus (LH). Two experiments (Keesey, Boyle, Kemnitz, & Mitchel, 1976) show the mirror image of the results with obese rats: a return of body weight to baseline after it has been artificially raised and lowered. Figure 11.3 shows the consequences of raising the body weights of LH rats. One of the LH group, at 79% of the weight of control animals, was force-fed to increase its body weight. Then it was permitted to feed ad libitum. Body weight promptly returned to that of the LH group from which the animal had been selected. The primary effect of the LH lesions is apparently on the body weight set point. As with hypothalamic obese animals, changes in food intake seem to be secondary to establishment of this new level of regulation.

A parallel experiment with food deprivation provided further evidence for the regulation of body weight in LH animals (Keesey et al., 1976). Figure 11.4 shows the usual body weights of these animals, which are 86% of the weights of a control group. Restriction of food intake further reduced their body weight to 80% of that of LH animals which had continued to feed ad libitum. Some of the animals in the non-lesioned control group were similarly deprived of food and similarly lost weight. When the animals were allowed free access to food,

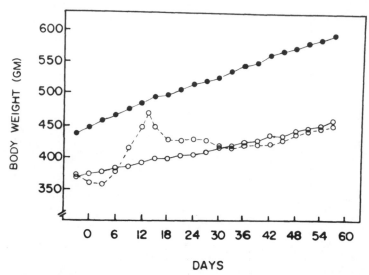

FIGURE 11.3   Reinstatement of anorexia in a lateral-hypothalamic-lesioned rat by means of force feeding. An animal selected from the lesioned group (open circles) was force-fed until its body weight approached that of the control group (closed circles). When it returned to ad libitum feeding, body weight fell to its previous level. (Keesey et al., 1976).

the body weights of both deprived groups, lesioned and unlesioned, promptly returned to the levels of their nondeprived controls.

Figure 11.4 shows how closely the pattern of weight change of the lesioned animals parallels that of the non-lesioned animals. Both regained at the same rate and took the same number of days to reach the levels of their nondeprived controls. The only difference between the LH and the normal animals was in the level of the body weights which each defended.

These experiments indicate that LH animals regulate their body weights, and they are compatible with the theory that LH lesions *lower* a body weight set point. They do not, however, test the theory in the same manner as the experiment illustrated in Figure 11.2 tested the parallel theory that ventromedial hypothalamic lesions *elevate* a body weight set point. Such a test would require that body weight be lowered to the level to be achieved by the LH lesion and then finding that the lesion produces no further weight loss. Precisely this outcome is depicted in Figure 11.5. It shows the changes in body weight produced by LH lesions in rats of normal weight and in those in which body weight had been reduced by food deprivation. Following the lesion, the body weight of the normal-weight animals fell to 93% of its previous value and then returned to a steady state. Following the lesion, the body weight of the food-deprived animals, however, showed a dramatic and paradoxical *increase* in body weight, a most unusual response to LH lesions. When an animal's body weight climbed to 93% of

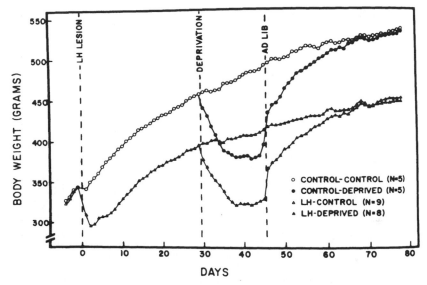

FIGURE 11.4   Recovery of body weight in lateral-hypothalamic-lesioned and control animals following a period of food restriction. Body weight of lesion-deprived and control-deprived groups was first reduced to 80% of the value each normally maintained. When returned to ad libitum feeding, body weights of each group returned to levels of the non-deprived groups (Keesey et al., 1976).

control values, it returned to a steady state. Lesions of the LH apparently establish a new and lower body weight set point; changes in food intake appear to be secondary to the establishment of this new level of regulation.

Anorectic Agents

A recent study has shown that anorectic agents seem to act precisely like LH lesions; they primarily lower a body weight set point and only secondarily suppress appetite (Levitsky, Strupp, & Lupoli, 1981). The experimental paradigm in this study closely paralleled that of Keesey's. They first deprived rats of food so as to reduce their body weight. The anorectic agent, fenfluramine, was then administered to these rats and to a control group whose body weight had remained at its baseline value.

Figure 11.6 shows the usual response of rats given fenfluramine at their normal body weight—decrease in body weight. Thereafter, weight increased slowly, parallel to that of the control rats, but at a lower level. By contrast, rats which had previously lost weight showed no drug-induced suppression of appetite. Instead, their food intake and body weight *increased* during the first few days on fenfluramine. When their body weight reached that of rats which had received

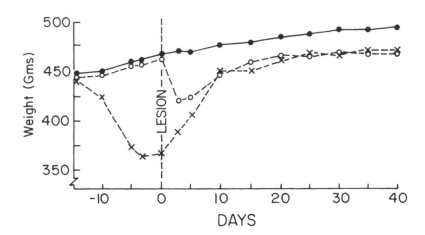

FIGURE 11.5   Body weight of control and lateral-hypothalamic-lesioned rats as a function of weight at time of lesioning. Solid circles refer to rats fed ad lib. Open circles refer to rats fed ad lib prior to lesioning. Xs refer to rats whose body weight had been reduced to 80% of control values by partial starvation prior to lesioning. (Redrawn from Keesey et al., 1976.)

fenfluramine at normal body weight, weight gain decreased to the same slow rate. It was as if their weight increased to the level set by that particular dose of fenfluramine. When fenfluramine was discontinued, the body weights of both groups of fenfluramine-treated rats rapidly increased toward control levels. These effects are not confined to fenfluramine, but occur also with d-amphetamine, an agent whose pharmacological and behavioral actions differ radically from those of fenfluramine (Levitsky et al., 1981).

Levitsky's experiment with fenfluramine is remarkably similar to Keesey's experiment with brain lesions, illustrated in Figure 11.5. They differ only in the reversibility of the manipulation. Surgical lowering of the set point is irreversible; pharmacological lowering is reversible. In each case, food intake is determined by pressures to reach a new set point. When this new set point is higher than the current weight, the usual response to both LH lesions and to anorectic agents (anorexia) is reversed. Under both circumstances, animals overeat!

Hervey and Parabiosis

An old experiment by Hervey (1959) provides additional support for the regulation of food intake and the existence of body weight set points. Hervey rendered rats parabiotic by opening the peritoneal cavities and suturing the cut edges of muscle and peritoneum to form artificial Siamese twins. The circulation of the members of the pair was sufficiently crossed to permit the exchange of plasma

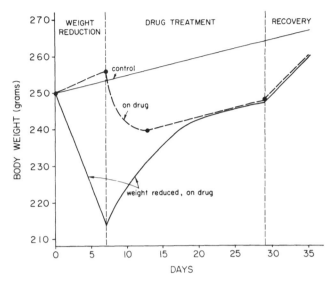

FIGURE 11.6 Increase in body weight during administration of "appetite-suppressant" medication. Following a period of weight reduction, rats gained weight when fed ad libitum even though receiving fenfluramine. When body weight reached that of rats which had received fenfluramine without prior weight reduction, rapid weight gain ceased. Body weights of both groups of rats rapidly returned toward control values when fenfluramine was discontinued. (Adapted from Levitsky et al., 1981.)

between the two at a rate of about 1% per minute. Under normal circumstances, each rat regulated its body weight. One rat was then made hyperphagic and obese by lesions in the ventromedial hypothalamus. The other rat responded in a dramatic manner: It drastically curtailed its food intake and, in some cases, even died of starvation. While body fat increased from 12% to 50% in the obese rats, it fell from 12% to less than 2% in their "twins."

Hervey suggested that satiety factors produced in the lesioned animal crossed into the unlesioned animal and decreased its food intake. A corollary interpretation is that the total body weight, or body fat, of the two animals was regulated. If the body fat of one animal was increased, that of the other animal was decreased in compensation.

Faust and Body Fat

Increasing body fat in one of a pair of parabiotic rats led to a decrease in the other. Decreasing body fat in a rat by lipectomy, conversely, leads to a compensatory increase in body fat. Some of the strongest evidence for the regulation of body fat comes from studies of lipectomy. Liebelt, Ichinoe, & Nicholson,

(1965) were the first to show that surgical removal of body fat in rats and mice was followed by compensatory growth of the remaining adipose tissue.

Faust, Johnson, & Hirsch, (1977) determined the mechanism for this compensatory growth of adipose tissue following lipectomy and, in the process, learned how body fat is linked to the control of eating behavior. They showed that the increase in body fat following lipectomy was accomplished by an increase in the size of individual fat cells; there was no increase in fat cell number. After lipectomy, particularly when receiving a palatable high-fat diet, rats increased their food intake, their body weight, and the size of their fat cells. When the size of the fat cells reached a maximum, however, food intake decreased and weight gain ceased, even if the lost body fat had not been totally restored. The regulation of body fat is evidently determined by, and secondary to, the regulation of the size of individual fat cells. If the capacity of these cells to store fat is exceeded, regulation of total body fat following lipectomy does not occur. So, in the final analysis, the regulation of body weight (and body fat) depends on the regulation of fat cell size, and the critical determinant of a body weight set point is the set point for fat cell size.

Fantino and Hoarding

An important new contribution to our understanding of the regulation of body weight has recently been made by Fantino's study of hoarding behavior (Fantino & Cabanac, 1980; Fantino, Faion, & Rolland, in press). Hoarding constitutes a specialized and remarkably quantifiable response to food deprivation and weight loss. Until the introduction of the study of hoarding behavior, information about body-weight set points could be deduced only from the body weight itself. This limitation has meant that information about set points can be determined only when the body weight is in equilibrium, and we can know nothing about quantitative departures from the set point. Such quantitative information can readily be obtained, however, from the measurement of hoarding behavior at various levels of body weight below the set point.

Figure 11.7 shows the remarkable responsiveness of the hoarding behavior of rats to decreases in body weight (Fantino & Cabanac, 1980). The loss of 30% of body weight is associated with intense hoarding behavior, and the intensity of this behavior decreases in proportion to the restoration of body weight. A quantitative representation of this regulation is depicted in Figure 11.8 which plots amount hoarded against body weight during periods of weight gain and weight loss (Fantino et al., in press). Rats do not hoard food when they are fed ad libitum, but begin to do so as soon as they lose weight from food deprivation. The amount hoarded is directly proportional to the amount of weight lost, and, with severe weight loss, can reach enormous quantities—two kilograms in three hours.

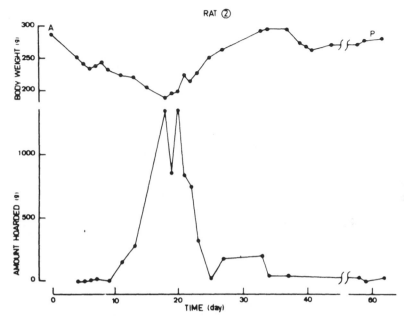

FIGURE 11.7   Effect of losing and gaining weight on hoarding behavior in the
rat (Fantino & Cabanac, 1980).

According to the hoarding model, the body-weight set point is that weight at
which the amount hoarded reaches zero in the regression of amount hoarded on
body weight. Figure 11.8 shows the exquisite sensitivity with which hoarding
behavior responds to decreases in body weight below the set point defined in
this manner.

Fantino and his colleagues (Fantino et al., in press) have used the hoarding
model to determine the body-weight set point at varying food intakes and body
weights, in an effort to determine whether these changes reflect changes in the
set point. Two factors known to modify food intake and body weight were
studied: the cafeteria diet, which induces dietary obesity, and the appetite sup-
pressant, d-fenfluramine. Animals received either a diet of laboratory chow or
the highly palatable cafeteria diet, and either a placebo or fenfluramine. The
results are shown in Figure 11.9 which plots the difference in grams between
the body weight of the animals while feeding ad libitum and the set point as
determined by the hoarding model. In the chow-fed, placebo-treated rats, hoarding behavior began following a weight loss of less than 10 grams, suggesting
that the body weight of these rats was at its set point when food deprivation
began. By contrast, hoarding behavior of the chow-fed, fenfluramine-treated rats
did not begin until they had lost at least 60 grams. The hoarding model thus

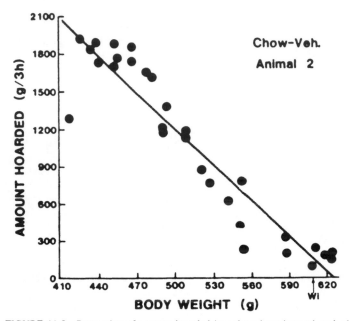

FIGURE 11.8   Regression of amount hoarded in a three-hour interval on body weight. Loss of weight below a threshold of about 620 grams results in a linear increase in amount hoarded (Fantino et al., in press).

suggests that fenfluramine lowered a body weight set point, just as the earlier experiment by Levitsky et al. (1981) had done.

A different picture is provided by rats fed a cafeteria diet. These rats did not begin to hoard until they had lost at least 50 grams of body weight. The hoarding model suggests that the body weight of the cafeteria-diet rats is at least 50 grams above its set point. Figure 11.9 also shows that the cafeteria-diet rats are at least 75 grams overweight in comparison to their chow-fed controls. Part of the excess weight of the cafeteria-diet rats is apparently above the set point and is thus not regulated, while another part is below the set point and *is* regulated.

Administering fenfluramine to cafeteria-diet rats significantly increased the extent of their weight loss before hoarding occurs, much as with chow-fed rats.

These results suggest that the highly palatable diet induced a dietary obesity, which included both a regulated and a nonregulated component. How much of the obesity is regulated and how much is not regulated may depend on the duration of the diet. Dietary obesity is totally reversible after a short time on a cafeteria diet, whereas it may become permanent after a longer time on a cafeteria diet. The mechanism of this transformation has been established. Both Mandenoff, Lenoir, and Apfelbaum (1982) and Faust, Johnson, Stern, and Hirsch (1978) have shown that a short period of cafeteria diet induces an increase in fat cell size, whereas longer periods on such diets result also in an increase in

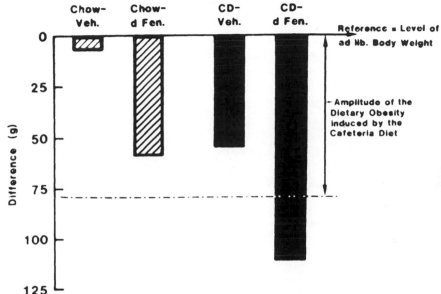

FIGURE 11.9   Difference (in grams) between the mean ad libitum body and the set point for energy regulation (required for the initiation of hoarding) following treatment with d-fenfluramine on chow and cafeteria diets (Fantino, Faion & Rolland, in press).

fat cell number. Once the number of fat cells has increased, the obesity becomes irreversible and subject to regulation at an elevated body-weight set point.

IMPLICATIONS FOR BEHAVIOR THERAPY AND PHARMACOTHERAPY

Four problems encountered in the treatment of obesity, noted above, can be interpreted in terms of set-point theory: dropping out of treatment, symptoms during treatment, limited weight losses, and regaining of weight lost in treatment. Two other implications of the theory can be drawn from a recent large-scale, controlled clinical trial.

The trial was undertaken to determine the relative effectiveness of behavior therapy and pharmacotherapy, the two leading treatments for obesity. It assessed the effects of behavior therapy alone, pharmacotherapy (with fenfluramine) alone, and their combination in 98 obese women during 6 months of treatment and at a one-year follow-up (Craighead, Stunkard, & O'Brien, 1981). These three conditions were compared with each other and with two control groups, a waiting-list control and a "doctor's-office-medication control group" which received traditional office treatment for obesity. The patients averaged 63% overweight, their median age was 47, and all were of middle socioeconomic status.

Figure 11.10 shows that the patients in all treatment groups lost significantly more weight than did those in the waiting-list control group, who gained 1.3 kg. Weight losses of the pharmacotherapy (14.5 kg) and combined-treatment patients (15.3 kg) did not differ significantly, and both exceeded the weight losses of the behavior therapy patients (10.9 kg, $p < 0.01$). Patients in the doctor's-office-medication control group lost only 6.0 kg, significantly less than the 14.5 kg lost by the pharmacotherapy patients ($p < .05$), even though the drug dosage in the two groups was the same.

A one-year follow-up of all of the patients in the three major treatment conditions showed a striking reversal in the relative efficacy of the treatments.

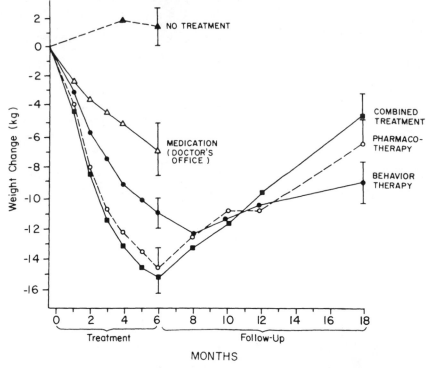

FIGURE 11.10   Weight changes during six-month treatment and 12-month follow-up. The three major treatment groups lost large amounts of weight during treatment: behavior therapy, 10.9 kg; pharmacotherapy, 14.5 kg; and combined treatment, 15.3 kg. Behavior therapy group regained weight slowly; pharmacotherapy and combined-treatment groups rapidly. No-treatment group gained weight; doctor's-office-medication group lost 6.0 kg. Vertical lines represent 1 SEM (Craighead et al., 1981).

Far less weight was regained by behavior therapy patients than by pharmaco-therapy and combined-treatment patients. At one year, behavior therapy patients had regained only 1.9 kg, for a net weight loss from the beginning of treatment of 9.0 kg. By contrast, pharmacotherapy patients had regained 8.2 kg, for a net loss of only 6.3 kg, and the combined-treatment patients regained even more weight (10.7 kg), for an even smaller net loss—4.6 kg. The long-term results strongly favored behavior therapy alone over the two conditions that utilized pharmacotherapy.

The implications of set-point theory for the results of pharmacotherapy are clear. As we have noted, laboratory research has shown that fenfluramine acts primarily by lowering a body-weight set point and only secondarily by sup-pressing appetite (Fantino et al., in press; Levitsky et al., 1981). When fen-fluramine was discontinued in the trial, the body-weight set point of the patients returned to its pre-treatment level. Powerful biological pressures to gain weight to this higher level were thus released, resulting in the rebound in body weight.

These practical results, supported by the results of laboratory research suggest a radical revision of prescribing practices for "appetite-suppressant" medication: Do not use it unless you are prepared to use it indefinitely.

Important clinical implications can also be drawn from the effects of behavior therapy. The excellent maintenance of weight loss confirms the efficacy of this treatment modality and raises the question of how behavior therapy acts. Does it, for example, lower a body-weight set point? The answer is far from obvious and includes at least three possibilities:

1. Behavior therapy may lower a body-weight set point. A promising candidate for such a mechanism is the increase in physical activity which forms an important part of behavioral weight-loss programs. Whether or not increased physical activity can actually lower a body-weight set point is currently the subject of research. Should this research show that physical activity can lower a body-weight set point, it would provide an important rationale for a treatment measure that is still, in part, a matter of faith.

Another candidate for a lowering of a set point by behavior therapy is mod-ification of dietary habits. Behavioral programs place considerable emphasis on lowering the high-fat content of the typical American diet. If high-fat diets promote obesity in humans, as they do in experimental animals, it seems rea-sonable that lowering the fat content of the diet might limit its obesity-promoting effect.

2. Behavior therapy may have no effect on the body-weight set point. It may help a patient to maintain his or her body weight below its set point simply by providing the skills to live in a state of semi-starvation. The intensity of this starvation may vary, depending on the tolerance for fluctuations below the body-weight set point. If, for example, body weight is very tightly regulated, a reduc-tion of 10.9 kg below a set point, as in the present study, may be an onerous

task. It is quite possible, however, that there is considerable tolerance about the set point and that a loss of 10.9 kg would produce only modest pressures to restore weight to its higher, regulated level.

3. A third mechanism of action of behavior therapy is one rendered more plausible by Fantino's research (Fantino & Cabanac, 1980; Fantino et al., in press). Lowering the fat content of the diet may act to control obesity by limiting that component of dietary obesity that Fantino has shown to be not regulated (or not yet regulated). This component is the one that results from an increase in fat cell size, before any increase in fat cell number has occurred. This third mechanism has intuitive appeal and seems to fit the experience of many graduates of behavioral programs who have lost weight and maintained their weight losses without evidence that they are coping with semi-starvation.

It seems quite possible that these three mechanisms are not mutually exclusive and that more than one of them is at work in successful behavioral weight-control programs.

SUMMARY

There is strong reason to believe that body weight is regulated, for it not only remains at a relatively constant level, but it is also defended at that level against environmental challenges. Regulation occurs not only among animals of normal weight, as has long been believed, but also among obese animals. They are obese, it is argued, because the set point, about which their body weight is regulated, is elevated.

The evidence for regulation of body weight is vast and growing. It includes studies of animals made obese by lesions in the ventromedial hypothalamus, as well as animals made thin by lesions in the lateral hypothalamus. Studies of appetite-suppressant medication provide evidence for regulation via its apparent mechanism of action—lowering a body-weight set point. Studies of parabiotic rats and of lipectomized animals support the idea of regulation by demonstrating compensatory decreases and increases in body fat in response to experimentally induced changes in body fat. The study of hoarding in animals provides a quantitative model for estimating body-weight set points and their modification in response to interventions as varied as high-fat diets and pharmacotherapy.

Evidence for regulation of body weight in humans is derived from a study of starved volunteers (Keys et al., 1950) and from a study of overfed volunteers (Sims & Horton, 1968). In each case, when the subjects were allowed free access to food, their body weights rapidly returned to normal.

The idea of the regulation of body weight helps to explain four traditional problems in the treatment of obesity: dropping out of treatment, symptoms during treatment, limited weight losses, and regaining of weight lost during treatment. In each case, the problem can be ascribed to the attempt to reduce body weight in the face of opposing physiological regulations. Another clinical problem—the transiency of the effects of appetite-suppressant medication—is susceptible to similar explanation. Reasons for the relative success of behavior therapy of obesity are considered in the light of the regulation of body weight.

REFERENCES

Adolph, E. F. (1947). Urges to eat and drink in rats. *American Journal of Physiology, 151*, 110–125.

Cohn, C., & Cohn, J. D. (1962). Influence of body weight and body fat on appetite of "normal" lean and obese rats. *Yale Journal of Biology and Medicine, 34*, 598–607.

Craighead, L. W., Stunkard, A. J., & O'Brien, R. (1981). Behavior therapy and pharmacotherapy of obesity. *Archives of General Psychiatry, 38*, 763–768.

Cruce, J. A. F., Greenwood, M. R. C., & Johnson, P. R., et al. (1974). Genetic vs. hypothalamic obesity: Studies of intake and dietary manipulation in rats. *Journal of Comparative and Physiological Psychology, 87*, 295–301.

Fantino, M., & Cabanac, M. (1980). Body weight regulation with a proportional hoarding response in the rat. *Physiology and Behavior, 24*, 939–942.

Fantino, M., Faion, F., & Rolland, Y. (in press). Body weight set point modifications induced by cafeteria diet and d-fenfluramine: Study in rat using hoarding behavior. *American Journal of Physiology.*

Faust, I. M., Johnson, P. R., & Hirsch, J. (1977). Surgical removal of adipose tissue alters feeding behavior and the development of obesity in rats. *Science, 197*, 393–396.

Faust, I. M., Johnson, P. R., Stern, J. S., & Hirsch, J. (1978). Diet-induced adipocyte increase in adult rats: A new model of obesity. *American Journal of Physiology, 235*, E279–E286.

Fenichel, O. (1945). *The psychoanalytic theory of neurosis.* New York: W. W. Norton.

Hamilton, C. L. (1969). Problems of refeeding after starvation in the rat. *Annals of the New York Academy of Sciences, 157*, 1004–1017.

Hervey, G. R. (1959). The effects of lesions in the hypothalamus in parabiotic rats. *Journal of Physiology, 154*, 336–352.

Hoebel, B. G., & Teitelbaum, B. (1966). Weight regulation in normal and hypothalamic hyperphagic rats. *Journal of Comparative and Physiological Psychology, 61*, 189–193.

Kaplan, H. I., & Kaplan, H. S. (1957). The psychosomatic concept of obesity. *Journal of Nervous and Mental Disease, 125*, 181–201.

Keesey, R. E., Boyle, P. C., Kemnitz, J. W., & Mitchel, J. S. (1976). The role of the lateral hypothalamus in determining the body weight set point. In D. Novin, W. Wyrwicka, & G. A. Bray (Eds.), *Hunger: Basic mechanisms and clinical implications* (pp. 87–96). New York: Raven Press.

Keys, A., Brozek, J., Henschel, A., Mickelson, D., & Taylor, H. L. (1950). *The biology of human starvation.* Minneapolis: University of Minnesota Press.

Levitsky, D. A., Strupp, B. J., & Lupoli, J. (1981). Tolerance to anorectic drugs: Pharmacological or artifactual. *Pharmacology and Biochemsitry of Behavior, 14*, 661–667.

Liebelt, R. A., Ichinoe S., & Nicholson, N. (1965). Regulatory influences of adipose tissue on food intake and body weight. *Annals of the New York Academy of Sciences, 131*, 559–582.

Mandenoff, A. T., Lenoir, T., & Apfelbaum, M. (1982). Tardy occurrence of adipocyte hyperplasia in cafeteria-fed rat. *American Journal of Physiology, 242*, 349–351.

Mrosovsky, N., & Powley, T. L. (1977). Set points for body weight and fat. *Behavioral Biology, 20*, 205–223.

Odum, E. P. (1960). Pre-migratory hyperphagia in birds. *American Journal of Clinical Nutrition, 8,* 621–629.

Pengelley, E. T., & Fisher, K. C. (1963). The effect of temperature and photoperiod on the yearly hibernating behavior of captive golden-mantled ground squirrels. *Canadian Journal of Zoology, 41,* 1103–1120.

Sims, E. A. H., & Horton, E. S. (1968). Endocrine and metabolic adaptation to obesity and starvation. *American Journal of Clinical Nutrition, 21,* 1455–1470.

Stunkard, A. J. (1957). The "dieting depression." Incidence and clinical characteristics of untoward responses to weight reduction regimes. *American Journal of Medicine, 23,* 77–86.

Stunkard, A. J. (1975). From explanation to action in psychosomatic medicine: The case of obesity. *Psychosomatic Medicine, 37,* 195–236.

Stunkard, A. J. (1982). Anorectic agents lower a body weight set point. *Life Sciences, 30,* 2043–2055.

AUTHOR INDEX

A

Abbot, F. K., 149, 153, *155*
Abd-El-Samie, Y., 5, *26*
Abe, H., 41–42, *44, 46*
Abood, L. G., 76, *93*
Ackerman, S. H., 166, 168, 169, 171, *173, 174*
Adachi, A., 54, *56*
Adachi, S., 87, *92*
Adair, L. S., 8, *24, 28*
Adams, N., 85, *97*
Adcock, J., 105, 107, *109, 110*
Ader, R., 164, *173*
Adler, W. H., 77, *96*
Adolph, E. F., 190, *205*
Adrian, T. E., 152, *159*
Agnati, L. F., 74, *88*
Agunod, M., 167, 171, *173*
Ahlman, H., 8, *28, 73, 93*
Ahn, B. T., 101, *110*
Aibara, S., 22, *29*
Akdamar, K., 11, *25*
Akil, H., 67, 69–70, 73, 80, *88*, 92, *98*, 106, *112*, 115, *131*
Albanese, V., 11, *29*
Albert, L. H., 87, *91*
Alexander, F. G., 138, *155*
Allen, J., 77, *92*
Allen, M., *32*

Almy, T. P., 141, 149, 152, 153, *155*
Alpers, D. H., 144, 147, 148, *155*
Altamirano, M., 5, *24*
Ambrose, W. W., 1, *26*
Ament, M. E., 34, *48*, 166–67, 171, *173, 174*
Amir, S., 124, 126, *129*
Amirian, D. A., 5, *30*
Amit, Z., 124, 126, *129*
Anand, R., 87, *96*
Andersson, S., 13, *24*
Andrews, P. L. R., 14, *24*
Angus, J. A., 3, *24*
Annitto, W., 128, *135*
Antelman, S. M., 124, *129*
Apfelbaum, M., 127, 128, *129, 133*, 200, *205*
Appelbaum, M., 86, *93*
Appelboom, T., 76, *98*
Aprison, M., 108, *110*
Arancibia, S., 108, *109*
Arcomano, A., 118, *132*
Arimura, A., 6, 11, *25, 41, 47*
Armstrong, S., 125, *129*
Arndorfer, R. C., 141, *156*
Arnold, J., 85, *97*
Aronchick, C. A., 15–17, 21–22, *24, 26*
Arrigo-Reina, R., 106, *110*
Assenmacher, I., 108, *109*
Astier, H., 108, *109*
Atkinson, M., 142, *155*
Atkinson, R. L., 128, *129*

207

Atrens, D. M., 127, *129*
Atweh, S. F., 73, 83, *88,* 115, *129*
Aures, D., 169, *173*
Awouters, F., 81, 84, *88*
Ayalon, A., 5, *30*
Azar, A. P., 115, 117, 118, 122, 127, *135*

B

Bacon, F., 137, *155*
Baigts, F., 127, 128, *129*
Bailo, M., 126, *131*
Baird, A. W., 4, *24*
Ballenger, J. C., *109*
Banerjee, U., 71, *88*
Bankhurst, A. D., 77, *93*
Banks, W. A., 104, *112*
Barajas, L., 2, *28*
Baranetsky, N. G., 79, *94*
Barbero, G. J., 154, *160*
Barbour, H. G., 85, *90*
Barchas, J. D., 67, *98,* 119, *133*
Barclay, G., 164, *173*
Bardakjian, B. L., 150, *159*
Baron, J. H., 11, *24,* 44, *45*
Barraclough, C. A., 79, *88*
Barth, E., 2, *28*
Barth, H., 2, 4, *28*
Bartness, T. J., 63, *65*
Basu, P., 139, 150, *160*
Battenberg, E., 67, 69, *88*
Battersby, C., 15, *24*
Bauer, B. G., *89*
Bauer, K., *93*
Bauer, R. F., 8, 9, *24, 32*
Baum, M. J., 78, *95*
Bauman, J., 80, *98*
Bayon, A., 67, 69, *88*
Beattie, A. D., 144, *156*
Beaumont, W., 163, *173*
Becker, K. L., 106, *109*
Befrits, R., 11, *24*
Belitala, G., *90*
Bell, P. R. F., 15, *24*
Bell, T. A., 15, *30*
Bellinger, L. L., 116, *129*
Belluzzi, J. D., 127, *135*
Belsheim, M. R., 82, *92*
Benjamin, S. B., 142, *155*
Bennett, J. R., 142, *155*
Bennett, W., 175, *186*

Berglindh, T., 3, *24*
Berka, C., 124, 125, *133*
Berle, B., 149, 152, *155*
Bernardis, L. L., 51, *56,* 116, *129*
Berntson, G. B., 124, 125, *133*
Berntson, G. G., 120, *133*
Bernz, J. A., 63, *64*
Berson, S. A., 35, *47*
Bertierre, M. C., 127, 128, *129*
Berzas, M. C., 116, 128, *131*
Besev, G., *93*
Besser, G. M., 80, *95*
Besterman, H. S., 152, *155*
Beubler, E., 84, *88*
Bhakthavatsalam, P., 116–20, 122, 125, 126, *129, 134*
Bialowas, J., 124, 127, *130, 135*
Bianco, F. C., 79, *88*
Billington, C. J., 86, *94*
Bitar, K. N., 6, *30,* 42, *47,* 82, *88*
Black, J. W., 3, *24*
Blackburn, A. M., 44, *45*
Blair, E. L., 15, *24*
Blalock, J. E., 78, *88*
Blaney, R., 139, *160*
Blankstein, J., 80, *88*
Blaschke, T. F., 76, *96*
Bläsig, J., 87, *89,* 121, 123, *129*
Blendis, L., 144, *157*
Bloom, A. A., 149, *155*
Bloom, F. E., 67, 69, 76–78, *88, 91,* 121, 124, 128, *134*
Bloom, S. R., 14, *29,* 36, 37, 44, *45, 47,* 104, *110,* 152, *155, 159*
Bodnar, R. J., 124, *130*
Bogoch, A., 81, *90*
Bogoch, E. R., *160*
Bolman, R. M. III, 34, 42, 45
Bolme, P., 74, *88*
Bonanni, A., 78, *96*
Bond, J. H., 148, *158*
Bonfils, S., 8, *24*
Bonnevie, O., 144, *159*
Bonoma, C., 8, *28*
Booth, D. A., 51, *56,* 127, *130*
Bortoff, A., 145, *161*
Bosman, F. T., 144, *158*
Bowen, S. R., 72, *97*
Bowes, K. L., *160*
Bowie, D. L., 78, *95*

Boyle, P. C., 193–96, *205*
Bradley, R., 74, *88*
Bradshaw, J. E., 124, *135*
Brady, J. P., 22, *26*, 79, *88*
Brady, J. V., 22, *29*
Brand, D. L., 142, 143, *155*
Brandeis, L., 116, 122, *134*
Brands, B., 86, *89*
Brandt, J., 73, *97*
Brantl, V., 87, *89*
Bray, G. A., 86, *97*, 119, *130*
Brazeau, P., 40, *45*
Brett, L. P., 53, *56*
Brief, D., 62, *64*
Briggs, J. E., 87, *95*
Britt, L. G., 15, *30*
Broccardo, M., 83, *89*
Brodie, D. A., *89*
Brooks, F. P., 1, 7, 8, 10, 12, 14–19, 21–22, *24, 25, 26, 28, 31, 32*
Brooks, J. W., 71, *97*
Brown, B. H., 150, *160*
Brown, D. M., 86, *93*
Brown, D. R., 84, *89, 94*
Brown, J. C., 43, 44, *45, 47*
Brown, J. D., *45*
Brown, M., 2, 21, *30, 31*, 79, 81, *96, 97* 105, 106, 108, *111*
Brown, M. A., 22, *28*
Brown, M. R., 22, *28*
Brown, O., 118, 122, *132*
Brown, Z. W., 124, 126, *129*
Browne, R., 67, 69, *88*
Brown-Sequard, C. E., 101, *109*
Brownstein, M. J., 67, *92*
Brozek, J., 191, 204, *205*
Bruch, H., 177, 183, *186*
Bruni, J. F., 79, *89*
Brutus, M., 124, *130*
Bueno, L., 82, *90*, 150, *155*
Bukhave, K., 84, *88*, 151, *155*
Bunnett, N. W., 32, *37*, 38, 41, *45, 47*
Burgis, V., 125, *130*
Burgus, R., 40, *45*
Burks, T. F., 71, 82, 83, *88, 89, 91, 93, 95, 96*, 105, *111*
Burns, G. M., 151, *156*
Burt, D. R., 108, *111*
Buscino, G. A., 80, *97*
Butcher, M., 40, *45*

Butland, R. J., 72, *89*
Butler, R. C., 139, *160*
Butterfield, W. J. H., 139, *160*
Byrne, W. J., 34, *48*, 167, 171, *173, 174*

C

Cabanac, M., 198, 204, *205*
Calam, J., 164, *173*
Callahan, B. M., 101, *110*
Calvet, M. C., 78, *89*
Cameron, N., 183, 184, *186*
Campbell, D., 149, 150, 153, *158*
Campbell, E. H. G., 13, *25*
Campbell, G. A., 79, 80, *92*
Campbell, R. G., *64*
Candeletti, S., 106, *110*
Cannon, V. B., 50, *56*
Cannon, W. B., 152, *155*
Capelari, J., 102, *110*
Capone, R. J., 74, *99*
Caputo, G., 11, *29*
Card, W. I., 144, *156*
Carleton, J. L., 63, *65*
Carlson, G. M., 150, *160*
Carlson, H. E., 79, 87, *94, 95*
Carlson, N. R., 52, *56*
Carmen, J. S., *109*
Carpenter, F. G., 72, *97*
Carr, D. H., 7–9, *25*
Carr, K. D., 123, *130*
Carraway, R. E., 44, *46*
Casper, R. C., 128, *135*
Castell, D. O., 142, *155, 156*
Castellanos, F. X., 116, 128, *131*
Cetel, N. S., 80, *89*
Champagnat, J., 72, *90*
Champion, P., 151, *156*
Chang, D., 13, *24*
Chang, J. K., 74, *98*
Chang, K., 117, 119, 122, *132, 134*
Chang, R. J., 79, *94*
Charcot, J. M., 138
Chariot, J., 84, *96*, 106, *111*
Chaudhary, N. A., 138, 146, 147, 149, 151, 152, 154, *156*
Chavkin, C., 86, *89*
Chayvialle, J. A., 42, 43, *48*
Chen, H. T., 79, 80, *92*
Chernick, V., 72, *89*
Cheszkowski, M., 85, *92*

Chew, C. S., 4, *28*
Chew, P., 7, 36, 37, *47*
Chey, W. H., 145, *156, 161*
Chey, W. Y., 21–22, *24*, 145, 152, *156, 157, 161*
Chhabra, R., 178, *187*
Chiba, T., 41–42, *44, 46*
Chihara, K., 41–42, *46*
Chin, P., 124, *129*
Ching, M., 79, *89*
Cho, D., 80, *98*
Choi, H., 101, *110*
Chou, S. N., 101, *110*
Chowdhury, A. R., 151, 152, *156*
Chretien, M., 67, *95*
Christensen, C. W., 78, *95*
Christensen, J., 150, *156*
Christensen, K. C., 14, *25*
Christensson, I., 69, *98*
Christiansen, J., 13, *29*, 85, *95*
Christie, D. L., 34, *48*
Christofides, N. D., 44, *45*, 152, *159*
Cicero, T. J., 79, *89*
Clark, B., 7, 36–38, *45, 47*
Clark, W. G., 71, *89*
Clouse, R. E., 140, 143, *156*
Clouter, C., 139, *161*
Cobb, S., 138, *161*
Cochin, J., 71, *96*
Coffman, J. D., 74, *89*
Coghill, N. F., 144, *157, 161*
Cohen, B. R., 140, *156*
Cohen, M. E., 147, *161*
Cohen, M. R., 87, *89*
Cohen, R. A., 74, *89*
Cohen, R. M., 87, *89*
Cohen, S. C., 82, *98*, 142, 150, *156, 158, 160*
Cohn, C., 190, *205*
Cohn, J. D., 190, *205*
Coil, J. D., 18, *25*
Collins, R. J., 78, *93*
Collu, R., 104–6, 108, 109, *111*
Conlon, J. M., 41, *47*
Connell, A. M., 140, 148, 149, 151, 152, *156, 157, 159*
Cooke, A., 164, *173*
Cooper, C. W., 34, *45*
Cooper, K. A., 10, *30*
Cooper, P. H., 34, 54, *57*
Cooper, S. J., 127, *130*

Corazziari, E., 40, *46*
Corbet, H. J., 38, *45*
Corcoran, P., 83, *97*
Costa, E., 104, *111*
Costa, F., 106, *110*
Costa, M., 81, *91*
Cote, J., 67, *95*
Coulomb, P., 150, *155*
Cousins, L. M., 167, 171, *173*
Cowan, A., 71, 72, *89, 90*
Cowley, Y. M., 14, *26, 90*
Coy, D. H., 69, 70, 78, 80, 85, *92, 95, 98*, 106, *112, 115, 131*
Craighead, L. W., 201, 202, *205*
Crean, G. P., 13, *25*, 144, *156*
Crocket, A., 2, *25*
Cross, B. A., 121, *134*
Crowley, T. J., 79, *90*
Cruce, J. A. F., 128, *130*, 192, *205*
Csendes, A., 35, *46*
Cuello, A. C., 67, 69, *90*
Culp, D. J., 4, *25*
Cumming, J. D., 9, *25*
Cushin, B. J., 60, *65*
Cushing, H., *109*, 163, *173*
Cytawa, J., 127, *130*

D

DaCosta, J. M., 147, *156*
Dafny, N., 78, *90*
Dahlstrom, A., 8, *28, 73, 93*
Dallman, M. F., 119, 126, *130, 136*
Dally, P., 148, *157*
D'Amato, R. J., 75, 76, *90, 92*
Daniel, D. R., 117, 122, *130*
Daniel, E. E., 81, *90*, 149, 150, 153, *156, 158, 159*
Darby, C., 139, 150, *160*
Davies, H. A., 142, 143, *156*
Davis, E. K., *32*
Davis, J. D., 62, *64*
Davis, J. M., 128, *135*
Davis, R. A., *25*
Davis, T. P., 83, *89*
Dawson, A. M., 146, *158*
Debas, H. T., 12, 19, 20, 22, *25, 26, 29, 31,* 35, 37, 38, 41, 44, *45, 47, 48*
DeBellis, M., 117, *133*
de Dombal, F. T., 144, *157*
Degertekin, H., 8, 11, *25*
Delaney, J. P., 15, *25*

Delawari, J. B., 151, *157*
Del Duca, T., 152, *157*
DeLeon, M. J., 87, *96*
Delitala, G., 79, 80, *90*
Deller, D. J., 149–52, 153, *159, 160*
Del Mazo, J., 35, *46*
del Milton, R. C., 37, 38, *45*
de Lourdes, M., 20, *27*
DeMeester, T. R., 141, 143, *158*
Denavit-Saubie, M., 72, *90*
Dent, J., 141, *156*
De Sarro, G. B., 71, *95*
Devilla, L., 79, 80, *90*
Devos, M., 127, *133*
Dewald, I., 104, *111*
Di Biaso, D., 80, *90*
Dietz, R., 74, *93*
DiMarino, A. J., Jr., 142, *156*
Dimirco, J. A., 19, *32*
Dininger, N. B., 79, *97*
Dinoso, V. P., 151, 152, *156, 157*
Dockray, G. J., 8, *25*, 34, 36, *46*, 164, *173*
Dodds, W. J., 141, *156*
Dodge, J. A., 151, *156*
Dohrn, R. H., 15, *30*
Donaldson, R. M., Jr., 4, *27*
Dotevall, G. J., 140, *156*
Doxey, J. C., 71, *90*
Doyle, D., 2, *25*
Dreifuss, J. J., 121, *134*
Drossman, D. A., 139, 146, 148, *156, 157*
Drugan, R. C., 119, *133*
Dryburgh, J. R., 43, *45*
Dubinsky, W. P., 34–35, *47*
Dubois, A., 85, *97*
Dubrasquet, M., 84, *96*, 105, 106, *110, 111*
Duka, Th., 115, 122, *130*
Dum, J., 127, *130*
Dunham, E. S., 85, *90*
Dupre, J., 43, *45*
Duranton, A., 82, *90*
Duthie, H. L., 150, *160*
Du Val, J. W., 6, *25*
Dvorkin, B., 122, *132*

E

Eades, C. G., 85, *93*
Ebert, M. H., 129, *131*
Ecknauer, R., 2, *25*
Edelman, N. H., 72, 73, *96*
Eden, N. K., 115, *133*

Edin, R., 8, 73, *93*
Edlin, R., *28*
Edwards, A. V., 37, *45*
Edward, F. C., 144, *157, 161*
Edwards, J. D., 125, *130*
Efendic, S., 8, *32*
Eisenman, A. J., 71, *97*
Elander, B., 3, *28*
Elde, R. P., 2, 7, 18, *28, 29, 30*, 69, 73, 81, 83, *90, 92, 97*
Elder, J. B., 13, *25*
Eldridge, F. L., 72, *93*
Elfvin, L.-G., 73, *97*
El-Gindi, M., 5, *26*
Ellingboe, J., 79, *90, 94*
Elshowihy, R. M., 73, *92*
Elson, M. K., 86, *94*
Elwin, C. E., 34, *46*
Emas, S., 13, *26, 27*
Engel, B. T., 148–49, 154, *157, 161*
Epstein, L. B., 78, *90*
Erskine, B., 179, *187*
Ertan, A., 11, *25*
Esler, M. D., 147, *157*
Eterno, R., 60, *65*
Euler, A. R., 167, 171, *173, 174*
Evans, J. M., 80, *95*
Evans, R., 106, *111*
Evered, M. D., 21, *26, 31*
Everett, S., 166–67, *174*
Ewald, C. A., 138

F

Facchinetti, F., 81, *91*
Facer, P., 14, *29*
Factor, A. D., 126, *131*
Faden, A. I., 74–76, *90, 91, 92, 95, 96, 98*
Fahrenkrug, J., 42, 44, *46*
Faiman, C., 80, *88*
Faion, F., 190, 192, 198–200, 203, 204, *205*
Famaey, J. P., 76, *98*
Fantino, M., 190, 192, 198–200, 203, 204, *205*
Farooq, O., 11, *26*
Farrar, J. T., 148, 149, *155, 157*
Farsang, C., 76, *96*
Faust, I. M., 198, 200, *205*
Feldberg, W., 71, 74, *88, 90*
Feldman, E. J., 34, *46*
Feldman, H. A., 73, *97*
Feldman, J. D., 76–78, *91*

Feldman, M., 10–11, 14, *26, 29, 30,* 36, *46,* 85, *90,* 171, *174*
Fellenius, E., 3, *28*
Fencl, V., 73, *97*
Feng, H. S., 15–18, 21–22, *24, 26, 28*
Fenichel, O., 189, *205*
Fennessy, M. R., 74, *90*
Ferguson-Segall, M., 128, *130*
Ferrari, J., 14, *29*
Ferrari-Taylor, J., 35, *47*
Ferri, S., 106, *110*
Ferris, S. H., 87, *96*
Feuerstein, G. Z., 74–75, *90, 91, 95*
Fielding, J., 138, 140, 146, *157*
Fielding, L. P., 15, *27*
Figlewicz, D. P., 62, *65*
Filart, R., 115, 117, 118, 122, 127, *135*
Filla, A., 83, *96*
Finkel, M., 141–42, *157*
Fioramonti, J., 150, *155*
Fischli, A., 70, 73, *98*
Fisher, A. E., 124, *129*
Fisher, K. C., 191, *206*
Fitzpatrick, M. L., 44, *45*
Flannigan, K. P., 101, 102, *111*
Fleischer, F., 117, 118, 124, 127, *131*
Flemstrom, G., 5, *26*
Fleshler, B., 142, *159*
Fletcher, D. R., 44, *45*
Florencio, H., 105, *110*
Flowers, S. H., 85, *90*
Flynn, J. J., 128, *130*
Foch, T. T., 175, *187*
Folkers, K., 13, *24*
Fordtran, J. S., 10, *30,* 34, 36, *46, 47, 48,* 171, *174*
Forte, J. G., 4, *25*
Forte, V. A., Jr., 73, *97*
Forti, D. M., 170, *174*
Franklin, P. A., 5–6, *27*
Frantz, A. G., 81, *91*
Frederickson, R. C. A., 79, *97,* 125, *130*
French, E. D., 67, 69, *88,* 124, *134*
French, J. D., 101, *110*
French, L. A., 101, *110*
Frexinos, J., 150, *155*
Friedman, M. I., 54, *57*
Friedman, R. H., 141, *156*
Fritsch, W. P., 14, *27*
Froelich, C. J., 77, *93*
Frohman, L. A., 51, *56*

Fugiwara, M., 22, *29*
Fujita, T., 34, 41–42, *46*
Fujiwara, M., 102, *111*
Fuke, H., 85, *98*
Fukushima, M., 87, *91*
Fumeron, F., 86, *93,* 128, *133*
Furness, J. B., 81, *91*
Fuxe, K. F., 74, *88*

G

Gaafer, M., 151, *156*
Gabel, R. A., 73, *97*
Gaehwiler, B. H., 121, *134*
Gaida, W., 74, *93*
Gaines, K. J., 15, *30*
Gale, R. P., 77, *97*
Galligan, J. J., 82, 83, *89, 91*
Gambert, S. R., 124, 127, *130*
Ganten, D., 74, *93, 97, 99*
Garabedian, M., 145, *157*
Garcia, J., 53, *56*
Garcia, R., 19, *32*
Garner, A., 5, *26*
Garrett, J. R., 2, *26*
Garthwaite, T. L., 124, 127, *130*
Garvey, T. Q., III, 19, *32*
Gavaerts, A., 76, *98*
Geary, N., 60, *64*
Gebhard, P. H., 78, *92*
Gebhard, R. L., 88, *94*
Geddes, D. M., 72, *89*
Geibel, V., 87, *96*
Geumei, A., 5, *26*
Gen, M. C., 72, *91*
Genazzani, A. R., 81, *91*
Gerhardt, D. C., 142, *155*
Gessa, G. L., 78, 79, *91, 96*
Ghatei, M., 36, 37, *47,* 104, *110*
Ghazarossian, V. E., 69–70, *98*
Gibbs, J., 52, *57,* 59, 60, 62, 63, *64, 65,* 115, *130*
Gibson, M. J., 128, *130*
Gillespie, G., 13, *25*
Gillespie, J. E., 13, *25*
Gillies, M., 142, *157*
Gillis, R. A., 17–19, *26, 29, 32*
Gilman, S. C., 76–78, *91*
Gintzler, A. R., 81, *91*
Gioffré, M., 11, *29*
Giordano, G., 79, *90*

Giusti, M., 79, *90*
Glanzman, D. L., 53, *56*
Glass, G. B. J., 167, 171, *173*
Glick, Z., 86, *97*
Glossi, F. B., 152, *157*
Glusman, M., 124, *130*
Go, V. L. W., 83, *97*
Godiwala, T., 11, *25*
Goetz, F. C., 88, *94*
Goland, R. S., 81, *91*
Golanska, E. M., 41, *45*
Gold, M. S., 128, *135*
Gold, R. M., 121, *134*
Goldberg, S., 142, *158*
Goldman, C. K., 117, *130*
Goldman, J. K., 51, *56*
Goldman, M. S., 141–42, *157*
Goldstein, A., 69–70, 72, 73, 79, 80, 83, 86, 87, *89, 91, 92, 98,* 106, *112,* 115, *131*
Goldstein, M., 2, *30,* 73, 81, *97*
Goldstone, J., 15, *27*
Goltzman, D., 106, *111*
Gomez, J., 148, *157*
Gonella, J., 83, *96*
Goodman, R. R., 115, 122, *130*
Goodrich, C. A., 71, *88*
Gosnell, B. A., 63, 65, 86, *94,* 115, 116, *130*
Goto, Y., 8, 19, 20, 22, *26, 29, 31,* 41–42, *44, 46,* 107, 108, *111*
Goulston, K. J., 147, *157*
Gowdey, C. W., 86, *89*
Gowdey, W., 115, 116, 121, *135*
Goyal, R. K., 81, 82, *96*
Grace, M., 19, *28,* 72, 86, *94*
Graham, D. Y., 142, *157*
Gramsch, C. H., 127, *130*
Grand, E. R., 15, *24*
Grand, R. J., 170, *174*
Grandison, L., 86, *91,* 115, 116, *130*
Graziani, L. A., 34–35, *47*
Greenwood, M. R. C., 192, *205*
Greetham, R. B., 9, *25*
Gregg, J. A., 145, *157*
Gregory, R. A., 8, *25,* 34, *46*
Greider, M. H., 34, *46*
Gresser, I., 78, *89*
Grevert, P., 87, *91*
Grijalva, C. V., 54, *57,* 101, 109, *110*
Grill, H. J., 53, 55, *56*
Grinker, J. A., 118, *135*
Grohman, L. A., *56*

Groot, K., 11, *25*
Gross, C. W., 15, *30*
Gross, E. R., 72, *89*
Grossman, A., 80, *95*
Grossman, M. I., 11–13, *25, 26, 31,* 34–36, 40, 44, *46, 47, 48,* 164, *173*
Grossman, S. P., 79, 118, *130*
Grundy, D., 9, *26*
Gudmand-Hoyer, E., 144, *159*
Guerkin, S., 152, *155*
Guidotti, A., 86, *91,* 115, 116, *130*
Guillemin, R., 40, *45,* 67, 69, 79, 88, *96,* 124, 128, *134*
Guilleminault, C., 76, *96*
Gunion, M. W., 21, 22, *26, 31,* 128, *131*
Gunne, L. M., 71, *91, 93*
Gurin, J., 175, *186*
Gurll, N. J., 75, 76, *96, 98*
Guth, P. H., 15, *26*
Gutierrez, J. G., 152, *156, 157*

H

Hagen, T. C., 124, 127, *130*
Haggitt, E. C., 143, *158*
Haglund, U., 3, *28*
Hakanson, R., 169, *173*
Hall, W. H., 22, *26,* 165, *174*
Hamel, D., 22, *29,* 108, *111*
Hamilton, C. L., 190, *205*
Hammer, N. J., 117, 118, 122, *132*
Hammer, R. A., 44, *46*
Hammond, P., 139, 150, *160*
Handi, I. A., 151, *156*
Handwerger, B. A., 86, *93*
Hanker, J. S., 1, *26*
Hankins, W. G., 53, *56*
Hansteen, R. W., 79, *91*
Harada, T., 166–67, *174*
Hardy, F. E., Jr., 19, *29*
Harmon, J. W., 19, *32*
Harper, A. A., 7, *26*
Harrell, C. E., 125, *130*
Harris, V., 41, 42, *47*
Harty, R. F., 5–6, *27, 31*
Harvey, R. F., 152, *157*
Harvey, R. H., 151, *157*
Hass, W., 76, *93*
Hassanein, M. A., 151, *156*
Hassen, A. H., 74–75, *91*
Hatton, J. D., 121, *134*

Hauser, H., 119, 126, *131*
Hawke, D., 7, 36, *47*
Hayshi, S., 15, *29*
Heaton, K. W., 139, 140, 144, *158, 160*
Helander, H. T., 13, *27*
Heldsinger, A., 3, *32*
Hellemans, J., 142, *160*
Hendrix, T. R., 144, *160*
Hengels, K. S., 14, *27*
Henke, P., 101, *110*
Henrichs, I., 88, *97*
Henricksen, S. J., 67, 69, *88*
Henriksen, F. W., 43, *46*
Henry, J. L., 79, *91*, 113, 128, *131*
Henschen, A., 87, *89*, 191, 204, *205*
Herb, R. W., 22, *26*
Herberman, R. B., 77, *91*
Herman, B., 86, *92*
Herman, C. P., 178–86, *187*
Hermann, G. E., 54, *56*, 127, *131*
Hermann, K., 74, *93*
Hernandez, D. E., 105–7, *109, 110, 111*
Herrman, J. B., 71, *91*
Hersey, S. J., 4, *28*
Hershkowitz, M., 78, *98*
Hershman, J. M., 79, 87, *94, 95*
Hervey, G. R., 196, *205*
Herz, A., 69, 82, *93, 97*, 115, 121–23, 127, *129, 130*
Hester, S. E., 22, *28*
Hicks, M. I., 36, *47*
Hill, O. W., 144, *157*
Hiller, J., 116, 122, *134*
Hinkle, L. E., 152, *155*
Hinkle, L. E., Jr., 63, *65*, 149, 153, *155*
Hirano, T., 11, *27*
Hirning, L. D., 83, *89*
Hirsch, J., 175, *187*, 198, 200, *205*
Hirschfeld, J. W., 142, *158*
Hirschowitz, B. I., 13, *27*
Hirst, M., 86, *89, 98*, 115, 116, 120, 121, *131, 135*
Hislop, I. G., 147, *157*
Hoaki, Y., 124, *135*
Hodes, Z., 108, *110*
Hoebel, B. G., 115, 120–22, 126, *133, 135*, 191, 193, *205*
Hofer, M. A., 9, 171, *173*
Hoffer, B. J., 121, *134*
Hogan, W. J., 141, *156*

Hokfelt, T., 2, 7, 8, *28, 30*, 69, 73, 81, 83, *90, 91, 92, 93, 97, 98*
Holaday, J. W., 75, 76, *90, 92, 96, 98*, 119, *131*
Holden, H. T., 77, *91*
Holden, R. J., 144, *156*
Holdstock, D. J., 148, *157*
Holland, A., 88, *97*
Hollister, L. E., 79, *92*
Hollt, V., 69, *93*
Holst, J. J., 8, 27, 37, 42, 44, *46, 47*
Holst, S. S., 13, *29*
Hood, L., 83, *91*
Hopkins, D. A., 20, *31*
Hor, L., 86, *93*, 115, 119, 121–23, *132*
Horita, A., 108, *110*
Horowitz, L., 148, *157*
Horrocks, J. C., 144, *157*
Horton, E. S., 191, 204, *206*
Horton, P. F., 141, *158*
Hoshino, K., 102, *110*
Howard, J. M., 82, *92*
Hsiao, S., 63, *65*
Huidobro-Toro, J. P., 71, *92*
Hunkapiller, M., 83, *91*
Hunt, P. S., 140, *157*
Hunt, R. H., 151, *157*
Hunter, G. C., 15, *27*
Hunter, J. O., 151, *158*
Hyman, P. E., 166–67, *174*
Hyson, R. L., 119, *133*

I

Ichinoe, S., 197–98, *205*
Ida, Y., 124, *135*
Ieiri, T., 79, 80, *92*
Iimori, K., 124, *135*
Ikeda, H., 62, *65*
Impicciatore, M., *46*
Improta, G., 83, *89*
Imura, H., 41, *44*
Inagama, T., 171, *174*
Ingelfinger, F. J., 142, *157*
Inoue, M., 171, *174*
Inoue, Y., 41–42, *46*
Inturrisi, C. E., 87, *91*
Isaza, J., 35, *47*
Ise, H., 15, *32*
Isenberg, J. I., 11, *26*, 34–36, *46, 47*, 164, *174*
Ishi, K., 15, *29*

Ishikawa, T., 19, *27*
Ismail-Beigi, F., 141, *158*
Isom, G. E., 73, *92*
Issa, I., 5, *26*
Issac, L., 169, *174*
Iversen, L. L., 37, *47*
Iversen, S. D., 115, *134*

J

Jackson, I. M. D., 87, *92*
Jackson, L., 79, *97*
Jacobowitz, D. M., 104, *111*, 128, *130*
Jacobs, A., 140, *158*
Jacobs, D. M., 169, *174*
Jacobson, E., 143, *158*
Jaloweic, J. E., 86, *92*
James, B., 80, *98*
James, W. B., 144, *156*
Jamison, K. R., 79, *94*
Janssen, P. A. J., 81, 84, *88*
Jansson, G., 15, *27*
Jawaharlal, K., 115, *135*
Jensen, S. L., 8, *27*, 42, 44, *46*
Jerome, C., 60, 62, *65*
Jessell, T. M., 37, *47*
Jhanwar-Uniyal, M., 117–19, 121, 122, 124–27, *131, 132, 135*
Joffe, S. N., 2, *25*
Johansson, C., 11, *24*
Johansson, O., 69, 73, *90, 91*
Johnson, J. R., 167, 169, *174*
Johnson, L. F., 141, 143, *158, 159*
Johnson, L. R., 2, 7, *25, 28*, 167, 169, *174*
Johnson, P. R., 192, 198, 200, *205*
Jones, C. M., 138, *161*
Jones, D. B., 142, 143, *156*
Jones, F. A., 148, 149, 151, *156*
Jones, J. G., 121, *131*
Jones, V. A., 151, *158*
Jorgensen, S. P., 43, *46*
Jörnall, H., 104, *110*
Jornvall, H., 40, *47*
Jurkowlaniec, E., 127, *130*
Jurkowski, M., 124, *135*

K

Kadekaro, M., 2, 20, *27*
Kadowaki, S., 41–42, *44, 46*
Kaiya, H., 87, *92*

Kalia, M., 15,16, *27*
Kanarek, R., 117, 122, *133*
Kanazawa, I., 37, *47*
Kandasamy, S. B., 71, *92*
Kang, S. H., 101, *110*
Kao, P. C., 83, *97*
Kapadia, C. R., 4, *27*
Kaplan, H. I., 177, *187*, 189, *205*
Kaplan, H. S., 177, *187*, 189, *205*
Karteszi, M., 120, *131*
Kasbekar, D. K., 17–19, *29*
Kastin, A. J., 78, 87, *95*, 104, *112*, 113, 116, 128, *131, 134*
Kato, Y., 41, *44*
Kauffman, G. L., 7, *29*, 41, *45*
Kavaliers, M., 120, *131*
Kaveh, R., 3, *32*
Kay, A. W., 13, *25*
Kay, N., 77, *92*
Kaye, W. H., 129, *131*
Keesey, R. E., 51, *56*, 193–96, *205*
Kelly, D. D., 124, *130*
Kelly, K. A., 145, *158*
Kemali, D., 80, *97*
Kemnitz, J. W., 193–96, *205*
Kenney, N. J., 115, *133*
Kerdelhue, B., 120, *131*
Kern, F., 149, 152, *155*
Keuhnle, J., *94*
Kewenter, J., 8, *28*, 73, *93*
Keys, A., 191, 204, *205*
Khachaturian, H., 69, 70, 73, 80, *88, 92, 98*, 106, *112*, 115, 116, *131*
Kiang, J. G., 74, *92*
Kidd, C., 7, *26*
Kihl, B., 13, *27*
Kiley, N., 149, 150, *160*
Kim, C. H., 101, *110*
Kim, J. K., 101, *110*
Kim, M. S., 101, *110*
King, B. M., 116, 128, *131*
Kinsey, A. C., 78, *92*
Kirkegaard, P., 13, *29*, 85, *95*
Kirkpatrick, G. S., 140, *158*
Kirschgessner, A., 118, 122, *132*
Kissileff, H. R., 63, *65*
Kitagawa, K., 38, *48*
Klajner, F., 178, *187*
Klee, W. A., 87, *99*
Klein, K. B., 22, *27*
Klier, M., 88, *97*

Kneip, J., 19, *28*, 72, 86, *94*
Knigge, U., 37, *47*
Knight, S. E., 15, *27*
Knill-Jones, R. P., 144, *156*
Knittle, J. L., 175, *187*
Knoturek, S. J., *28*
Knuhtsen, S., 8, *27*, 37, 42, 44, *46, 47*
Knutson, U., 11, *27*
Kobashi, M., 54, *56*
Kobayashi, R., *45*
Kobayashi, S., 34, *46*
Kobberling, J., 80, *93*
Kodaira, H., 11, *25*
Koelz, H. R., 4, *28*
Kohlerman, N. J., 54, *56*
Kohno, Y., 124, *135*
Konishi, S., 85, *92*
Konturek, S. H., 151, *158*
Konturek, S. J., 7, 85, *92*
Kopajtic, T. A., 122, 123, *136*
Kopin, K. J., 75, *95*
Kovacs, T. O. G., 37, 38, *45*
Kraft, K., 74, *93*
Kreuning, J., 144, *158*
Krieger, D. T., 67, 74, *92*, 103, *110*, 119,
    126, 128, *130, 131*
Kubek, M., 108, *110*
Kuehnle, J. C., 79, *90*
Kuhar, M. J., 73, 83, *88, 95*, 106, *111, 112*,
    115, 116, 122, 123, *129, 130, 132, 134*,
    136
Kuiper, G., 144, *158*
Kulkosky, P. J., 52, *57*, 60, *64*
Kunos, G., 76, *96*
Kusano, M., 15, *29*
Kusche, J., 2, *28*
Kushima, K., 87, *91*
Kyosola, K., 2, *28*

L

LaBrie, F., 67, *95*
Lahann, T. R., 108, *110*
Lahti, R., 78, *93*
Laidlaw, J. M., 139, *160*
Lake, C. R., 129, *131*
Lam, S. K., 36, *47*
Lamki, L., 83, *97*
Lanciault, G., 8, *28*
Landor, J. H., 35, *47*
Lane, W. H., 36, *47*
Lang, R. E., 74, *93*

Lanthier, D., 115, 116, 120–21, *132, 135*
Larsson, L. I., 41, 42, 44, *46, 47*
Lasiter, P. S., 53, *56*
Lasser, R. B., 148, *158*
Latimer, M. R., 149, 150, 153, *158*
Latimer, P. R., 139, 149–51, 153, 155, *158*
Laubie, M., 74, *93*
Lauffenburger, M., 22, *31*, 108, *111*
Lautt, W. W., 54, *56*
Law, P.Y., 119, *131*
Lawson, E. E., 72, *89, 93*
Leake, R. D., 167, 171, *173, 174*
Lechago, J., 2, *28*
Lechner, R. J., 75, 76, *96, 98*
Leclerc, R., 67, *95*
Lee, A., 74, *98*
Lee, K. T., 145, *161*
Lee, K. Y., 145, *156, 161*
Leeman, S. E., 44, *46*
Lehtinen, V., 140, *158*
Leibowitz, S. F., 86, *93*, 113–28, *129, 130,*
    131, 132, 133, 134, 135, 136
Leith, D. E., 73, *97*
LeMagnen, J., 52, *56*, 126, 127, *133*
Lendorf, A., 85, *95*
Lennard-Jones, J. E., 138, 152, *158, 159*
Lenoir, T., 200, *205*
Lenz, H. J., 22, *28*, 35, *47*
Lenz, H. S., 22, *28*
Leonard, A. S., 101, *110*
Leppaluoto, J., 67, *88*
Lesiege, D., 21, *28*, 108, *111*
Leth, R., 3, *28*
Levin, B. E., 117, 118, 121, 124, 127, 128,
    131, 133
Levin, S. R., 7, *29*, 79, *94*
Levine, A. S., 19, 22, *28, 29*, 52, *56*, 60, *65*,
    72, 85, 86, 88, *93, 94*, 106, *111*, 113–16,
    120, 122, 124, 126, 129, *130, 134*
Levine, R., 108, *111*
Levitsky, D. A., 195–97, 200, 203, *205*
Levitt, M. D., 148, *158*
Lewis, J. W., 77, *97*
Lewis, M. E., 69, 73, *88, 92*, 115, 116, 128,
    131, 133
Lewis, T. H. C., 144, *161*
Li, C. H., 67, 78, *90, 98*, 119, *131*
Libby, L., 127, *133*
Lic, C. H., *131*
Lichtenberger, I., 167, 169, *174*
Lichtenberger, L. M., 34–35, *47*

Lichtenstein, S. S., 118, 128, *133*
Liebelt, R. A., 197–98, *205*
Liebeskind, J. C., 77, *97*
Liebowitz, S. F., 52, 53, *56*
Lilienfeld, A., 148, *158*
Lin, M. T., 71, *93*
Lind, J. F., 150, *159*
Lindberg, B., *93*
Lindholm, E., 101, 109, *110*
Lindman, J., 144, *158*
Lindstrom, L. H., *93*
Ling, N., 40, *45*, 67, 69, 79, *88, 96*, 105, *110*, 124, *134*
Linkens, D.A., 150, *160*
Lionetti, F. J., 76, *93*
Liotta, A. S., 67, *92*, 128, *130*
Lis, M., 67, *95*
Ljungdahl, A., 69, 73, 83, *91, 92*
Logan, D., 8, *29*
Loh, H. H., 119, *131*
Lombardi, D. M., 18, *28*
London, R. L., 142, *158*
Long, D. M., 101, *110*
Long, J. F., 14, *28*
Long, R. G., 44, *45*
Lopez, R., 167, 171, *173*
Lopkor, A., 76, *93*
LoPresti, P., 149, *155*
Lorber, D. H., 151, 152, *156*
Lorber, S. H., 152, *156*
Lorenz, W., 2, 4, *28*
Lotter, E. C., 62, *65*
Lotti, G., 79, *90*
Lotti, V. J., *89*
Lottspeich, F., 87, *89*
Louis-Sylvestre, J., 52, *56*
Lovitz, A. J., 139, *157*
Lowery, P. J., 72, *91*
Lowney, L. I., 83, *91*
Lowy, M. T., 86, 88, *93*, 113–16, 120, 122, 126, 129, *134*
Lucas, R. W., 144, *156*
Luciano, M., 128, *134*
Luft, R., 8, *32*
Luhby, A. L., 167, 171, *173*
Lundberg, J. M., 7, 8, *28, 30*, 73, *91, 93, 97*
Lundgren, O., 15, *27*
Luparello, T. J., 101, *110*
Lupoli, J., 195–97, 200, 203, *205*
Lustman, P. J., 140, 143, *156*

Lynch, W. C., 127, *133*
Lyrenas, S., *93*

M

MacFarlane, I. R., 72, *89*
MacLennan, A. J., 119, *133*
McCabe, J. T., 117, *133*
McCaleb, M. L., 118, 127, *134*
McCarthy, P. S., 86, *96*
McClearn, G. G., 175, *187*
McDonald, T. J., 36, 37, *47*, 104, *110*
McDougal, J. N., 71, *93*
McGivern, R.F., 120, 124, 125, *133*
McGuigan, J. E., 5, *27, 31, 32*, 34, 35, *46, 47*
McIsaac, R. L., 15, *27*
McKay, L. D., *57, 62, 65*, 115, *133*
McKee, D. C., 139, *157*
McKenna, R. J., 184, *187*
McLaughlan, P., 151, *158*
McLaughlin, P. J., 77, *99*
McLean, S., 115, 120–22, 126, *133*
McManus, N. H., 78, *90*
McMichael, H. B., 146, *158*
McQueen, D. S., 72, *93*
Madansky, D. L., 72, *89*
Madden IV, J., 119, *133*
Maeda-Hagiwara, M., 107, 108, *110*
Mahklouf, G. M., 6, *25*
Maickel, R. P., 86, *93*
Maico, D. G., 5, *27*
Maier, S. F., 119, *133*
Main, I. H. M., 4, *24*
Maire, F. W., 101, *110*
Maj, M., 80, *97*
Makhlouf, G. M., 6, 7, 22, *30*, 42, *47*, 82, *88*
Makhlouf, J. E., 7, *30*
Makino, T., 80, *95*
Makman, M. H., 122, *132*
Malagelada, J.-R., *22, 23, 31, 83, 97*, 145, *159*
Maley, B., 18, *29*
Mame Sy, T., 127, 128, *129*
Mandenoff, A. T., 86, *93*, 127, 128, *129, 133*, 200, *205*
Manning, A. P., 144, *158*
Manshardt, J., 125, *133*
Mansour, E. J., 74, *99*
Mara, S. G., 106, *111*
Marfaing-Jallat, P., 127, *133*

Margolin, S., 82, *93*
Margules, D. L., 86, *93*, 113, 128, *130*, *133*
Marinescu, C., 118, 128, *133*, *135*
Marino, E., 71, *95*
Marino, L., 117, *130*
Marki, W., 21, *31*
Marks-Kaufman, R., 117, 122, *133*
Marques, P. R., 71, *93*
Marshall, S., 79, *89*
Martin, C. E., 78, *92*
Martin, D., 142, 143, *155*
Martin, G. E., 117, 124, 127, *133*
Martin, J. S., 9, *31*
Martin, W. R., 71, 85, *93*, *97*
Martindale, R., 7, *29*
Martinson, J., 15, *27*
Mash, D. C., 125, *133*
Mason, D. T., 74, *99*
Mason, J. W., 22, *29*
Matarazzo, S. A., 150, *160*
Mather, F., 11, *25*
Mathews, P. M., 77, *93*
Matsukura, S., 41–42, *44*, *46*
Matsushima, R., 20, *31*
Matsushima, S., 20, *31*
Mauk, M. D., 116, 128, *131*
Maxwell, V., 44, *47*, 164, *173*
Mayer, G., 80, *93*
Mayer, J., 49, *56*
Mayer, N., 87, *95*
Maysinger, D., 69, *93*
Mazzocchi, G., 79, *90*
Mehraein, P., 69, *93*
Meis, P. J., 167, *174*
Meites, J., 79, 80, *89*, *92*, 122, *136*
Melchiorri, P., 83, *89*
Melendez, R. L., 37, *47*
Mello, N. K., 79, *90*, *94*
Mellow, M., 143, *158*
Melmed, S., 79, 87, *94*, *95*
Melvin, J. A., 107, *110*
Mendeloff, A. I., 140, 148, *158*
Mendelson, J. H., 79, *90*, *94*
Menezes, C. E., 102, *110*
Menguy, R., 145, *156*, *161*
Mensah, P. A., 53, *56*
Mermod, J. J., 106, *111*
Meshkinpour, H., 152, *156*
Messini, B., 152, *157*
Messini, M., 152, *157*
Mesulam, M. M., 15, 16, *27*

Metcalf, G., 71, *90*, *98*
Meyer, E. R., 79, *89*
Meyerson, B. J., 79, *94*
Mezey, E., 120, *131*
Micali, B., 11, *29*
Miceli, D., 127, *133*
Mickelson, D., 191, 204, *205*
Mignon, M., 8, *24*
Mikos, E., 85, *92*
Miller, G. C., 76, 78, *95*
Miller, J. M., 71, *96*
Miller, L. J., 145, *159*
Miller, N. E., 117, *135*
Miller, R. A., 171, *174*
Miller, R. J., 81, 84, *89*, *91*, *94*
Milner, R. J., 76–78, *91*
Minty, F. M., 21, *26*
Mir, P., 87, *96*
Misiewicz, J. J., 148–51, *157*, *159*, *160*
Mitchel, J. S., 193–96, *205*
Miyoshi, A., 171, *174*
Mogard, M., 38, 43, *45*
Mohri, K., 2, *28*
Moisset, B., 128, *133*
Moller, S., 43, *46*
Möllman, K.-M., 144, *159*
Monk, M., 148, *158*
Monteleone, P., 80, *97*
Moody, F. G., 8, *32*
Moody, T., 104, *111*
Moore, D. F., *109*
Moore, J. G., 11, 12, *29*
Mori, K., 41–42, *46*
Morita, K., 87, *92*
Morley, J. E., 19, 22, *28*, *29*, 60, *65*, 72, 77–80, 85–88, *92*, *93*, *94*, *95*, 106, *111*, 113–16, 120, 122, 124, 126, 129, *130*, *134*
Morley, S. E., 52, *56*
Morris, A. F., 144, *158*
Morrison, J. F. B., 7, *29*
Moss, I. R., 72, *95*
Moss, R. L., 121, *134*
Motoki, D., 11, *29*
Moult, P. J., 80, *95*
Moura, J. L., 102, *110*
Mrosovsky, N., 51, *56*, 192, *205*
Mucha, R. F., 115, *134*
Muehlethaler, M., 121, *134*
Muraki, T., 80, *95*
Muramatsu, I., 102, *111*
Murari, G., 106, *110*

Murphy, D. L., 87, *89*
Murphy, M. R., 78, *95*
Murray, S., 86, *94*
Murrell, T. G. C., 149, 151, *159*
Mutt, V., 36, 37, 40, 43, *45, 47*, 104, *110*
Muurhainen, N. E., 63, *65*
Myers, B. M., 78, *95*
Myers, R. D., 117, 118, 124, 127, *133, 134*

N

Naber, D., 129, *131*
Naccari, F., 71, *95*
Nagasaki, N., 124, *135*
Nagler, R., 142, 143, *159*
Najam, N., 86, *92*
Nakagawa, R., 124, *135*
Nakamura, K., 15, *29*
Nakamura, T., 15, *30*
Nakata, Y., 38, *48*
Namba, M., 87, *92*
Narasimhachari, N., 128, *135*
Nargi, M., 83, *89*
Nemeroff, C., 105–07, *109, 110, 111*
Neugebauer, E., 2, *28*
Nicholson, N., 197–98, *205*
Nicks, R., 142, *157*
Nicolaidis, S., 62, *65*
Nielsen, O. V., 8, *27*, 37, 42, 44, *46, 47*
Niemeck, W., 22, *29*
Niemegeers, C. J. E., 81, 84, *88*
Nijima, A., 11, *27*
Nikoomanesh, P., 143, *159*
Nilaver, G., 70, 73, *98*
Nilsson, G., 2, 7, 8, *28, 30*, 35–37, *47*, 69, 73, 81, 83, *92, 93, 97*, 104, *110*
Nisbett, R. E., 177, 179, 182, *187*
Nistico, G., 71, *95*
Norgren, R., 18, *25*, 53, 55, *56*, 60, 62, *65*
Norland, C. C., 147, 163
Norman, W. P., 17–19, *26, 29, 32*
Novin, D., 49, 50, 54, *56, 57*, 101, 108, 109, *110, 111*, 127, *131*
Nozawa, M., 41, *44*
Nyberg, F., *93*

O

O'Brien, C. P., 128, *134*
O'Brien, R., 201, 202, *205*
O'Donohue, T., 104, *111*
Odum, E. P., 191, *205*

Ohe, K., 171, *174*
Oken, M. M., 72, *94*
Oku, J., 86, *97*
Olbe, L., 3, 8, 10, 11, 13, *27, 28, 29, 31*
Oldendorf, W. H., *65*
Olesen, M., 37, *47*
Olmsted, M. P., 181–83, *187*
Olsen, P. S., 13, *29*, 85, *95*
Olson, G. A., 87, *95*, 113, 116, 128, *131, 134*
Olson, L., 121, *134*
Olson, R. D., 87, *95*, 113, 116, 128, *131, 134*
Oltmans, G. A., 128, *134*
Oomura, Y., 54, *56, 57*)
Oppenheimer, R. L., 119, *132, 134*
Orbach, S., 183, *187*
Orlando, R. C., 105–7, 109, *110, 111*
Orloff, M. O., 38, *45*
Orloff, M. S., 37, 38, *45, 47*
Ormsbee, H. S., III, 19, *29, 32*
Orr, W. C., 141, *159*
Ortaldo, J. R., 77, *91*
Osaka, M., 85, *92*
Osumi, Y., 19, 22, *27, 29*, 102, *111*
Ouyang, A., 142, *158*

P

Packman, P. M., 79, *95*
Pagani, F. D., 17–19, *29*
Pagani, F. P., 18, *26*
Paglietti, E., 78, 79, *91, 96*
Paintal, A. S., 7, *29*
Painter, N. S., 151, 152, *159*
Palkovits, M., 73, 120, *131*
Palmer, M. R., 121, *134*
Panksepp, J., 86, *92*
Panula, P., 104, *111*
Pappas, T. N., 8, 22, *29*, 37, 38, *45*
Park, J. H., 6, *31*
Parke, J., 101, *110*
Parr, D., 79, *95*
Parrini, D., 81, *91*
Pasi, A., 69, *93*
Pasqualini, C., 120, *131*
Passaro, E., Jr., 164, *174*
Pasternak, G. W., 76, *92*
Patton, H. D., 101, *110*
Pavlov, I. P., 152, *159*
Pawlik, W., 85, *92*

Pearse, A. G. E., 14, *29*
Pearson, J., 116, 122, *134*
Peck, J. W., 50, *56*, 175, *187*
Pedersen, L., 146, *160*
Pederson, R. A., 43, *45*
Peitsch, W., 167, 169, *174*
Pekary, A. E., 87, *95*, 108, *111*
Pelikan, E. W., 71, *96*
Pelletier, G., 67, *95*
Peña, A. S., 146, *159*
Pengelley, E. T., 191, *206*
Penick, S. B., 63, *65*
Percival, H. G., 9, *25*
Pert, A., 104, *111*
Pert, C. B., 78, 83, *95*, 104, *111*, 116, 122, 128, *132, 133, 134*
Pescor, F. T., 85, *93*
Peters, M. N., 14, *29*
Peters, R. H., 128, *131*
Petersen, B., 85, *95*
Petrie, D. J., 141, *156*
Petta, M., 78, *96*
Petterson, G., 8, *28*, 73, *93*
Pevnick, J., 80, *98*
Pfaffman, C., 53, 55, *56*
Pfeiffer, A., 75, *95*
Pfeiffer, E. F., 88, *97*
Pickar, D., 87, *89*, 129, *131*
Pilot, M. L., 143, *159*
Piris, J., 145, *159*
Pi-Sunyer, F. X., 63, *65*
Pittman, Q. J., 121, *134*
Plakovits, M., *95*
Plekss, O. J., 82, *93*
Plotnikoff, N. P., 76, 78, *95*
Polak, J. M., 14, *29*
Polish, E., 22, *29*
Polivy, J., 178–86, *187*
Pomeroy, W. B., 78, *92*
Pontes, F. A., 149, 151, *159*
Pontzer, C. H., 124, 127, *130*
Pope, II, C. E., 141–43, *155*
Porreca, F., 83, *95*, 105, *111*
Porreca, R., 83, *96*
Porte, D., Jr., *57*, 62, *65*
Porter, R. W., 101, *110*
Posner, B. I., 20, *32*
Post, R. N., *109*
Pottash, A. L. C., 128, *135*
Powell, D. W., 84, *96*, 139, 146, 149, *157, 159*

Powley, T. L., 19, *32*, 51, *56*, 178, *187*, 192, 205
Pradayrol, L., 40, 42, 43, *47, 48*
Prange, A. J., 105–7, 109, *110, 111*
Prange, J., 107, *109*
Preshaw, R. M., *29*, 35, *48*
Preston, D. M., 152, *159*
Prigge, W. F., 88, *94*
Probst, S. J., 9, *31*
Puhakka, H., 140, *158*
Puurunen, S., 22, *29*

Q

Quarantotti, B. P., 78, 79, *91, 96*
Quartermain, D., 127, *130*
Quigley, M. E., 80, *89, 96*

R

Raleigh, M., 129, *131*
Rambaud, J. C., 152, *155*
Ramirez-Gonzalez, M. D., 76, *96*
Raney, R. B., 101, *110*
Rasch, M. S., Jr., 141–42, *157*
Rask-Madsen, J., 84, *88*, 151, *155*
Rattan, S., 81, 82, *96*
Rattray, J. F., 74, *90*
Rea, M., 108, *110*
Read, A. E., 152, *157*
Read, N. W., 139, *159*
Recant, L., 128, *134*
Reed, E. W., 147, *161*
Reed, J. D., 14, 15, *24, 30*
Reel, G. M., 5, *32*
Rees, J. M. H., 71, *98*
Rees, L. H., 80, *95*
Rees, W. D. W., 145, *159*
Reeve, J. R., 7, 36–38, *45, 47, 48*
Rehfeld, J. F., 2, 7, 8, 11, 14, *27, 28, 30, 31*, 81, *97*
Reid, L. D., 127, *135*
Reid, R. L., 80, *96*
Reimann, H.-J., 2, *28*
Reimann, H. S., 2, *28*
Reinberg, A., 120, *131*
Reisberg, B., 87, *96*
Reker, D., 80, *98*
Remolina, C., 72, 73, *96*
Remond, G., 74, *93*
Renny, A., 82, *98*
Reyes, F. I., 80, *88*
Reynell, P. C., 146, *160*

Reynolds, D. G., 75, 76, *96, 98*
Rhodes, J., 142, 143, *156*
Ribet, A., 40, 42, 43, *47, 48*
Ricci, M., 152, *157*
Rice, P. E., 125, *134*
Richard, C. W., 67, *98*
Richardson, C. T., 10, 22, *30*, 34, 36, *47, 48,* 171, *174*
Richardt, L., 2, *28*
Richelson, E., *23, 31*
Richter, J. A., 121, *131*
Riddell, R. H., 142, *159*
Ritchie, J., 148, *159*
Rivier, C., 79, *96*, 124, *134*
Rivier, J. E., 21, 22, *28, 31*, 37, 38, 40, *45, 47*, 104–6, 108, *111*, 119, *135*
Rizzo, A., 106, *111*
Robinson, M. G., 141, *159*
Rockhold, R., 74, *97*
Rodin, J., 178, 182, *187*
Rogers, J., 128, *134*
Rogers, R. C., 54, *56*
Rohde, H., 2, *28*
Rokeaus, A., 44, *47*
Roland, C. R., 118, 119, 122, 125, 126, *131, 132, 134*
Rolland, Y., 190, 192, 198–200, 203, 204, *205*
Roman, C., 83, *96*
Roossin, P., 118, *132*
Ropert, J. F., 80, *96*
Rosato, E. F., 13, *30*
Rosato, F. E., 13, *30*
Rose, M. E., 78, *90*
Rosell, S., 13, *24*
Rosenfeld, G. C., 2, *25*
Rosenfeld, J. P., 125, *134*
Rosenfeld, M. G., 106, *111*
Rosenn, M., 118, *132*
Rosow, C. E., 71, *96*
Ross, L., 146, *161*
Ross, S. A., 43, *45*
Rossier, J., 67, 69, *88*, 124, 128, *134*
Roth, H. P., 142, *159*
Roth, J. L. A., 141, *159*
Rothchild, J. A., 79, *95*
Rotiroti, D., 71, *95*
Rotter, J., 164, *173*
Rouiller, D., 42, *47*
Rowlands, E. N., 148, 149, *156*
Roze, C., 8, *24*, 84, *96*, 105, 106, *110, 111*

Rubin, J., 143, *159*
Rubin, P., 76, *96*
Rubin, W., 146, *161*
Ruby, E. B., 80, *96*
Rukebusch, Y., 150, *155*
Ruppel, M., 101, *110*
Rusiniak, K. W., 53, *56*
Ruvio, B. A., 75, 76, *92*

S

Sachs, G., 4, *28*
Saffouri, B., 6, 7, *25, 30*, 42, *47*
Said, S., 2, 7, 8, *28, 30*, 73, 81, *93, 97*
Saitta, F. P., 11, *29*
Sakae, K., 22, *29*
Samloff, I. M., 14, *27*, 164, *173, 174*
Samuelsson, K., 11, *24*
Sanders, D. J., 14, 15, *24, 30*
Sanders, M. J., 5, *30*
Sandler, R. S., 139, *157*
Sandman, C. A., 124, 125, *133*
Sanger, D. J., 86, *96*, 113–15, *134*
Santen, R. J., 80, *96*
Santiago, T. V., 72, 73, *96*
Sapperstein, R. L., 169, *174*
Sapru, 74
Sarna, S. K., 149, 150, 153, *158, 159*
Sarson, D. L., 152, *155*
Satomi, H., 15, *32*
Saunders, W., 116, *136*
Savaki, H., 20, *27*
Savoie, R. J., 101, *110*
Sawchenko, P. E., 54, *57*, 106, *111*, 119, 121, 127, *134, 135*
Sawyer, C. H., 79, *88*
Saxena, Q. B., 77, *96*
Saxena, R. K., 77, *96*
Scarpelli, E. M., 72, *95*
Schachter, S., 182, 185, *187*
Schainker, B. A., 79, *89*
Schallert, T., 101, 102, *110, 111*
Schally, A. V., 78, 85, 92, *95*
Schapiro, H., 15, *30*
Schaz, K., 74, *97*
Schiff, M., 163
Schlemmer, R. F., 128, *135*
Schlor, K.-H., 74, *97*
Schlusselberg, D., 2, *30*
Schmierer, G., 63, *65*
Schmitt, H., 74, *93*
Schneider, C., 63, *65*

Schubert, M. L., 6, 7, 22, *30*, 115, 122, *130*
Schubert, P., 115, 122, *130*
Schulman, J. L., 63, *65*
Schultzberg, M., 2, *30*, 73, 81, *91, 97*
Schulz, R., 82, *97*
Schusdziarra, V., 40–42, *47*, 88, *97*
Schuster, M. M., 139, 140, 142, 143, 148–49, *159, 161*
Schwartz, J. M., 76–78, *91*
Sclafani, A., 127, *135*, 185, *187*
Scoles, V., 72, 73, *96*
Scoto, G., 106, *110*
Scott, P., 115, *135*
Scratcherd, T., 7, 9, 14, *24, 26*
Secrist, D. M., 164, *174*
Seelig, L. L., Jr., 2, *30*
Segal, D., 67, 69, *88*
Segawa, T., 38, *48*
Seiger, A., 121, *134*
Seino, Y., 41–42, *44, 46*
Seizinger, B. R., 69, *93*
Sekiguchi, T., 141, *156*
Semkin, E., 164, *173*
Senay, E., 108, *111*
Sessions, J. T., Jr., 139, 146, *157*
Shaar, C. J., 79, *97*
Shafer, R. B., 86, 88, *94*
Sharif, N. A., 108, *111*
Shavit, Y., 77, *97*
Shaw, B., 15, *24*
Shaw, J. E., 8, *28*
Shaw, S. E., 8, *24*
Shea-Donohue, P. T., 85, *97*
Shibasaki, T., 128, *134*
Shibuya, H., 128, *133*
Shimizu, N., 54, *56, 57*
Shimonura, Y., 86, *97*
Shindledecker, R. D., 168, *173*
Shinsako, J., 119, *136*
Shiraishi, T., 20, 21, *30, 31*
Shirakawa, H., 87, *92*
Shirakawa, T., 171, *174*
Shively, J. E., 7, 36, *47*
Shor-Posner, G., 115, 117, 118, 122, 127, *132, 135*
Short, G. M., 5, *32*
Shorthouse, M., 151, *158*
Shulkes, A., 44, *47*
Shumway, G. S., 101, *110*
Sibbitt, W. L., 77, *93*
Siegel, C. I., 148, *158*

Siggins, G. R., 67, 69, *88*
Silva, O. L., *109*
Silvis, S. E., 19, 22, *28, 29*, 85, 88, *94*, 106, *111*
Simansky, K. J., 60, *65*
Simantov, R., 78, *98*
Simard, P., 104–6, 108, 109, *111*
Simon, E. J., 116, 122, 123, *130, 134, 135*
Simon, J., 35, *47*
Simon, W., 74, *97*
Simpson, A., 20, 21, *31*
Simpson, R., 79, *90*
Sims, E. A. H., 191, 204, *206*
Siviy, S. M., 127, *135*
Sjodin, I., 140, *156*
Sjodin, L., 8, 13, *24, 31*
Skirboll, L., 18, *26*
Skyring, A., 142, *157*
Sladen, G. E., 142, *159*
Slangen, J. L., 117, 124, *135, 136*
Sleisinger, M. H., 146, *161*
Sloan, J. W., 71, *97*
Slochower, J., 184, *187*
Smallwood, R., 150, *160*
Smiley, T. B., 140, *157*
Smith, B., 147, *160*
Smith, C. L., 139, *161*
Smith, E., 15, *26*
Smith, E. M., 78, *88*
Smith, G. P., 22, *31*, 52, *57*, 59, 60, 62–64, *64, 65*, 115, *130*, 165, *174*
Smythe, G. A., 124, *123*
Smythies, J., 74, *88*
Snager, G., 15, *24*
Snape, W. J., Jr., 82, *98*, 142, 150, *158, 160*
Snider, R. H., *109*
Snyder, S. H., 83, *95*, 106, *111*, 115, 116, 122, *130, 132, 134*
Soares, E. C., 35, *48*
Sokaloff, L., 20, *27*
Soliman, K. F. A., 125, *133*
Soll, A. H., 2–6, *25, 30, 31*, 35, *48*, 164, 165, *174*
Solomon, T. E., 40, 44, *46, 47*, 164, *173*
Sowell, J. G., 72, *97*
Spencer, J., 11, *31*
Speroni, E., 106, *110*
Spiegel, D., 22, *27*
Spiegelhalter, D., 144, *156*
Spindel, E., 5, *31*
Spiro, H. M., 142, 143, *159*

Spirtes, M. A., 78, *95*
Squillari, V., 119, 122, *132*
Stacher, G., 63, *65*, 140, 143, *160*
Stachowiak, M., 124, *135*
Stadil, F., 14, *25*, *31*
Stanghellini, V., 83, *97*
Stanley, B. G., 115–17, 120–22, *130*, *132*, *135*
Stanley, D. A., 107, *110*
Stark, R. I., 81, *91*
Steardo, L., 80, *97*
Stein, L., 127, *135*, *136*
Stein, L. J., 62, *65*
Stein, L. S., *57*
Steinberg, V., 34, *46*
Steinbrook, R. A., 73, *97*
Steinringer, H., 63, *65*
Stenquist, B., 11, *31*
Stern, J. S., 200, *205*
Sternbach, H. A., 128, *135*
Stevenson, J. A. F., 50, 51, *57*
Stewart, J. S., 152, *155*
Stock, G., 74, *97*, *99*
Stone, R. T., 154, *160*
Storms, M. D., 179, *187*
Straus, E., 35, *48*
Streaty, R. A., 87, *99*
Stroiber, R., 115, 122, *130*
Strunz, U. T., 35, *48*
Strupp, B. J., 195–97, 200, 203, *205*
Stuckey, J. A., 62, *65*
Stumpf, H., 74, *99*
Stunkard, A. J., 128, *134*, 189, 190, 201, 202, *205*, *206*
Su, C. Y., 71, *93*
Sugano, K., 6, *31*
Sullivan, A. C., 128, *133*
Sullivan, M. A., 150, *160*
Sullivan, S. N., 14, *29*, 82, 83, *92*, *97*
Sun, E. A., 82, *98*
Susini, C., 42, 43, *48*
Sutherland, W. H., 81, *90*
Svedlund, J., 140, *156*
Svensson, S. O., 13, *27*
Swanson, L. W., 106, *111*, 119, 127, *135*
Szechtman, H., 78, *98*, 124, *129*

T

Taché, Y., 21, 22, *26*, *28*, *29*, *31*, 104–9, 111
Tachibana, S., 83, *91*

Takahushi, K., 15, *32*
Takeuchi, K., 87, *92*, 167, 169, *174*
Takeuchi, Y., 20, *31*
Taminato, T., 41–42, *44*, *46*
Tan, L., 81, *98*
Tanaka, M., 124, *135*
Tanaka, T., 87, *92*
Tansy, M. F., 9, *31*
Tapia-Arancibia, L., 108, *109*
Tapper, E. J., 1, *26*
Tasler, J., 85, *92*
Taylor, B., 138
Taylor, I., 150, *160*
Taylor, I. I., 34, *48*, 139, 150, *160*
Taylor, I. L., 85, *90*, 164, *173*, 191, *205*
Tchakarov, L., 76, *96*
Teitelbaum, B., 191, 193, *205*
Tempel, D., 115, 117, 122, 127, *135*
Tepperman, B. L., 21, *26*, *31*, 35, *48*
Tepperman, F. S., 86, *98*, 115, 116, 121, *135*
Terenius, L., 2, 7, 8, *28*, *30*, 69, 73, 79, 81, 83, *90*, *92*, *93*, *94*, *97*, *98*, 116, *136*
Terman, G. W., 77, *97*
Ternes, J. W., 128, *134*
Teschemacher, H., 87, *89*
Texter, E. C., Jr., 139, *160*
Thach, J. S., 22, *29*
Thayson, E. H., 146, *160*
Thoa, N. B., 104, *111*, 128, *130*
Thompson, D. G., *23*, *31*, 139, *160*
Thompson, W. G., 139, 140, 144, 147, *158*, *160*
Thompson, W. J., 2, 22, *25*
Thon, K., 2, *28*
Thornhill, J. A., 86, *89*, 116, *136*
Thornton, J., 63, *65*
Thorpe, V., 14, *30*
Timo-Iaria, C., 2, 20, *27*
Toates, F. M., 49–51, *57*
Tokunaga, Y., 80, *95*
Toris, J., 127, *135*
Tracy, H. S., 8, *25*
Tracy, J. J., 34, *46*
Tretter, J. R., 118, 122, 128, *132*, *133*
Troidl, H., 2, 4, *28*
Truelove, S. C., 138, 146, 147, 149, 151, 152, 154, *156*, *159*, *160*
Tseng, L. F., 119, *131*
Tsuda, A., 124, *135*
Tsunoo, A., 85, *92*
Tulin, M., 149, 152, *155*

Turner, A. J., 38, *45, 47*
Tusjta, M., 85, *98*
Tyalor, H. L., 204, *205*

U

Ueki, H., 87, *92*
Uhl, B. R., 106, *111*
Unger, R. H., 41, 42, *47*
Unger, T., 74, *93, 97, 99*
Unnerstall, J. R., 122, 123, *136*
Urban, I., 121, *134*
Urquhart, J., 8, *28*
Urquhart, S., 8, *24*
Uvnäs-Wallensten, K., 8, *28, 32*

V

Vagne, M., 36, 37, *47*, 104, *110*
Vaillant, C., 36, *46*
Vaille, C., *96*, 106, *111*
Valas Boas, M., 102, *110*
Valdman, A. V., 72, *91*
Vale, W. W., 21, 22, *28, 31*, 40, *45*, 79, 84,
    96, 105, 106, 108, *111*, 119, *135*
Van der Gugten, J., 124, *136*
vander Wal, A. M., 144, *158*
VanderWeele, D. A., 50, *56*
Van Hee, R. H., 15, *32*
van Houten, M., 20, *32*
Vanhoutte, P. M., 15, *32*
Vantrappen, G., 142, *160*
Van Vugt, D. A., 79, *89*, 122, *136*
van Wimersma Greidanus, T. B., 70, 73, *98*
Vargish, T., 75, 76, *96, 98*
Vargo, T. M., 67, *88*
Varner, A. A., 79, *94*
Vatu, M. H., 14, *32*
Vaysse, N., 42, 43, *48*
Veldhuis, J. D., 79, *90*
Vella, R., 15, *27*
Venuti, A., 11, *29*
Veyola, L., 2, *28*
Vicentini, M., 20, *27*
Vigna, S. R., 36, *48*
Vincent, M., 74, *93*
Vincent, S. R., 69, *98*
Vinik, A., 3, *32*
Vining, R. F., 124, *135*
Volavka, J., 80, *98*
Volpicelli, N. A., 144, *160*
von Amerongen, F. K., 101, *110*

von Bergmann, G.¨, 137
von Strümpel, A., 138
von Vietinghoff-Riesch, F., 127, *129*
Voyles, N. R., 128, *134*
Vvnas-Wallenstein, K., 8, 73, *93*

W

Wadsworth, M. E. J., 139, *160*
Waldbillig, R. J., 63, *65*
Waldorp, T. G., 72, *93*
Walker, C. A., 125, *133*
Walker, J. M., 69, 73, *88*, 124, 125, 128,
    130, 133
Walker, W., 3, *32*
Waller, S. L., 148–150, *157, 160*
Walsh, J., 22, *31*
Walsh, J. G., *31*, 34, 41, *45*
Walsh, J. H., *7*, 8, 10–12, 14, *25, 26, 29,
    30*, 34–38, 40–44, *45, 46, 47, 48*, 85, *90*,
    167, 171, *173*
Walsh, J. I., 6, *25*
Walus, K. M., 85, *92*
Wangel, A. G., 149–53, *160*
Ward, S. J., 71, *98*
Wardlaw, S. L., 81, *91*
Warsh, S., 184, *187*
Watanabe, H., 107, 108, *110*
Watanabe, K., 107, 108, *110*
Watanabe, S., 87, *91*
Waterfall, W. E., 149, 150, 153, *158, 159*
Watkins, J. B., 170, *174*
Watson, S., *112*
Watson, S. J., 67, 69–70, 73, 80, *88, 92, 98*,
    106, *112*, 115, 116, *131*
Way, E. L., 71, *92*
Way, L. W., 15, *27*
Webb, J., 146, *158*
Webb, V. J., 22, *28*
Webster, D. R., *29*
Wei, E. T., 74, *90, 92, 98*
Weinberger, S. E., 73, *97*
Weiner, H., 171, *173*
Weiner, M. A., 9
Weingarten, H. P., 19, *32*
Weingartner, H., 87, *89*
Weinstein, Wm., *160*
Weir, G. C., 6, *25, 30*, 42, *47*
Weiss, G. F., 118, 128, *133*
Weitzman, R., 79, *94*
Weller, M.D.I., 75, *98*
Wells, D., 143, *159*

Wells, S. A., 34, *45*
Wesche, D. L., 125, *130*
Weser, E., 146, *161*
Wessel, J., 80, *93*
West, D. B., 62, *65*
Whalen, R. E., 78, *98*
Wheeler, E. O., 147, *161*
Whishaw, I. Q., 101, 102, *111*
White, B. V., 138, *161*
White, P. D., 147, *161*
Whitehead, R., 145, *159*
Whitehead, W. E., 148–49, *161*
Whitehorn, J. C., 63, *65*
Whitney, G., 63, *65*
Whorwell, P. J., 139, *161*
Wikler, A., 85, *93*
Wildecklund,. G., *93*
Wilkinson, C. W., 119, *136*
Willette, 74
Williams, A. W., 144, *161*
Williams, B. A., 71, *92*
Williams, F. E., 116, *129*
Williams, R. H., 115, *133*
Williford, D. J., 19, *32*
Willoughby, J. M. T., 142, *159*
Wilts, D. S., 141–42, *157*
Wingate, D. L., 139, *160*
Wingert, T. D., 79, *94*
Winklehner, S., 63, *65*
Winter, J. S. D., 80, *88*
Wise, C. D., 127, *136*
Wise, R. A., 127, *136*
Wolfe, M. M., 5, *32*
Wolosin, J. M., 4, *25*
Wong, H. C., 36, *46*
Wood, J. D., 62, 81, *98*
Wood, P., 106, *112*
Woodcock, A. A., 72, *89*
Woods, J. S., 115, 116, 121, 123, *131, 136*
Woods, S. C., *57*, 62, *65*, 115, *133*
Woodward, A. F., 19, *29*
Woodward, E. J., *2*, *30*
Workman, E., 151, *158*
Wright, D. J. M., 75, *98*
Wruble, L. D., 15, *30*
Wulff, H. R., 144, *159*
Wurtman, R. J., 125, *133*
Wuster, M., 82, *97*
Wybran, J., 76, *98*

Wynne, R. D. A., 14, *24*
Wyrwicka, W., 19, *32*

Y

Yajima, H., 38, *48*
Yalow, R. S., 35, *47, 48*
Yamada, T., 6, 7, *29, 31*, 88, *94*
Yamagishi, T., 44, *48*
Yamaguchi, I., 85, *98*
Yamaguchi, N., 167, 171, *173*
Yamamoto, T., 15, *32*
Yamashiro, Y., 151, *156*
Yang, H., 104, *111*
Yardley, J. H., 144, *160*
Yee, F., 118, 128, *133*
Yen, S. S. C., 80, *89, 96*
Yim, G. K., 88, 114–16, 120, 122, 126, 129, *134*
Yim, G. K. W., 86, *93*, 113, *134*
You, C. H., 145, *156, 161*
Young, E., 69, 73, *88*
Young, R. C., 59, 60, *65*
Young, S. J., 147, *161*
Young, W. S., 106, *112*, 115, 122, *130*
Younger, J. C., 179, *187*
Yu, P. H., 81, *98*
Yukimura, T., 74, *99*

Z

Zaborszki, L., 73, *95*
Zadina, J. E., 104, *112*
Zagata, M., 19, *27*
Zagon, I. S., 77, *99*
Zalewsky, C. A., 8, *32*
Zanoboni, A., 79, *99*
Zanoboni-Muciaccia, W., 79, *99*
Zanussi, C., 79, *99*
Zaterka, S., 35, *48*
Zecca, L., 79, *99*
Zelis, R., 74, *99*
Zerbe, R. L., 75, *95*
Zhu, W.-Y., 8, *25*
Zieglgansberger, W., 72, *90*
Zimmerman, E., 70, 73, *98*
Zinsmeister, A. R., 83, *97*
Zioudrou, C., 87, *99*
Zizolfi, S., 80, *97*

SUBJECT INDEX

A

Acetylcholine, 14, 42, 165
Acetylcholinesterase, 2
Active period, 126
Adenosine, 6
Adiposity, 51, 128, 175, 198
Adrenergic, 4
Afferent fibers, 8
Alpha-2 receptors, 122
Amygdala, 54
Anabolic, 178
Analgesia, 125
Anorectic agents, 195
Anorexia nervosa, 129, 177
Antagonists, 169
Anticipation, 178
Antral pH, 8
Antrum, 8
Anxiety, 138, 177
Aphagia, 50
Appetite, 175
Appetite regulation, 120
Appetite-suppressant medication, 203
Approach–avoidance conflict paradigm, 164
Asthma, 177
Atrophine, 170
Atropine, 3, 4, 6, 14, 15
Autonomic nervous system, 53

B

Bad breath, 140
β-endorphin, 124, 125, 127, 128
Betazole, 167
Bethanechol, 166, 168
Biological density, 182
Body weight, 51, 128, 175, 189
Bombesin, 6, 21, 41
Bowel disorders, 137
Bulimic binges, 129

C

Cafeteria diet, 199
Calcium, 2, 42
Calcium-dependent protein kinases, 3
Caloric density, 190
Canalicular membrane, 3
Cannula mapping, 122, 125
Carbachol, 3, 5
Catacholamines, 5, 14, 52
Cephalic-phase response, 178
Chemoreceptors, 7
Chloride bicarbonate, 5
Cholecystokinin, 52
Cholinergic neurons, 4
Cimetidine, 2, 165
Colon, 146–152
Conflicts, 190

Constipation, 139
Control, 49
Cortex, 53
Cranial nerves, 53
Cricopharyngeal contraction, 140
CSF β endorphin, 129
Cushing's disease, 128
Cyclic AMP, 2

D

Dark period, 125
Decerebration, 15
Depression, 189
Deprivation, 171
d-fenfluramine, 199
Diet, 175
Dieters, 178
Disinhibition, 185
Diuranal cycle, 124, 125
DMPP (1,1 dimethyl-4-phenylpiperazinium), 7
Duodenal ulcer, 11, 164
Duodenum, 13
Dyspepsia (heartburn), 138, 140, 144–146

E

Efferent mechanisms, 126
Electric shock, 164
Electrophysical, 126
Emotional disorder, 189, 190
Emotional state, 163
Endocrine secretion, 1
Endogenous opioid peptides, 14, 67–87, 106–
    108, 113–117, 119–129, 132
Endogenous secretagogues, 169
Enkephalins, 14
Environment, 181
Epinephrine, 14
Epithelial cells, 2, 5
Esophageal function, 140–144
Esophagostomies, 1
Exorphines, 88–89
Externality, 182
External stimuli, 49

F

Fat behavior, 176
Fat cell, 198, 201
Feeding, 49, 51, 53
Fenfluramine, 195

Food deprivation, 123, 126
Food intake, 50
Food restriction, 190
Force feeding, 190
Frustrations, 190
Fundic glands, 2

G

Gamma-aminobutyric acid (GABA), 5
Ganglion cells, 4
Ganglionic cholinergic blocker, 3
Gastroesphageal reflux, 140
Gastric acid, 140
Gastric erosions, 163
Gastric exocrine, 1
Gastric fistula, 163
Gastric receptors, 52
Gastrin, 164, 165
Gastrin cells, 2
Gastrin-cholecystokinin (CCK), 2
Gastrin-releasing peptide (GRP), 5
Genetic factors, 164
Genetic obesity, 128
Gland cells, 2
Globus, 11, 140
Glossal papollae, 140
Glucagon, 13
Glucocytopenia, 10
Glucoreceptors, 54
Glycemic, 52
Grieving, 140
Gustatory chemoreceptors, 52

H

Hexamethonium, 3, 7
Histamine, 165, 168
Hives, 177
Homeostatic imbalance, 126
Horading, 198
Hormonal reactions, 1, 178
Humoral agents, 52
Hunger, 126
Hyperphagia, 191, 197
Hyperplasis, 164
Hypoglycemia, 126
Hypopharnax, 140
Hypothalamus, 11, 50
Hypothalamic, 191
Hypothalamic area (LHA), 50

Hypothalamic limbic-system, 53
Hypothalamic paraventricular nucleus, 53
Hypothermia, 171
Hysteria, 123

I

Imitation, 179
Impromidine, 166, 168
Incentive, 49, 51
Insulin, 11, 52, 190
Insulin hypoglycemia, 10
Irritable bowel syndrome, 138–140
Isoproterenol, 4, 5

L

Lateral perifornical site, 124
Ligands, 165
Ligation, 8
Lipectomy, 197
Liver, 54
Luemen, 6
Luminal membrane, 5

M

Macronutrients, 127
Mechanoreceptors, 7
Medulla, 11, 53
Metabolic, 177
Met-enkephalin, 125
Methacholine, 6
Morphine, 126
Motivation, 185
Myenteric plexus, 4

N

Nadir, 11
Naloxone, 14, 115, 123, 128
Naltrexone, 128
Neural mechanisms, 1
Neurasthenia, 138
Neurocircuit, 121
Neuromodulator, 1
Neuropeptides, 14, 101–106
Neurotensin, 13
Neurotransmitter, 1, 14, 120
Norepinephrine, 5, 14, 15
Nucleus retroambigualis, 15, 16
Nutrient, 51

O

Obesity, 189
Opiate receptor, 120
Opioid neuropeptides, 14
Optic thalamus, 163
Oral dependency, 182
Oral stage, 189
Osmoreceptors, 7
Overeating, 178, 179, 180

P

Pain, 139
Palatability, 175
Pallidus, 11
Parabrachial nucleus (PBN), 53
Parabrachial taste units, 127
Paracrine messenger, 1
Parasympathetic nerves, 9
Parietal cells, 1, 8, 164–168
Parotid gland, 9
Pentagastrin, 11, 41, 165
Pepsinogen, 4, 14, 164
Peptic ulcer disease, 163–165
Peptides, 2, 52
Peripheral nervous system, 121
Peritoneal cavities, 196
Pirenzepine, 14
Pituitary-adrenal systems, 122
Pons, 53
Postnatal development, 164
Propranalol, 14
Protein, 126
Proton pump, 3
Psychoanalytic, 189
Psychogenic, 189
Psychogenic gastrointestinal disorder, 139
Psychosomatic, 177
Pulmonary parenchyma, 16
Pyloric antrum, 2
Pyloric ligation, 168

R

Radio-immunoassays, 7
Radioglands, 127
Repletion, 51
Reward systems, 127

S

Salivary, 2
Salivary responses, 178

Satiety, 175
Secretagogues, 164
Secretin, 169
Secretory cells, 14
Sensory functions, 54
Set point, 182, 198
Sham feeding, 10
Social influence, 179, 181
Solitary tract, 53
Somatogenic, 189
Somatostatin, 40, 41, 169
Spinal cord, 54
Splanchnic nerves, 7, 14
Splandic sympathetic branches, 53
Starvation, 192
Stereotype, 175
Stomach, 164
Stress, 123, 126, 177, 183
Submucosal plexus, 2
Substance P, 2, 41
Sucrose hyerphia, 127

T

Tactus solitarius, 15
Taste, 53

Taste aversion, 54
Temperature, 168, 171
Tetrodotoxin, 3
Thalamus, 53, 54
Tracheobronchial tree, 15
Treatment, 202

U

Ulcers, 104–105, 177
Underweight, 129
Ussing-chambers, 7

V

Vagal, 8
Vagal parasympathetic, 53
Vagi, 7
Vagotomy, 3, 13
Vagus nerve, 8, 163
Vasoactive intestinal polypeptide (VIP), 2, 42
Ventro-medial hypothalamic nuclei (VMH), 50

W

Weaning, 171
Weight loss, 129

Printed and bound by CPI Group (UK) Ltd, Croydon, CR0 4YY

17/10/2024

01775688-0010